HORMONAL REGULATION OF MAMMARY TUMORS

VOLUME II: PEPTIDE AND OTHER HORMONES

Edited by Benjamin S. Leung
Associate Professor of Obstetrics and Gynecology, and
Director for Reproductive Endocrinology/Oncology Research
University of Minnesota
Minneapolis, Minnesota, U.S.A.

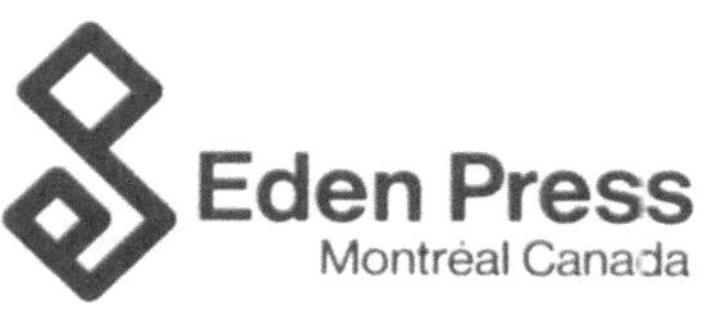

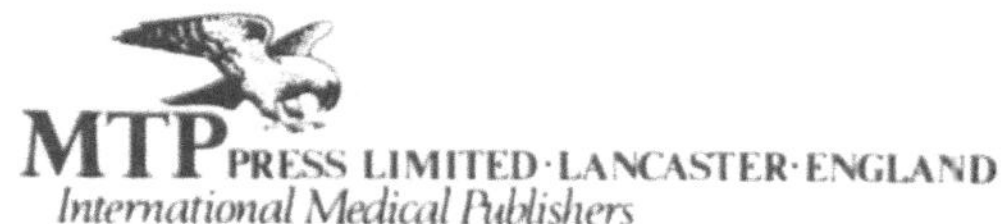

HORMONAL REGULATION OF MAMMARY TUMORS
Volume Two: Peptide and Other Hormones
edited by Benjamin S. Leung

PUBLISHED BY EDEN PRESS INC.

4626 St. Catherine St. West, Montreal, Canada H3Z 1S3
and
P.O. Box 51, St. Albans, Vermont, U.S.A. 05478

ISBN 978-94-011-8047-4 **ISBN 978-94-011-8045-0 (eBook)**
DOI 10.1007/978-94-011-8045-0

Softcover reprint of the hardcover 1st edition 1982

Published in U.K. and Europe by
MTP Press Limited
Falcon House, Cable Street, Lancaster, England

ISBN 978-94-011-8047-4

Dépôt légal – quatrième trimestre 1982
Bibliothèque nationale du Québec

LIST OF CONTRIBUTORS FOR VOLUME II

M.R. BANERJEE, Professor, Head, Tumor Biology Laboratory, School of Life Sciences, University of Nebraska-Lincoln, 210 Lyman Hall, Lincoln, Nebraska 68588.

YOON SANG CHO-CHUNG, Head, Cellular Biochemistry Section, Laboratory of Pathophysiology, National Cancer Institute, N.I.H., Building 10, Room 5B-38, Bethesda, Maryland 20205.

JEAN DJIANE, Laboratoire de Physiologie de la Lactation, INRA, 78350 Jouy-en-Josas, France.

NIVEDITA GANGULY, Tumor Biology Laboratory, School of Life Sciences, University of Nebraska, 201 Lyman Hall, Lincoln, Nebraska 68502

RANJAN GANGULY, Tumor Biology Laboratory, School of Life Sciences, University of Nebraska, 201 Lyman Hall, Lincoln, Nebraska 68502.

PHILIPPE GANDILHON, Centre de Recherches en Endocrinologie Moleculaire, Le Centre Hospitalier de l'Universite Laval, 2705 boulevard Laurier, Quebec, Quebec, Canada G1V 4G2.

RUSSELL HILF, Professor of Biochemistry, University of Rochester Medical Center, 601 Elmwood Avenue, Rochester, New York 14642.

HIDEO INOUE, Laboratory of Biochemistry and Metabolism, National Institute of Arthritis, Diabetes, Digestive Diseases and Kidney, National Instititutes of Health, Bethesda, Maryland 20205.

PAUL A. KELLY, Associate Professor, Centre de Recherches en Endocrinologie Moleculaire, Le Centre Hospitalier de l'Universite Laval, 2705 boulevard Laurier, Quebec, Quebec, Canada G1V 4G2.

FRANCES E. LELAND, Department of Biochemistry and Molecular Biology, University of Texas Medical School at Houston, P.O. Box 20708, Houston, Texas 77025.

BENJAMIN S. LEUNG, Associate Professor, Department Obstetrics and Gynecology, Director, Endocrine Oncology Research, Box 395 Mayo Memorial Building, 420 Delaware Street S.E., Minneapolis, Minnesota 55455.

NOZER M. MEHTA, Tumor Biology Laboratory, School of Life Sciences, University of Nebraska, 201 Lyman Hall, Lincoln, Nebraska 68502.

HIROSHI NAGASAWA, Experimental Animal Research Laboratory, Meiji University, Tama-ku, Kawasaki-shi, Kanagawa 214, Japan.

TAKAMI OKA, Senior Investigator, Laboratory of Biochemistry and Metabolism, National Institute of Arthritis, Diabetes, Digestive Diseases and Kidney, National Institutes of Health, Building 10, Room 9B-15, Bethesda, Maryland 20205.

JOHN W. PERRY, Laboratory of Biochemistry and Metabolism, National Institute of Arthritis, Diabetes, Digestive Diseases and Kidney, National Institutes of Health, Building 10, Room 9B-15, Bethesda, Maryland 20205.

JAMES A. RILLEMA, Professor of Physiology, Wayne State University School of Medicine, Gordon H. Scott Hall of Basic Medical Sciences, 540 East Canfield Avenue, Detroit, Michigan 48201.

ALZIRA A.M. ROSA, Centre de Recherches en Endocrinologie Moleculaire, Le Centre Hospitalier de l'Universite Laval, 2705 boulevard Laurier, Quebec, Quebec, Canada G1V 4G2.

RENE ST-ARNAUD, Centre de Recherches en Endocrinologie Moleculaire, Le Centre Hospitalier de l'Universite Laval, 2705 boulevard Laurier, Quebec, Quebec, Canada G1V 4G2.

TADASHI SAKAI, Laboratory of Biochemistry and Metabolism, National Institute of Arthritis, Diabetes, Digestive Diseases and Kidney, National Institutes of Health, Bethesda, Maryland 20205.

ROBERT P.C. SHIU, Protein and Polypeptide Hormone Laboratory, Department of Physiology, University of Manitoba, 770 Bannatyne Avenue, Winnipeg, Manitoba, Canada R3E 0W3.

DAVID A. SIRBASKU, Associate Professor, Department of Biochemistry and Molecular Biology, University of Texas Medical School at Houston, P.O. Box 20708, Houston, Texas, 77025.

GRACE Y. SUN, Associate Professor, Sinclair Comparative Medicine Research Farm and Biochemistry Department, University of Missouri, Columbia, Missouri 65201.

TOSHIYUKI TAKEMOTO, Laboratory of Biochemistry and Metabolism, National Institute of Arthritis, Diabetes, Digestive Diseases and Kidney, National Institutes of Health, Bethesda, Maryland 20205.

NOBUYUKI TERADA, Laboratory of Biochemistry and Metabolism, National Institute of Arthritis, Diabetes, Digestive Diseases and Kidney, National Institutes of Health, Bethesda, Maryland 20205.

BARBARA K. VONDERHAAR, Senior Investigator, Laboratory of Pathophysiology, National Cancer Institute, National Institutes of Health, Bethesda, Maryland 20205.

PREFACE

The concept that hormones influence tumor growth originated in 1889 with the proposal of Albert Schinzinger who suggested that breast cancer is related to the ovaries. Several years later, Sir George Beatson observed that remission of disseminated breast cancer could be achieved in premenopausal patients by performing bilateral oophorectomy. As a result of the contributions of Hedley Atkins, Charles Huggins and others, additive and ablative hormonal therapies have been widely used for the treatment of advanced breast cancers for several decades. Model systems to study the effects of hormones on growth and regression of breast tumors have been available for many years; however, the complexities of the hormonal environment have rendered *in vivo* studies difficult in man and experimental animals. Recently, the availability of long-term cultures of breast cancer cells has stimulated many investigators to use these cell lines to unravel the mechanisms of hormone action.

Because of the extreme diversity and complexity of advances regarding the endocrinology of the breast and breast cancers, a multi-authored review was deemed necessary. It has been gratifying to receive contributions from many noted scholars.

In Volume I of this monograph, the influence of steroid hormones and their antagonists upon normal and neoplastic tissues of the mammary gland are presented. In Volume II, the effects of peptide and other hormones are reviewed.

This monograph should provide stimulating reading for biochemists, endocrinologists, cell biologists and clinicians who are interested in the endocrinology of normal and neoplastic tissues of the breast, the underlying principles involving breast cancer growth and regression, and the applications of this information to future research and clinical care.

Benjamin S. Leung.

EDITOR

Benjamin S. Leung, Ph.D. is an Associate Professor of Obstetrics and Gynecology and Director for Reproductive Endocrinology/Oncology Research at the University of Minnesota, Minneapolis.

Dr. Leung graduated with a BS degree from Seattle Pacific College, Seattle in 1963. He was then appointed Research Scientist at the Pacific Northwest Research Foundation, Seattle, where he studied male reproductive endocrinology under Carl G. Heller, M.D., Ph.D.. He obtained his Ph.D. degree in Biochemistry at Colorado State University in 1969 and had his post-doctoral training in the discipline of steroid hormone action under the tutelage of Bert W. O'Malley, M.D. and Antony R. Means, Ph.D. at Vanderbilt University. From 1971 to 1976 he was Assistant Professor, and later Associate Professor, in the Department of Surgery, the Director for the Clinical Research Center Laboratory, the Director for Hormone Receptor Laboratory, and Affiliate Member in the Department of Biochemistry at the University of Oregon, Portland. Dr. Leung then served as the Senior Research Scientist and the Director of Research in the Department of Surgery at Cedar Sinai Medical Center, Los Angeles and has been a member of the faculty at the University of Minnesota since 1978.

Dr. Leung's major research interest is in the mechanisms of actions and interactions of steroid and peptide hormones in normal and neoplastic tissues of the mammary gland and uterus.

CONTENTS

1 ROLE OF PROLACTIN OR PLACENTAL LACTOGEN IN MAMMARY TUMOR DEVELOPMENT IN EXPERIMENTAL ANIMALS 1
Hiroshi Nagasawa
Introduction. 1
Prolactin or placental lactogen and mammary tumor development 1
Promotion by prolactin of mammary tumor development. 1
Promotion by prolactin of preneoplastic mammary gland lesions. 3
Promotion by placental lactogen of preneoplastic and neoplastic mammary gland development. 4
Difference in susceptibility to prolactin or placental lactogen between normal and neoplastic mammary glands. 4
Inhibition by prolactin of mammary tumor development 6
A mechanism of role of prolactin in mammary tumor development. 7
Stimulation by prolactin of mammary gland DNA synthesis, a primary factor for mammary tumor development 7
Synergism of prolactin and estrogen in mammary gland DNA synthesis 10
Species-difference in mammary gland DNA synthesis in response to prolactin 10
Factors which modulate mammary tumor development and prolactin secretion. 12
Perinatal hormonal exposure 12
Dietary fat. 12
Immunopotentiation 13
Role of prolactin in mammary tumor virus production. 14
Strain-difference in circulating levels of prolactin or placental lactogen and mammary gland susceptibility to it. 14
Strain-difference in hormone levels. 14
Strain-difference in mammary gland susceptibility to prolactin in mice. 15
Future prospects. 17
References. 17

2 PROLACTIN AND PROLACTIN RECEPTORS IN TUMOR DEVELOPMENT, GROWTH AND CELLULAR FUNCTIONS. 25
Paul A. Kelly, Jean Djiane, Philippe Gandilhon, Alzira A.M. Rosa, Rene St-Arnaud
Models of hormone-dependent mammary cancer. 25
Mice 25
Rats 26

In vitro systems. 28
Hormonal regulation of PRL receptors in normal tissue 28
Measurement of prolactin receptors 28
Receptor levels during pregnancy and lactation. 29
Up-regulation 29
Down-regulation 30
Hormonal regulation of receptors in mammary tumors. 32
DMBA-induced mammary tumors. 32
Regression of DMBA-induced tumors by RU16117 34
NMU-induced mammary tumors. 37
Organ culture of mammary tumors 45
Prolactin and human breast cancer 46
Evidence for role of prolactin 46
Prolactin receptors in human breast carcinoma 47
Summary and conclusions. 49
References 50

3 **STUDIES OF PROLACTIN RECEPTORS AND THE POSSIBLE PROLIFERATIVE ROLE OF PROLACTIN AND OTHER PITUITARY FACTORS IN HUMAN BREAST TUMOR CELLS** 63
Robert P.C. Shiu
References. 72
Acknowledgement. 76

4 **MODE OF ACTION OF PROLACTIN ON NORMAL AND NEOPLASTIC MAMMARY TISSUES** 77
James A. Rillema
Introduction. 77
Prolactin receptors. 77
Internalization of prolactin 78
Actions of prolactin at the plasma membrane 78
Sodium-potassium hypothesis 79
Calcium ions. 80
Polyamines, prostaglandins and cyclic nucleotides 81
Phospholipase A_2 82
Prostaglandins (PG) 82
Cyclic nucleotides 82
Polyamines. 83
Actions of prolactin on the proliferation of mammary cells. 83
References 85

5 GROWTH FACTORS FOR HORMONE-SENSITIVE TUMOR CELLS . . . 88
David A. Sirbasku, Frances E. Leland
Introduction . . . 88
Effects of known growth factors on mammary tumor cell proliferation . . . 89
Hormonally defined media . . . 89
Growth factor effects on cells cultured in collagen supported matrices . . . 90
Effects of other growth factors on mammary origin cells . . . 90
Effects of estrogens on growth factor activities for estrogen-responsive tumor cells . . . 91
New approaches to estrogen-responsive tumor growth . . . 91
Endocrine estromedin mechanism . . . 92
Paracrine and/or autocrine estromedin growth stimulation . . . 108
Platelet derived growth factors . . . 109
Platelet derived growth factors for mammary tumor cells . . . 110
Growth factors and growth control in normal versus malignant mammary cells . . . 113
Pituitary derived mammary cell growth factors . . . 115
Summary of new approaches to growth factor involvement in mammary tumor growth *in vivo* . . . 118
References . . . 118

6 PRIMARY AND PERMISSIVE ACTIONS OF INSULIN IN BREAST CANCER . . . 123
Russell Hilf
I. Direct actions of insulin on experimental mammary tumors . . . 123
A. Stimulation of growth: insulin-dependent tumors . . . 123
B. Inhibition of growth: insulin-responsive tumors . . . 124
C. Actions of insulin and relationship to tumor growth . . . 125
II. Facilitative effects of insulin on mammary tumors . . . 130
III. Estrogen-insulin interactions . . . 132
IV. Insulin and human breast cancer . . . 133
V. Conclusions . . . 133
Acknowledgement . . . 134
References . . . 134

7 EFFECT OF THYROID HORMONES ON MAMMARY TUMOR INDUCTION AND GROWTH . . . 138
Barbara K. Vonderhaar
Introduction . . . 138

Epidemiologic and clinical studies. 138
Animal studies 140
Mammary tumorigenesis 140
Normal mammary gland development 144
Possible mechanisms 147
References 148

8 MODE OF CYCLIC AMP ACTION IN GROWTH CONTROL 155
Yoon Sang Cho-Chung
Introduction. 155
Normal and neoplastic growth of the mammary gland 155
Intracellular content of cyclic nucleotides 155
Hormone-cyclic nucleotide interrelation 156
Mechanism of mammary tumor regression 158
Exogenous cyclic nucleotides. 158
Cyclic AMP receptor proteins 158
Antagonism between cyclic AMP and estrogen 162
Nuclear protein phosphorylation 163
Cyclic nucleotides in transformation 165
Cyclic AMP in reversion of malignancy 167
Conclusion 168
Acknowledgement 170
References 170

9 PROSTAGLANDINS, FATTY ACIDS AND PHOSPHOLIPIDS IN NORMAL AND NEOPLASTIC BREAST TISSUES 178
Grace Y. Sun, Benjamin S. Leung
Introduction. 178
Content of fatty acids and phospholipids 179
Normal mammary tissues 179
Mammary tumors 182
Metabolism of phospholipids 184
Normal mammary gland 184
Mammary tumors 188
Effects of dietary lipids 190
Mammary tumorigenesis and growth 190
Effect on tumor lipids 190
Effects of dietary carbohydrates. 191
Lipid inducers of cell transformation. 191
Fatty acid synthesis 191
Phospholipases and prostaglandins 193
Mammary gland lipids in response to hormonal regulation. . . . 194
Acknowledgement 197
References 198

10 POLYAMINES IN NORMAL AND NEOPLASTIC GROWTH OF MAMMARY GLAND 205
Takami Oka, John W. Perry, Toshiyuki Takemoto, Tadashi Sakai, Nobuyuki Terada, Hideo Inoue
Introduction. 205
Developmental changes in the synthesis and accumulation of polyamines in mammary gland 206
The control of polyamine biosynthesis during cell proliferation of mammary gland *in vitro* 207
The control of polyamine biosynthesis during differentiation *in vitro* 208
The functions of polyamines during mammary cell proliferation 213
Spermidine. 213
Putrescine 215
The role of polyamines in the differentiation of mammary gland 217
Milk protein synthesis 217
Spermidine and glucocorticoid action 218
The effect of spermidine on cellular components. 218
Differential actions of glucocorticoid and spermidine 220
Spermidine and cell-free translation of mammary mRNAs. . . . 221
Polyamine transport. 223
Concluding remark 224
References 225

11 HORMONE REGULATION OF CASEIN GENE EXPRESSION IN NORMAL AND NEOPLASTIC CELLS IN MURINE MAMMARY GLANDS 229
M.R. Banerjee, Ranjan Ganguly, Nozer M. Mehta, Nivedita Ganguly
I. Introduction 229
II. General macromolecular activity 230
III. Direct measure of casein mRNA 232
A. Specific translation activity 232
B. Hormonal regulation of $mRNA_{csn}$ translational activity . . . 232
IV. Purification of casein mRNA and synthesis of complementary DNA 233
V. Quantitative measurement of casein gene expression by the $cDNA_{csn}$ 235
A. Adrenal glucocorticoid influence on casein mRNA accumulation in mammary gland *in vivo* 235
B. Measurement of specific casein mRNA transcription. 236
C. Measurement of casein gene transcription. 238
VI. Hormonal modulation of casein gene transcription 240

VII. Casein gene expression in mammary tissue *in vitro* 242
A. Organ culture of pieces of mammary tissue from pregnant animals 242
B. The whole mammary organ in culture 242
VIII. Casein gene expression in a two-step culture model of the whole mammary organ 244
A. Measured by translational assay 244
B. Measured by molecular hybridization with $cDNA_{csn}$ probe . 245
IX. Simultaneous occurrence of morphogenesis and casein gene expression 249
X. Glucocorticoid is obligatory to casein gene expression 251
XI. Negative influence of progesterone on casein gene expression . . 256
XII. Cloning of $cDNA_{csn}$ 259
XIII. Mammary neoplasia and casein gene expression 264
A. In mammary cells transformed *in vivo* 266
B. In mammary cells transformed *in vitro* 267
XIV. Summary and comments 270
Acknowledgements 272
References 273

Chapter 1

ROLE OF PROLACTIN OR PLACENTAL LACTOGEN IN MAMMARY TUMOR DEVELOPMENT IN EXPERIMENTAL ANIMALS

Hiroshi Nagasawa

INTRODUCTION

It is unequivocal that prolactin is a most important hormone in experimental mammary tumorigenesis. Besides prolactin acts directly on mammary glands, recent studies have evidenced that the hormone also participates in mammary tumor virus production and that some factors which influence mammary tumorigenesis, such as perinatal hormonal exposure, nutrition and immune mechanism, modulate the pituitary prolactin secretion. Placental lactogen is also shown to play a role similar to prolactin in mammary tumor development as well as in several biological phenomena. The primary objective of this chapter is to summarize a number of pertinent studies on these problems in experimental animals.

Several interesting problems on the role of prolactin in mammary tumor progression, the interrelation between prolactin or placental lactogen and estrogen for mammary tumorigenesis and the receptors of these hormones as an index of normal and neoplastic mammary gland responsiveness will be discussed in the other chapters. Therefore, they will not be considered here. No report was available on the specific role of growth hormone on mammary tumor development, while it may play some role in the progression of established mammary tumors. In each section, the review articles are preferentially cited as references, if available. The readers can refer individual works from them.

PROLACTIN OR PLACENTAL LACTOGEN AND MAMMARY TUMOR DEVELOPMENT

Promotion by prolactin of mammary tumor development

Several studies have revealed that any factor which stimulates pituitary prolactin secretion or elevates circulating levels of the hormone, such as hypothalamic lesions, hypothalamic estrogen implantation, tranquilizer administration, normal and neoplastic pituitary grafting, prolactin injection, etc., can enhance the development of both spontaneous and carcinogen-induced mammary tumors in mice and rats (33), (59), (60). Furthermore, prolactin can promote mammary tumor development even in sex hormone-deficient, adreno-ovariectomized animals (59).

Administration of prolactin or pituitary grafting after adreno-ovariectomy stimulated the development of 7,12-dimethylbenz[a]-anthracene (DMBA)-induced mammary tumors in rats (Fig. 1) (26) or spontaneous mammary tumors in mice (Fig. 2) (65) to the level comparable to that of the control.

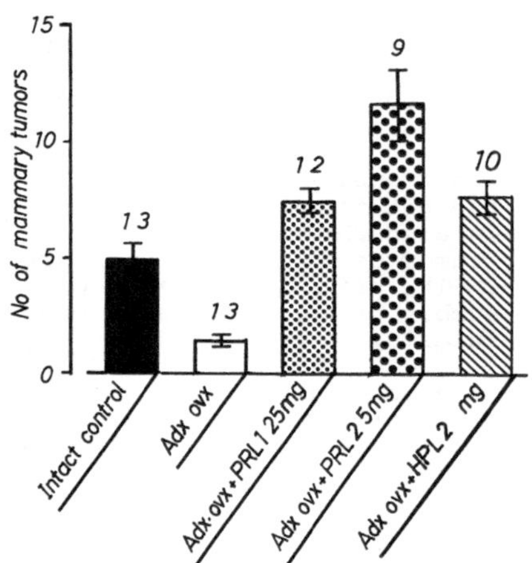

Figure 1.

Effects of adreno-ovariectomy and injection of prolactin or placental lactogen on the development of DMBA-induced mammary tumors in rats (means ± S.E.M.). Sprague-Dawley female rats bearing mammary tumors were given subcutaneous injections of each dose of ovine prolactin (PRL) or human placental lactogen (HPL) twice daily for 20 days beginning the following day of adreno-ovariectomy (adx·ovx). The number of newly developing tumors per rat was checked at the end of injection. Number of rats examined is indicated at the top of each column.

By contrast, treatments which induce hypoprolactinemia result in the inhibition of mammary tumor development. These are adreno-ovariectomy or administration of certain drugs, such as ergot alkaloids, cyclic imide derivatives, L-dopa, lyseric acid, etc. (33), (59), (60). An example is shown in Figure 2. Chronic administration of CB-154, a representative ergot alkaloid, inhibited markedly spontaneous mammary tumor incidence in mice (65).

All observations have substantiated that prolactin is the key hormone in mammary tumor development.

It was also found that daily injections of thyrotropic hormone releasing hormone (TRH) increased the number and size of DMBA-induced mammary tumors in rats. While the effects were abolished by CB-154, they were not affected by thyroidectomy (9). The results show that the development of this type of mammary tumors is largely dependent upon prolactin rather than thyroid hormone, both being stimulated the secretion by TRH.

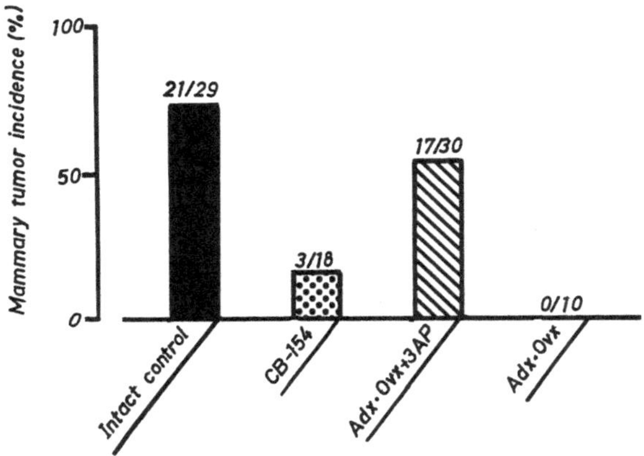

Figure 2.

Effects of adreno-ovariectomy and/or prolactin manipulation on the incidence of spontaneous mammary tumors in mice. C3H/He virgin mice received subcutaneous implantation of CB-154 or bilaterally adreno-ovariectomy (adx·ovx) and simultaneous grafting with 3 isologous pituitaries under the kidney capsules (3AP). The numbers at the top of each column show the number of mice with mammary tumors/ initial number of mice used.

Drosdowsky et al. (10) reported the stimulation by pituitary grafting of mammary tumor incidence (90 %) in mice which never develop spontaneous mammary tumors and the inhibition by brominated triphenylethylene (TBP) of this prolactin stimulating mammary tumor development associated with a significant decrease in pituitary prolactin secretion and prolactin receptor in normal mammary glands. They also found that TBP suppressed the development of spontaneous mammary tumors in mice (45a) and carcinogen-induced mammary tumors in rats (45b).

Promotion by prolactin of preneoplastic mammary gland lesions

Development and progression of preneoplastic mammary hyperplastic aleolar nodules (HAN) (16) are also primarily controlled by prolactin (57). The number and size of HAN were much decreased and the number of ghosts, remnants of regressed HAN, were increased by CB-154 injection. Normal mammary lobulo-alveolar system was also involuted by the treatment. On the other hand, the regression of HAN after adreno-ovariectomy was prevented or stimulated to the level higher than that of the intact controls by pituitary grafting (Fig. 3) (33), (57), (59). (60).

Another representative preneoplastic mammary gland lesion in mice is pregnancy-dependent mammary tumors (PDMT), which develop in some strains originated in Europe; GRS/A is a representative one (68). PDMT in GRS/A mice appear at the middle of pregnancy, progress with the advance of pregnancy, show peak sizes just before parturition and regress abruptly after parturition irrespective of lactation. More than 30 % of PDMT recur as malignant carcinomas at advanced ages (68). Development of this type of mammary tumors was reported to be suppressed by CB-154 (58). Pregnant GRS/A mice were injected subcutaneously once daily from day 17 to day 21 of pregnancy with 0.1 mg CB-154. At the end of injection, the incidence and average number per mouse of PDMT were 56 % and 1, respectively. On the other hand, those in the controls receiving vehicle only were 89 % and 1.7, respectively, which were significantly higher than those in the experimental mice. The results indicate that the development of PDMT is dependent upon prolactin.

Promotion by placental lactogen of preneoplastic and neoplastic mammary gland development

Placental lactogen, which resembles to prolactin in several biological actions (11), (43), (55) and participates quantitatively in normal mammary gland development during pregnancy (27), has the effects similar to prolactin on preneoplastic and neoplastic mammary gland development. It can increase the number of DMBA-induced mammary tumors in adreno-ovariectomized rats (Fig. 1) (28) and stimulate HAN formation in adreno-ovariectomized mice (Fig. 3) (66). Moreover, stimulation by progesterone of DNA synthesis of PDMT in GRS/A mice is markedly enhanced by placental lactogen (67).

Difference in susceptibility to prolactin or placental lactogen between normal and neoplastic mammary glands

As stated above, ovariectomy- or adreno-ovariectomy-induced regression of HAN is prevented or in some cases stimulated to the level higher than that of the control by pituitary grafting (63) or daily injections of human placental lactogen (66). However, these replacement therapies do not always prevent the involution of normal lobulo-alveolar system (Fig. 3).

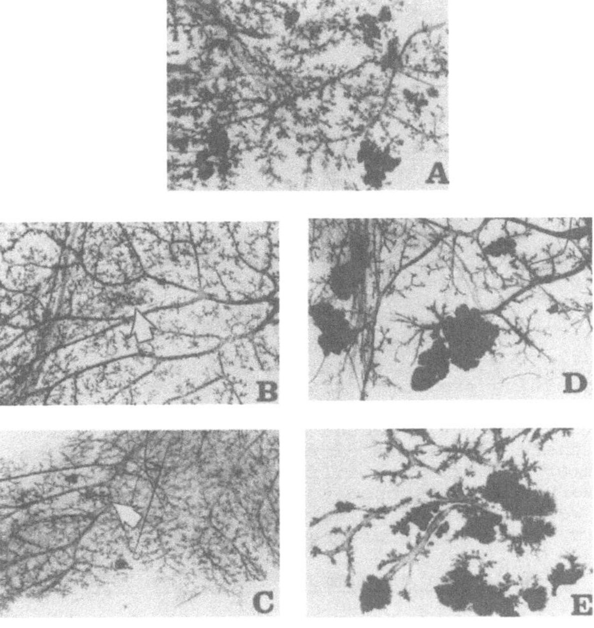

Figure 3.

Representative wholemount preparations of the third thoracic mammary glands of C3H/He mice receiving adreno-ovariectomy or manipulation of prolactin or placental lactogen (x5).

A. Intact control aged 7-8 months. Moderate lobulo-alveolar (L-A) system is maintained and several hyperplastic alveolar nodules (HAN) are found.

B. Mice given subcutaneous injections of 0.1 mg CB-154 for 40 days. L-A system regresses and there are no HAN. Ghosts, remnants of regressed HAN, are seen (indicated by the arrow).

C. Mice after 40 days of adreno-ovariectomy (adx·ovx). Mammary gland is similar to B.

D. Mice after 40 days of adx·ovx and grafting with 3 anterior pituitaries (3AP) each. Several huge HAN are seen, while L-A system is still involuted.

E. Mice ovariectomized and given subcutaneous injections of 0.5 mg human placental lactogen twice daily for 20 days. Mammary glands are similar to D and atypical end-buds and dilated ducts are observed.

This indicate that HAN appear to be much more susceptible to prolactin or placental lactogen or to have a higher growth potential in response to these hormones than do normal mammary glands. This concept has been confirmed by Bartley *et al.* (1) who examined the difference in nucleic acid synthesis in response to pregnancy, lactation or hypophysectomy between normal, preneoplastic and neoplastic mammary tissues in mice.

The difference in responsiveness to prolactin was also observed between normal mammary glands and DMBA-induced mammary tumors in rats (39). Rats bearing DMBA-induced mammary tumors were divided into two groups according to the growth rate of the first mammary tumors, the rapidly and the slowly growing groups which had tumors of more than 100 % and less than 20 % increase in size during 3 weeks after appearance, respectively. In the rapidly growing group, the tumor growth was stimulated by the single pituitary grafting in intact rats, but the treatment had no effect in adreno-ovariectomized rats. By contrast, in the slowly growing group, pituitary grafting prevented significantly the adreno-ovariectomy-induced regression of tumors, however, the tumor growth in intact rats was not affected by pituitary grafting. Meanwhile, there was little difference between host rats bearing mammary tumors with different growth potential in normal mammary gland response to these hormonal manipulation; the glands were involuted by adreno-ovariectomy and stimulated the growth by pituitary grafting.

Inhibition by prolactin of mammary tumor development

There are considerably less examples experimentally of inhibitory effects of prolactin on mammary tumorigenesis than those of stimulation. Nevertheless, there are certain endocrine conditions in which an increased secretion of this hormone is consistently inhibitory to the neoplastic process, especially in carcinogen-induced mammary tumorigenesis in rats. All treatments that stimulate pituitary prolactin secretion or elevate its circulating levels as described above, cause a marked inhibition of mammary tumor development, if they are given prior to carcinogen administration (60). While carcinogen-induced mammary tumors in rats appear to arise mostly from the ductal or end-bud elements of the glands, they are lost in the process of mammary gland proliferation which is stimulated by prolactin and it results in mammary gland refractoriness to carcinogens (22).

A MECHANISM OF ROLE OF PROLACTIN IN MAMMARY TUMOR DEVELOPMENT

Stimulation by prolactin of mammary gland DNA synthesis, a primary factor for mammary tumor development

A number of studies done mainly in my laboratory and Dr. Russo's laboratory in Detroit have revealed that mammary gland DNA synthesis around the time when carcinogenic agents act on the glands is a limiting factor for mammary tumor development (18), (22) and this synthesis has been demonstrated to be mostly controlled by prolactin (40). As presented in Figure 4, mammary gland DNA synthesis estimated by $[^3H]$thymidine incorporation was significantly higher on the afternoon of proestrus when pituitary prolactin surge was seen than on the 2nd day of diestrus in 50 days-old Sprague-Dawley rats. The number of DMBA-induced mammary tumors was significantly higher in the animals given a single intravenous injection of DMBA at proestrus than in the animals receiving DMBA at diestrus. Administration of CB-154, which inhibited prolactin surge at proestrus, resulted in the suppression of mammary gland DNA synthesis and DMBA-induced mammary tumorigenesis. On the other hand, in 90 days-old rats in which little difference was seen in mammary gland DNA synthesis between proestrus and diestrus, there was also no difference in mammary tumor development between rats given DMBA at proestrus and those receiving it at diestrus. Meanwhile, pre-stimulation of mammary gland DNA synthesis by prolactin injection increased the number of DMBA-induced mammary tumors(40).

The well-known stimulating effects of pituitary grafting on spontaneous mammary tumor development in mice is always preceded by the elevated mammary gland DNA synthesis (41).

Based on these experimental results, one of the roles of prolactin in mammary tumor development is considered to create mammary gland conditions favorable for the action of carcinogens through its stimulation of the rate of mammary gland DNA synthesis (Fig. 5: PRL-1) (20).

Both animals and human are constantly exposed to several kinds of carcinogenic agents throughout their lifetimes and it is impossible to escape from them. It appears, therefore, that the longer the total periods of low mammary gland DNA synthesis, the smaller the risk of mammary gland malignancy. From this point of view, it would be of much interest to study whether temporal inhibition of mammary gland DNA synthesis during a critical period would result in the prevention of mammary tumor development as much.

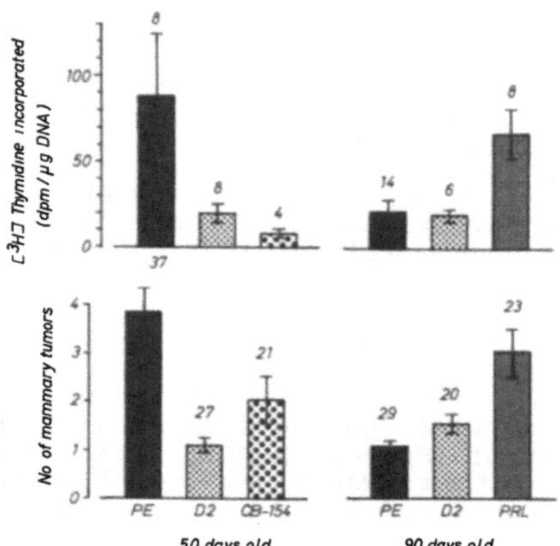

Figure 4

Relation between mammary gland DNA synthesis and development of DMBA-induced mammary tumors in Sprague-Dawley rats (means ± S.E.M.). DMBA was injected intravenously on the evening of proestrus (PE), on the 2nd day of diestrus (D2), after 30 or 24 hours of subcutaneous injection of CB-154 (1 mg) or ovine prolactin (PRL: 10 mg). The number of newly developing tumors per rat was checked until 26 weeks after DMBA injection. The number of rats used is indicated at the top of each column.

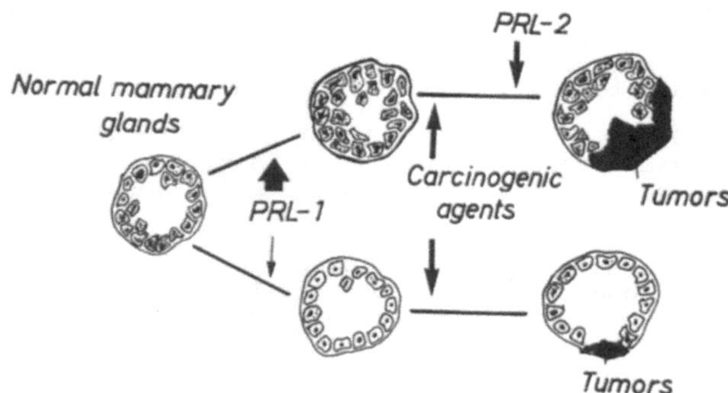

Figure 5

Scheme of the role of prolactin (PRL) in mammary tumor development. PRL-1 stimulates mammary gland DNA synthesis so that carcinogenic agents can act effectively. PRL-2 promotes the initial progression of mammary foci malignantly transformed by carcinogenic agents.

In order to check this possibility, the effects of temporal inhibition of mammary gland DNA synthesis in rats, which was generally high during young ages (peaks around 50 days) and declined with the advance of age, on spontaneous mammary tumor development was studied (23). The results are shown in Figure 6. Only 1 out of 30 or 3.3 % of rats given

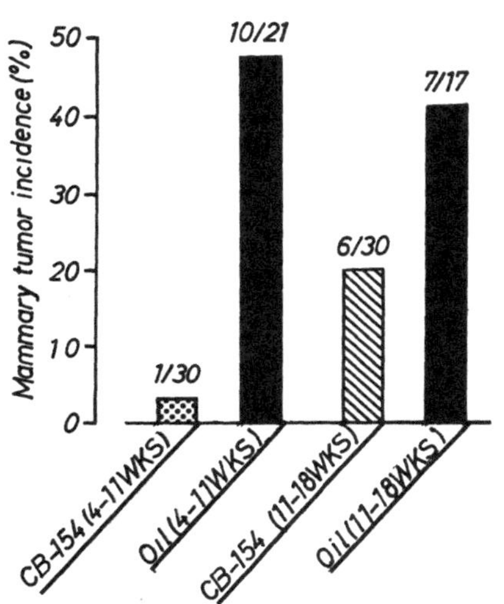

Figure 6

Prophylaxis of spontaneous mammary tumor development in rats at advanced ages by a temporal inhibition of mammary gland DNA synthesis through prolactin suppression during young ages. Sprague-Dawley virgin rats were given daily subcutaneous injections of 0.5 mg CB-154 for 7 weeks beginning 4 or 11 weeks of age. The controls received vehicle only. The number of rats bearing tumors at 20 months of age/ initial number of rats used are indicated at the top of each column.

daily subcutaneous injections of CB-154 for 7 weeks during 4-11 weeks of age developed mammary tumors until 20 months of age. On the other hand, mammary tumor incidence in rats injected with vehicle only was 47.6 % (10/21) at the same age. There was little difference in the onset age (> 14 months) and histologic type of mammary tumors between groups. The results indicate that a temporal suppression of mammary gland DNA synthesis during young ages which was induced by decline in circulating levels of prolactin contributed to the prophylaxis of spontaneous mammary tumor development at advanced ages.

Another role of prolactin in mammary tumor development is as a 'promoter' (Fig. 5: PRL-2). The character of prolactin as a promoter was well evidenced by a series of studies in late Prof. Furth's laboratory in New York (12). It was shown that when subcarcinogenic doses of carcinogens (chemicals, radiation or mammary tumor virus) were coupled with properly timed elevation in circulating levels of prolactin, the animals developed mammary tumors (Fig. 5), whereas hormone or carcinogens alone was ineffective. These have been confirmed and extended by Yokoro *et al.* (70), (71). They further provided the possibility of detection by prolactin of low-doses carcinogens and of persisting dormant mammary malignant foci (70).

Synergism of prolactin and estrogen in mammary gland DNA synthesis

While the relation between prolactin and estrogen in mammary tumor development will be discussed in the other chapters, only one problem is briefly discussed here. As already mentioned, mammary gland DNA synthesis is mostly controlled by prolactin. However, mammary gland DNA synthesis is very low during lactation (25), (30), (31) despite high circulating levels of prolactin in response to frequent suckling (30), (31). This was found to be primarily due to the low estrogen levels in the circulation during lactation, since supplement with estrogen resulted in the increase in mammary gland DNA synthesis. It was indicated that the action of estrogen in this process was to switch mammary gland cells over from the functional state to the proliferative state and that prolactin promoted mammary gland DNA synthesis when the functional activity was decreased by estrogen. Thus, estrogen probably increases DNA synthesis in lactating mammary glands both directly synergizing with prolactin and indirectly by suppressing mammary gland function and promoting the pituitary prolactin secretion (31).

Species-difference in mammary gland DNA synthesis in response to prolactin

Whereas pituitary grafting always enhances spontaneous mammary tumor development in mice, the same treatment before carcinogen administration inhibits the induction of mammary tumors in rats. This discrepancy is well accounted for by the different patterns of changes between species in mammary gland DNA synthesis in response to prolactin from the pituitary grafts (Fig. 7). After 20 days of pituitary grafting, the degree of mammary gland development observed in wholemount preparations was quite similar in mice (C3H/He) and rats (Sprague-Dawley). Meanwhile, mammary gland DNA synthesis in rats declined to less than a half by grafting, whereas the synthesis increased by 2 times in mice (19). Mammary glands in mice maintained the high synthesis after pituitary grafting (41), however, in mammary glands of rats, the differentiation, hypertrophy and mitotic rest would occur after temporal stimulation of mammary gland DNA synthesis by prolactin from the grafts (40). The cause of this species-difference is not understood at present.

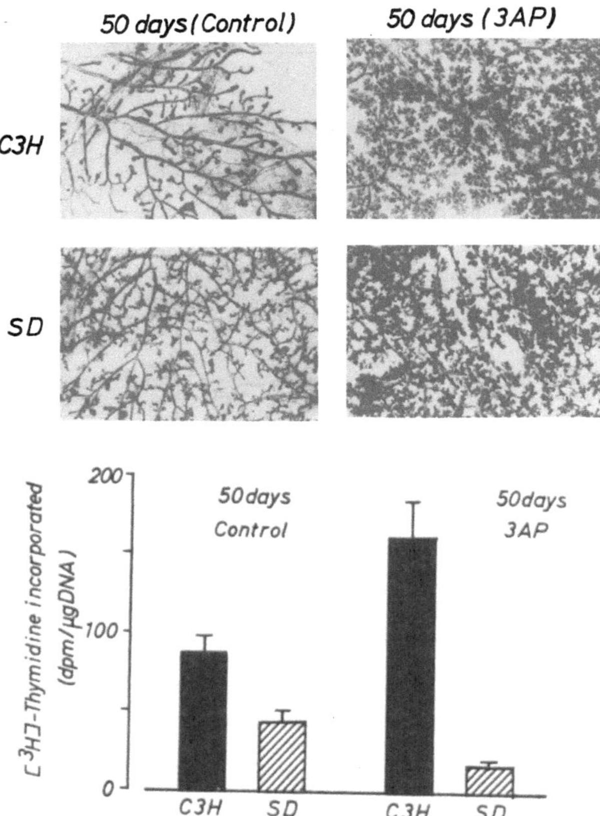

Figure 7

Changes in structure and DNA synthesis of mammary glands of mice and rats grafted with pituitaries. Thirty days-old C3H/He female mice and Sprague-Dawley (SD) female rats were grafted with 3 isologous anterior pituitaries each under the kidney capsules (3AP) and the right third and the bilateral inguinal mammary glands were used for wholemount evaluation and DNA synthesis, respectively, after 20 days of grafting or at 50 days of age. Number of animals is 8 each.

FACTORS WHICH MODULATE MAMMARY TUMOR DEVELOPMENT AND PROLACTIN SECRETION

Perinatal hormonal exposure

Exposure of mammals to hormones or drugs during pregnancy sometimes results in profound consequence in the offspring. Perinatal treatment with estrogen, progesterone, androgen or even prolactin not only induces sometimes irreversible changes in hypothalamus-pituitary-ovarian system but also influences spontaneous and carcinogen-induced mammary tumor development. While the effects vary according to the time and period of treatment and to the species and strains employed (17), neonatal treatment with hormones generally stimulates spontaneous mammary tumor development in mammary tumor virus-expressed mouse strains.

From the view point of primary importance of prolactin in mammary tumor development, plasma prolactin levels were determined in BALB/cfC3H female mice receiving daily subcutaneous injections of diethylstilbestrol (DES: 5 or 20 μg), estradiol-17β (E2: 20 μg), testosterone (T: 20 μg) or ovine-prolactin (20 μg) for the first 5 days of postnatal life. At about 2, 7 and 15 months of ages, plasma prolactin levels in mice treated with DES, E2 or prolactin were comparable to those in the controls at proestrus/estrus and usually higher than the levels at metestrus/diestrus. Treatment with T usually results in the significant elevation of plasma prolactin levels than the other treatment and the control (24). These observations indicate that enhanced mammary tumor development in female mice exposed neonatally to hormones is partly attributable to the stimulation by the treatment of pituitary prolactin secretion. This stimulation of prolactin secretion in neonatally hormone treated mice is wholly ovarian-dependent (38).

Whereas 5β-dihydrotestosterone (5β-DHT) is generally considered to be biologically inactive and is not aromatized by enzymes, daily injections of 5β-DHT (200 μg) for the first 5 days of postnatal life induced the promotion of pituitary prolactin secretion associated with the enhancement of both normal and neoplastic mammary gland development (61).

Dietary fat

It is established that diets can influence the development of some types of tumors and that mammary tumorigenesis is stimulated by high dietary fat (21), (45), (56). One of the enhancing effects of high fat diet on mammary tumor development may be mediated through its alteration of hypothalamic and pituitary function, especially prolactin secretion, although not conclusive. Chan and Cohen (5), (7) found that rats fed high fat (20 % corn oil) diet after carcinogen administration developed mammary tumors earlier and in greater numbers than rats fed low fat (5 %) diet. Stimulated tumor development by high fat diet was completely prevented by CB-154. Importance of prolactin in enhanced mammary tumor development by dietary fat has further been confirmed (6), (8). However, it should also be noted that if prolactin has a role in this process, it may sometimes has only a permissive effect on the tumor promoting action of dietary fat and alternatively that responsiveness of the individual tumor cells to hormones would increase (4).

Immunopotentiation

Both immunity and hormones are the essential factors for maintenance of homeostasis, the disorder of which is a cause of several diseases including tumors. The importance of immune mechanism in mammary tumorigenesis has recently been stressed in experimental animals and human. Nevertheless, no information was available on the interrelation between immunity and hormones on mammary tumor development. As a possible step to evaluate this relation, Nagasawa _et al_. (35) examined the effects of _Nocardia rubra_ cell wall skeleton (CWS), a potent immunopotentiator, on spontaneous mammary tumor development and pituitary prolactin secretion in SHN virgin mice. Once a week subcutaneous injections of CWS beginning 60 days of age inhibited significantly mammary tumor incidence until 11 months, but not at 12 months of age. The results imply the efficacy and the limit of immunopotentiation on protection of spontaneous mammary tumor development in mice which are largely controlled by genetical factors. In consonant with mammary tumor results, plasma prolactin levels were significantly declined by CWS at 4 months of age when no mice developed mammary tumors yet, but not at 9-12 months of age in mice bearing tumors. While mammary gland DNA synthesis was significantly suppressed by CWS treatment, little difference was observed in the synthesis between groups after supplement with prolactin. This indicates that mammary gland responsiveness to prolactin was not impaired by CWS.

Similar decline in serum prolactin levels associated with the inhibition of DMBA-induced mammary tumor development was observed in rats given CWS (36).

These results have demonstrated that prophylaxis by immunopotentiation of mammary tumor developemnt is partly due to its inhibitory effect on pituitary prolactin secretion.

ROLE OF PROLACTIN IN MAMMARY TUMOR VIRUS PRODUCTION

Mammary tumor virus (MTV) (2), (14) is an essential factor for mammary tumor development in mice. While prolactin alone has little effects on MTV production, synergistic effect of insulin, prolactin and glucocorticoids on MTV production has been reported *in vitro* in both cultured normal (69) and neoplastic (53), (54) mammary cells. Nusse *et al*. (44) also found that mammary tumorigenic hormone combination such as progesterone, estrogen and prolactin enhanced MTV protein production in mammary glands.

STRAIN-DIFFERENCE IN CIRCULATING LEVELS OF PROLACTIN OR PLACENTAL LACTOGEN AND MAMMARY GLAND SUSCEPTIBILITY TO IT

Strain-difference in hormone levels

Because of the primary importance of prolactin in mammary tumorigenesis, there may be any difference in pituitary prolactin secretion between strains in mice and rats with various mammary tumor potential.

Pituitary prolactin levels determined by disc electrophoresis were significantly higher in C3H/He female mice than in C57BL/6 mice during the virginal and pregnant stages. On the other hand, no strain-difference existed in the levels before and after suckling during lactation (64). The pituitary prolactin cells in these strains of mice were also examined by stereological morphometry with an electron microscopy (46).

Development of radioimmunoassay of mouse prolactin made it possible to measure more sensitively the pituitary and plasma levels of the hormone. No consistent patterns in either pituitary or circulating levels of prolactin were found between C3H and C57BL strains under various conditions (48), (50), (51). No distinct tendency was also observed in plasma prolactin levels between SHN and SLN mice which were segregated from the same basal stock and were different largely in mammary tumor potential; the level was significantly higher in SHN than in SLN during the virginal stage, but the opposite was the case on day 19 of pregnancy (42). No difference in the level was seen after 30 minutes suckling both on days 4 and 9 of lactation (32). Pituitary, serum and urine concentrations of prolactin were also compared between several strains of mice with varying incidence of mammary tumors (49), (52). There appears again no direct relationship between mammary tumor potential and circulating levels of prolactin.

In the experiment of mice in which the number of placentae was adjusted to 1-12 on day 8 of pregnancy, the number and weight of placentae had positive correlations with both DNA content and the rating for lobulo-alveolar development of mammary glands on day 19 of pregnancy (27). This suggest that placental mammotropic hormones including placental lactogen would contribute quantitatively to mammary gland growth during pregnancy in mice. However, there was little difference between C3H/He and C57BL/6 mice in the mammotropic activity of placental extracts either on day 4 or day 19 of pregnancy despite large difference in normal and neoplastic mammary development (62).

These results do not negate the importance of prolactin in mammary tumor development, but may suggest a moderate rate of prolactin secretion may be sufficient to permit tumor development. They also imply that the susceptibility of mammary glands to prolactin is another important factor for mammary tumor development.

On the contrary, some reports in rats have shown that there are apparent strain-difference in basal prolactin levels in the circulation at diestrus; the levels in strains susceptible to DMBA were higher than those in strains resistant to DMBA (3), (13). Furthermore, in DMBA susceptible Sprague-Dawley rats, DMBA significantly stimulated prolactin surge on the afternoon of proestrus at any cycle after DMBA administration, but not in DMBA insusceptible Wistar rats. The results show that there is a specific and transient hormonal deregulation in a DMBA susceptible strain of rats (15).

Strain-difference in mammary gland susceptibility to prolactin in mice

It has been evidenced in female mice that mammary gland growth in response to pituitary grafting was much greater in high mammary tumor strains (C3H/He and SHN) than in low mammary tumor strains (C57BL/6 and SLN) in wholemount preparations (37), (42). However, these *in vivo* studies have provided no evidence as to whether prolactin secreted from the grafts stimulates mammary gland growth directly or indirectly through its luteotropic effects on ovaries. Moreover, in the wholemount observation, no information is available on the dynamic aspect of mammary gland responsiveness, which is of most importance for mammary tumorigenesis (29). To clarify these problems, we have examined mammary gland DNA synthesis of SHN and SLN strains when cultured in the defined medium (Fig. 8) (34). Mammary glands from immature female mice of each strain were cultured in the medium containing insulin, aldosterone, prolactin, growth hormone, estrogen and progesterone or the medium deficient of prolactin. After the culture, each gland was further incubated with [^{3}H]thymidine under the same

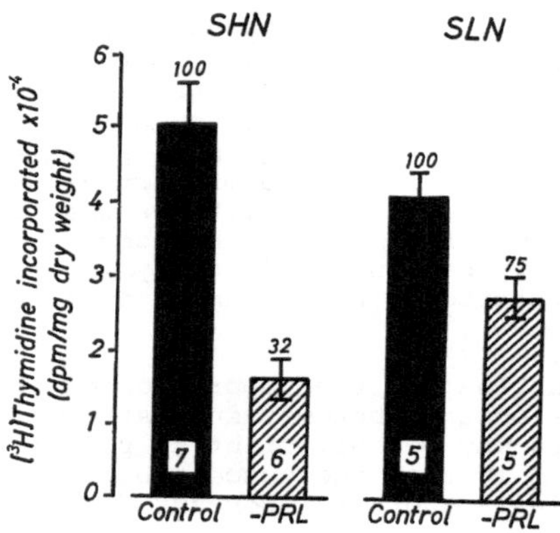

Figure 8

Difference between SHN and SLN strains of mice in the direct effect of prolactin on mammary gland DNA synthesis (means ± S.E.M.). The 2nd thoracic mammary glands from 32-35 days-old female mice injected subcutaneously with estradiol-17β (E2: 1 µg/ml) and progesterone (1 mg/ml) for 3 days were cultured in the Waymouth medium containing insulin (5 µg/ml), aldosterone (1 µg/ml), growth hormone (5 µg/ml), E2 (1 ng/ml) and progesterone (1 µg/ml) with (control) or without (-PRL) ovine-prolactin (5 µg/ml) for 6 days at 37 °C under constant gassing with 95% O_2-5% CO_2. At the termination of culture, each gland was further incubated for 2 hours in the medium containing 2.5 µCi [^{3}H]thymidine and the same hormones as in the preceding culture. The percentage against the value of the control and the number of glands used are presented at the top and the bottom of each column, respectively.

hormonal conditions. There was no significant difference between strains in mammary gland DNA synthesis of the controls cultured in the medium containing all hormones. While the synthesis declined significantly in mammary glands of both strains when cultured in the absence of prolactin, the degree was much more marked in SHN strain than in SLN strain (32 % vs 75% of the respective controls).

These observations have demonstrated that SHN mice with higher potential for both normal and neoplastic mammary gland growth are superior to SLN with lower potential not only in static state but also in dynamic aspect of mammary gland response to prolactin.

Since no distinct differences in the pituitary and placental mammotropic hormone levels in the circulation were generally found between high and low mammary tumor strains of mice, mammary gland susceptibility to mammotropic hormones, especially prolactin, would be of much importance in mammary tumor development as well as normal mammary gland growth.

FUTURE PROSPECTS

Whereas a number of *in vivo* and *in vitro* studies have been designed to evaluate the role of prolactin in human breast cancer, the results are still controversial. Despite well-known species- specificity in protein hormones, ovine- or bovine-prolactin has often been used for the experiments in human breast cancer. This may be a cause of confused results. Furthermore, all of these studies are on the effects of hormones (prolactin) on 'progression' of established breast cancers, but not on their 'initiation' or 'development'. Hormonal control of these two process is not always similar or quite different as seen in spontaneous mammary tumors in mice; preneoplastic and neoplastic transformation of mammary glands in mice is wholly dependent upon hormones, especially prolactin, however, the progression of established tumors is autonomous.

There would be no large difference between experimental animals and human in the role of prolactin or placental lactogen in mammary gland malignancy and its initial development. Thus, the unequivocal key role of these hormones in experimental mammary tumor development should provide sufficient impetus for vigorous efforts toward defining the role of these hormones in the development of human breast cancer.

REFERENCES

1. Bartley JC, Barber S, Abraham S. Rate of nucleic acid synthesis in mammary hyperplastic alveolar nodule outgrowths and transplanted adenocarcinomas in pregnant and lactating mice. Cancer Res 34: 2571-2575, 1974.

2. Bentvelzen P, Hilgers J. Murine mammary tumor virus. pp 311-355 in *Viral Oncology*, ed G Klein. Raven Press, New York, 1980.

3. Boyns AR, Buchan R, Cole EN, Forrest APM, Griffiths K. Basal prolactin blood levels in 3 strains of rats with differing incidence of 7,12-dimethylbenz(a)anthracene induced mammary tumours. Eur J Cancer 9: 169-171, 1973.

4. Cave WT Jr, Dunn JT, MacLeod RM, Effect of iodine deficiency and high-fat diet on N-nitrosomethylurea-induced mammary cancers in rats. Cancer Res 39: 729-734, 1979.

5. Chan PC, Cohen LA. Effect of dietary fat, antiestrogen and antiprolactin on the development of mammary tumors in rats. J Natl Cancer Inst 52: 25-30, 1974.

6. Chan PC, Cohen LA. Dietary fat and growth promotion of rat mammary tumors. Cancer Res 35: 3384-3386, 1975.

7. Chan PC, Didato F, Cohen LA. High dietary fat, elevation of rat serum prolactin and mammary cancer. Proc Soc Exp Biol Med 149: 133-135, 1975.

8. Chan PC, Head JF, Cohen LA, Wynder EL. Influence of dietary fat on the induction of mammary tumors by N-nitrosomethylurea associated hormone changes and differences between Sprague-Dawley and F344 rats. J Natl Cancer Inst 59: 1279-1283, 1975.

9. Chen HJ, Bradley CJ, Meites J. Stimulation of growth of carcinogen-induced mammary cancers in rats by thyrotropin-releasing hormone. Cancer Res 37: 64-66, 1977.

10. Drosdowsky M, Edery M, Guggiari M, Montes-Rendon A, Rudali G, Vives C. Inhibition of prolactin-induced mammary cancer in C3Hf(XVII) mice with the trans isomer of bromotriphenylethylene. Cancer Res 40: 1674-1679, 1980.

11. Forsyth IA. The comparative study of placental lactogenic hormones: A review. pp 49-67 in Lactogenic Hormones, Fetal Nutrition, and Lactation, eds JB Josimovich, M Reynolds, E Cobo. Wiley & Sons, New York, 1974.

12. Furth J. The role of prolactin in mammary carcinogenesis. pp 233-248 in Human Prolactin, eds JL Pasteels, C Robyn. Am Elsevier Publ Co, New York, 1973.

13. Hawkins RA, Drewitt D, Freedman B, Killin E, Jenner DA, Cameron EHD. Plasma hormone levels and the incidence of carcinogen-induced mammary tumours in two strains of rat. Br J Cancer 34: 546-549, 1976.

14. Hilgers J, Bentvelzen P. Interaction between viral and genetic factors in murine mammary cancer. Adv Cancer Res 26: 143-195, 1978.

15. Kerdellhue B, El Abed A. Inhibition of preovulatory gonadotropin secretion and stimulation of prolactin secretion by 7,12-dimethylbenz(a)anthracene in Sprague-Dawley rats. Cancer Res 39: 4700-4705, 1979.

16. Medina D. Preneoplasia in breast cancer. pp 47-102 in

Breast Cancer Vol 2, ed WL McGuire. Plenum Publ Corp, New York, 1978.

17. Mori T, Nagasawa H, Bern HA. Long-term effects of perinatal exposure to hormones on normal and neoplastic mammary growth in rodents: A review. J. Environ Path Toxicol 3: 191-205, 1980.

18. Nagasawa H. Mammary gland DNA synthesis as a limiting factor for mammary tumourigenesis (Forum). IRCS Med Sci 5: 405-408, 1977.

19. Nagasawa H. Causes of species difference in mammary tumourigenesis: Significance of mammary gland DNA synthesis. Med Hypotheses 5: 499-510, 1979.

20. Nagasawa H. Prolactin: Its role in the development of mammary tumours. Med Hypotheses 5: 1117-1121, 1979.

21. Nagasawa H. Nutrition and breast cancer. IRCS Med Sci 8: 786-791, 1980.

22. Nagasawa H. Causes of age-dependency of mammary tumour induction by carcinogen in rats. Biometrics 34: 9-11 1981.

23. Nagasawa H, Morii S. Prophylaxis of spontaneous mammary tumorigenesis by temporal inhibition of prolactin secretion in rats at young ages. Cancer Res. 41: 1935-1937, 1981.

24. Nagasawa H, Mori T, Yanai R, Bern HA, Mills KT. Long-term effects of neonatal hormonal treatments on plasma prolactin levels in female BALB/cfC3H and BALB/c mice. Cancer Res 38: 942-945, 1978.

25. Nagasawa H, Vorherr H. Rat mammary deoxyribonucleic acid synthesis during the estrous cycle, pregnancy, and lactation in relation to mammary tumorigenesis. Am J Obstet Gynecol 127: 590-593, 1977.

26. Nagasawa H, Yanai R. Effect of prolactin or growth hormone on growth of carcinogen-induced mammary tumors of adreno-ovariectomized rats. Int J Cancer 6: 488-495, 1970.

27. Nagasawa H, Yanai R. Quantitative participation of placental mammotropic hormones in mammary development during pregnancy in mice. Endocrinol Jpn 18: 507-510, 1971.

28. Nagasawa H, Yanai R. Effect of human placental lactogen on growth of carcinogen-induced mammary tumors in rats. Int J Cancer 11: 131-137, 1973.

29. Nagasawa H, Yanai R. Some discrepancies between the use of DNA synthesis and wholemount preparations as indices of mammary gland response to pituitary mammotrophin. J Endocrinol 67: 303-304, 1975.

30. Nagasawa H, Yanai R. Mammary nucleic acids and pituitary prolactin secretion during prolonged lactation in mice. J Endocrinol 70: 389-395, 1976.

31. Nagasawa H, Yanai R. Effects of oestrogen and/or pituitary grafts on nucleic acid synthesis in the mammary glands of lactating mice. J Endocrinol 77: 319-323, 1978.

32. Nagasawa H, Yanai R. Mammary gland prolactin receptor and pituitary prolactin secretion in lactating mice with different lactational performance. Acta Endocrinol (Kbh) 88: 94-98, 1978.

33. Nagasawa H, Yanai R. Normal and abnormal growth of the mammary gland. pp 121-159 in _Physiology of Mammary Glands_, eds A Yokoyama, H Mizuno, H Nagasawa. Jap Sci Soc Press/ Univ Park Press, Tokyo/Baltimore, 1978.

34. Nagasawa H, Yanai R. The _in vitro_ mammary gland response to mammotropic hormones in mice with different mammary tumorigenesis. Eur J Cancer 17: 503-509, 1981.

35. Nagasawa H, Yanai R, Azuma I. Suppression by _Nocardia rubra_ cell wall skeleton of mammary DNA synthesis, plasma prolactin level, and spontaneous mammary tumorigenesis in mice. Cancer Res 38: 2160-2162, 1978.

36. Nagasawa H, Yanai R, Azuma I. Inhibitory effect of _Nocardia rubra_ cell wall skeleton on carcinogen-induced mammary tumorigenesis in rats. Eur J Cancer 16: 389-393, 1980.

37. Nagasawa H, Yanai R, Iwahashi H, Fujimoto M, Kuretani K. Difference in mammary gland susceptibility to prolactin between a high and a low mammary tumor strains of mice. Endocrinol Jpn 14: 351-356, 1967.

38. Nagasawa H, Yanai R, Jones LA, Bern HA, Mills KT. Ovarian dependence of the stimulatory effect of neonatal hormone treatment on plasma levels of prolactin in female mice. J Endocrinol 79: 391-392, 1978.

39. Nagasawa H, Yanai R, Nakajima Y. Response to adreno-ovariectomy and/or pituitary grafting of carcinogen-induced mammary tumors in rats with different growth potential. Eur J Cancer 16: 1345-1350, 1980.

40. Nagasawa H, Yanai R, Taniguchi H. Importance of mammary gland DNA synthesis on carcinogen-induced mammary tumorigenesis in rats. Cancer Res 36: 2223-2226, 1976.

41. Nagasawa H, Yanai R, Taniguchi H. Reduction by pituitary grafts of mammary tumor age. Its variability in a high mammary tumor strain of mice. Effects of mammary DNA synthesis. Eur J Cancer 12: 1017-1019, 1976.

42. Nagasawa H, Yanai R, Taniguchi H, Tokuzen R, Nakahara W. Two-way selection of Swiss albino mice for mammary tumorigenesis: Establishment of new two strains (SHN and SLN). J Natl Cancer Inst 57: 425-430, 1976.

43. Nagasawa H, Yanai, R, Yamanouchi K. Inhibition of pituitary prolactin secretion by human placental lactogen in rats. J Endocrinol 71: 115-120, 1976.

44. Nusse R, Michalides R, Boot LM, Röpcke G. Quantification of mouse mammary tumor virus structural protein in hormone induced mammary tumors of low mammary tumor mouse strains. Int J Cancer 25: 377-383, 1980.

45. Reddy BS, Cohen LA, McCoy D, Hill P, Weisburger JH, Wynder EL. Nutrition and cancer. Adv Cancer Res 32: 237-345, 1980.

45a. Rudali G, Vives CI, Guggiari M, Montes-Rendon A. Mammary carcinogenesis in (C3HxRIII)F1 mice which receive the trans isomer of a brominated triphenylethylene. Biomedicine 33: 126-128, 1980.

45b. Rudali G, Montes-Rendon A, Assa R. Inhibition of mammary carcinogenesis of dimethylbenzanthracene treated rats with a brominated triphenylethylene. Biomedicine 31: 142-146, 1979.

46. Sasaki S, Iwami Y, Sano M. Strain-difference in prolactin cells of mouse anterior pituitary between high and low mammary tumor strains by stereological morphometry with an electron microscope. Okajimas Folia Anat Jpn 55: 341-350, 1979.

47. Sinha YN, Baxter SR. Metabolism of prolactin in mice with a high incidence of mammary tumours: Evidence for greater conversion into a non-immunoassayable form. J

Endocrinol 81: 299-314, 1979.

48. Sinha YN, Salocks CB, Lewis UJ, VanderLaan WP. Influence of nursing on the release of prolactin and GH in mice with high and low incidence of mammary tumors. Endocrinology 95: 947-54, 1974.

49. Sinha YN, Salocks CB, VanderLaan WP. Prolactin and growth hormone levels in different inbred strains of mice: Patterns in association with estrous cycle, time of day, and perphenazine stimulation. Endocrinology 97: 1112-1122, 1975.

50. Sinha YN, Salocks CB, VanderLaan WP. Circulating levels of prolactin and growth hormone and natural incidence of mammary tumors in mice. J Toxicol Environ Health 1 (Suppl): 131-160, 1976.

51. Sinha YN, Selby FW, VanderLaan WP. The natural history of prolactin and GH secretion in mice with high and low incidence of mammary tumors. Endocrinology 94: 757-764, 1974.

52. Sinha YN, Vlahakis G, VanderLaan WP. Serum, pituitary and urine concentrations of prolactin and growth hormone in eight strains of mice with varying incidence of mammary tumors. Int J Cancer 24: 430-437, 1979.

53. Svec J, Hlavayova E, Matoska J, Thurzo V. Conditions for hormone-stimulated expression of endogenous C57Bl strain-associated mammary tumor virus genome. Neoplasma 28: 539-550, 1979.

54. Svec J, Links J. Mouse mammary tumor virus production stimulated by hormones and polyamines in cells grown in semisynthetic in vitro conditions. Int J Cancer 19: 249-257, 1977.

55. Talamantes F, Ogren L, Markoff E, Woodard S, Phylogenetic distribution, regulation of secretion, and prolactin-like effects of placental lactogens. Fed Proc 39: 2582-2587, 1980.

56. Vorherr H. Breast Cancer pp 37-54. Urban-Schwarzenberg, Baltimore and Munnich, 1980.

57. Welsch CW. Prolactin and the development and progression of early neoplastic mammary gland lesions. Cancer Res 38: 4054-4058, 1978.

58. Welsch CW, Goodrich-Smith M, Brown CK, Wilson M.

Inhibition of mammary tumorigenesis in GR mice with 2-bromo-α-ergocryptine. Int J Cancer 24: 92-96, 1979.

59. Welsch CW, Meites J, Prolactin and mammary carcinogenesis. pp 71-92 in Endocrine Control of Neoplasia, eds RK Sharma, WE Criss. Raven Press, New York, 1978.

60. Welsch CW and Nagasawa H. Prolactin and murine mammary tumorigenesis: A review. Cancer Res 37: 951-963, 1977.

61. Yanai R, Mori T, Nagasawa H. Long-term effects of prenatal and neonatal administration of 5β-dihydrotestosterone on normal and neoplastic mammary development in mice. Cancer Res 37: 4456-4459, 1977.

62. Yanai R, Nagasawa H. Mammary growth and placental mammotropin during pregnancy in mice with high or low lactational performance. J Dairy Sci 54: 906-910, 1971.

63. Yanai R, Nagasawa H. Enhancement by pituitary isografts of mammary hyperplastic nodules in adreno-ovariectomized mice. J Natl Cancer Inst 46: 1251-1255, 1971.

64. Yanai R, Nagasawa H. Pituitary prolactin and growth hormone levels during different reproductive states in mice with a high and a low lactational performance. Horm Behav 2: 73-82, 1971.

65. Yanai R, Nagasawa H. Inhibition of mammary tumorigenesis by ergot alkaloids and promotion of mammary tumorigenesis by pituitary grafts in adreno-ovariectomized mice. J Natl Cancer Inst 48: 715-719, 1972.

66. Yanai R, Nagasawa H. Enhancement by human placental lactogen of mammary hyperplastic nodules in ovariectomized mice. Cancer Res 33: 1642-1644, 1973.

67. Yanai R, Nagasawa H. Importance of progesterone in DNA synthesis of pregnancy-dependent mammary tumors in mice. Int J Cancer 18: 317-321, 1976.

68. Yanai R, Nagasawa H. Development and growth of pregnancy-dependent and -independent mammary tumors in GR/A strain of mice and their interrelationship. Gann 69: 25-30, 1978.

69. Yang J, Enami J, Nandi S. Regulation of mammary tumor virus production by prolactin in BALB/cfC3H mouse mammary epithelial cells in vitro. Cancer Res 37: 3644-3647, 1977.

70. Yokoro K, Nakano M, Ito A, Nagao K, Kodama Y, Hamada K. Role of prolactin in rat mammary carcinogenesis: Detection of carcinogenicity of low-dose carcinogens and of persisting dormant cancer cell. J Natl Cancer Inst 58: 1777-1783, 1977.

71. Yokoro K, Sumi C, Ito A, Hamada K, Kanda K, Kobayashi T. Mammary carcinogenic effect of low-dose fission radiation in Wistar/Furth rats and its dependency on prolactin. J Natl Cancer Inst 64: 1459-1466, 1980.

Chapter 2

PROLACTIN AND PROLACTIN RECEPTORS IN TUMOR DEVELOPMENT, GROWTH AND CELLULAR FUNCTIONS

Paul A Kelly, Jean Djiane, Philippe Gandilhon, Alzira A.M Rosa, Rene St-Arnaud

The importance of prolactin (PRL) in the development and growth of the mammary gland and experimental mammary tumors is clearly established. Prolactin, however, does not act alone in its stimulatory action on normal mammary development nor in its role as an initiator or co-inducer of mammary tumors. A number of other hormones such as estrogens, progesterone, glucocorticoids, thyroid hormones, insulin and growth hormone have been shown to be important for full development and action of the mammary gland (21) and are undoubtedly of great importance in the evolution and maintenance of mammary tumors.

In this chapter, we will describe various models of hormone-dependent breast cancer, the hormonal regulation of prolactin receptors in normal and neoplastic tissue and the role of prolactin in human breast cancer.

MODELS OF HORMONE-DEPENDENT MAMMARY CANCER

Several reviews on prolactin and breast cancer have appeared (38, (39), (40), (65), (69), (71), (88), (93), (94), (114), (128). Spontaneous mammary tumors appear in a high percentage of rats 24 months of age or older. These tumors are usually a single fibroadenoma (88). Multiparous rats have been observed to have a higher incidence of spontaneous tumors than nulliparous animals (129). The positive role of prolactin in the development of these spontaneous tumors has been clarified by several studies. Welsch et al. (126) observed that rats receiving multiple pituitary homographs, which produce elevated prolactin levels, had a greater incidence of spontaneous mammary tumors than did the control rats. The same group also showed that median eminence hypothalamic lesions which increased plasma prolactin levels in female rats also markedly increased spontaneous tumor development (129). The continued growth of established spontaneous mammary tumors can be rapidly reversed and regression induced by administration of ergot drugs which lower plasma prolactin levels (102). These data indicate that the spontaneous mammary tumors of the rat are prolctin-dependent, increasing in incidence with increased prolactin levels and regressing where prolactin levels decline.

Mice

Similar studies linking prolactin to mammary tumorigenesis in mice have also been reported. In a review by Welsch and

Nagasawa (128), the authors point out, in contrast to what occurs for the majority of mammary tumors of the rat, that tumors at the developmental stages are prolactin-dependent, but that advanced mammary tumors of most strains of mice become independent of prolactin.

A direct role of prolactin in the development of mammary tumors in mice has clearly been shown by a series of studies involving the grafting of pituitaries under the kidney capsule, a condition which leads to an increased secretion of prolactin (80, 89). Several reports of ergot-induced suppression of prolactin secretion in pituitary grafted mice have shown a marked reduction in mammary tumor incidence (37) (131). Other means of increasing plasma prolactin levels, either by reserpine (77) or direct administration of ovine PRL (11), also led to an increase in the incidence of mammary tumors in mice.

Most strains of mice are capable developing mammary tumors with a relatively high incidence including C3H/He, BALB/C, SHN, C3Hf, GR, etc. Nagasawa (90) has recently proposed that elevated prolactin levels result in an increase in the frequency of cell division in the normal mammary gland, a condition which is essential for later expression of tumor development. The fact that the more advanced stages of tumor development in mice appear to be independent of prolactin has led many investigators to the conclusion that the mouse tumor system more closely reflects the pattern of breast cancer development in humans.

Rats

The mammary carcinoma induced in the rat by dimethylbenzanthracene (DMBA) has been the most widely accepted model of hormone-dependent breast cancer (54). Estrogens and prolactin have been shown to be important in the development and growth of these mammary tumors. In fact, procedures that reduce circulating levels of prolactin (hypophysectomy, ergot drugs) have been shown to reduce the number and size of these tumors (14), (46), (69), (88), (93), (94), (101), (114), (128). Teller et al. (115) compared the effect of eight prolactin-inhibiting ergot alkaloids or ergoline derivatives for their ability to inhibit DMBA-induced mammary tumors. They found an arrangement of three groups of compounds in terms of antitumor activity: high (ergocryptine and Deprenon), intermediate (ergocornine, Lysenyl, Dironyl and Lergotrile), and low (CB-154 and 6605-VUFB). It should be mentioned that these data, especially for the effectiveness of CB-154, are at variance with a number of published reports (14), (46), (101), as well as data from our laboratory which have described this prolactin-inhibiting compound as very effective in preventing new tumor growth as well as inducing regression of establish tumors. Agents which increase plasma prolactin levels, such as adrenalectomy (16), pregnancy (86), pituitary homografts (125) or tumors (70) and neuroleptic agents (93), (100), (127) have a positive influence in tumor growth. Tumors can also be reinitiated in hypophysectomized rats by the exogenous administration of prolactin (93). The predominant role of prolactin in DMBA tumor growth has been shown by studies in which estrogen receptors were blocked with an antiestrogen, and tumor growth could be reinitiated by simply increasing prolactin levels (82).

The importance of prolactin in DMBA-induced mammary tumors was confirmed by the finding that there is a direct correlation between serum prolactin levels and the susceptibility of various strains of rats to the carcinogen (12). These data, taken together with numerous other reports correlating increased prolactin levels with enhanced tumor growth and reduced prolactin levels with an inhibition of tumor growth (see reviews), indicate a direct positive influence of prolactin on DMBA-induced mammary tumors.

Prolactin has also been reported to have an inhibitory influence on tumor development, dependent upon the time the animals are exposed to elevated prolactin levels. Welsch et al. (125) reported that rats implanted with four pituitaries under the kidney capsule 30 days prior to the injection of DMBA failed to cause tumor growth and, in fact, led to a 27% reduction in the incidence and a 62% decline in the number of these carcinogen-induced tumors. Several other stimuli which increase prolactin secretion if given prior to DMBA treatment have an inhibitory effect on tumor development in rats (128). In addition, agents which increase plasma prolactin levels can either have no effect or result in a reduced incidence and delayed appearance. Therefore, although the role of prolactin is predominantly stimulatory, the specific role, either stimulatory or inhibitory, should also be taken into account when evaluating the hormonal response of a tumor.

In addition to DMBA, other chemical carcinogens have been utilized to study hormone-dependent cancer. Methycholanthrene was found to successfully induce mammary tumors in rats and these tumors were shown to be hormone-dependent. Gullino et al. (42) have reported the development of mammary tumors induced by nitrosomethylurea (NMU). These tumors appear to differ from DMBA-induced mammary tumors in that they metastasize, as do human carcinomas, and, therefore, may represent a better model to study human tumorigenesis in experimental animals. Recently, NMU-induced tumors have been characterized in our laboratory (120), (121) as well as by other groups (118), (124).

In vitro systems

In an attempt to uniformize the methodological approach to the study of breast cancer, several groups have attempted to develop long-term cultures of mammary tumors. For experimental tumors, reports have appeared on the use of tissue explants (79), (105) of DMBA tumors which responsed to prolactin in terms of an increase in estrogen receptor concentrations following exposure of the explants to prolactin in the medium.

Another group showed that DMBA-induced tumors in short-term incubations responsed to both estradiol and prolactin equally by an increase in [^{3}H]-leucine incorporation, but together the two hormones acted synergistically (78). Chan et al. (15) reported a monolayer culture system of DMBA tumor cells. However, the response of this system to estradiol and prolactin was not the same as is observed in vivo. Similarly, organ culture of DMBA tumors yielded variable responses to estrogen and prolactin (92). We are currently using short-term (24-48h) explant cultures to investigate the role of various hormones on both hormone receptor regulation as well as DNA synthesis and casein and lactalbumin production.

HORMONAL REGULATION OF PRL RECEPTORS IN NORMAL TISSUE

The mammary gland is the primary target organ of prolactin. This tissue was in fact chosen for the development of a radioreceptor assay for lactogenic hormones (112). Prolactin receptors from the rabbit mammary gland were subsequently characterized (108), solubilized and purified (109). One of the actions of prolactin in the mammary gland is the production of milk proteins. In both rabbit (26) and rat (84) mammary gland, prolactin has been shown to stimulate the production of casein messenger RNA. Antiserum prepared against purified prolactin receptors has been shown to inhibit by more than 90% the binding of [^{125}I]prolactin to rabbit mammary tissue (111) as well as preventing the prolactin-induced synthesis of casein from rabbit mammary explants (110). These studies demonstrate the functional importance of the binding of prolactin to a specific receptor as the central event leading to hormone action.

Measurement of prolactin receptors

For the quantitation of receptor levels in a tissue, crude plasma membrane fractions are prepared by differential centrifugation, and ovine prolactin is iodinated to a low specific activity (48-80 μCi/μg). Prolactin binding is assayed by incubating receptors with labeled PRL in the absence or presence of excess unlabeled PRL and is often reported as a percent of the total counts added. In addition, saturation or displacement curves can be carried out on representative membrane preparations and the data transformed into Scatchard plots (106) which yield affinity constants and binding capacities of the membrane.

In addition to the classical approach to measure prolactin receptors which involves differential centrifugation of a tissue homogenate and subsequent binding to the particulate membrane fraction, alternative approaches which utilize small biopsy determinations have emerged. Costlow et al. (19) reported prolactin binding using 0.5 mm tissue slices of tumor tissue. Even smaller samples can be utilized if frozen "microslices" are used (50). This involves cutting 20 μm slices of tumor on a cryostat and incubation of approximately 8 slices (0.5 mm^2) with [^{125}I]-ovine prolactin as described for membrane fractions (62). Ongoing studies in our laboratory indicate that this technique is applicable to repeated determinations in the same tumor as well as for localization of receptors using autoradiography (34).

Receptor levels during pregnancy and lactation

The concept that hormone receptors are not static systems, but change with the physiological state of the animal is important in terms of the control of cellular activity. Recently, we measured prolactin receptors in the mammary gland of rabbits which had been pretreated for a 36-hour period with the dopamine agonist CB-154 (Sandoz, Basle, Switzerland) to lower circulating prolactin (32). Measurement of receptor levels revealed a gradual increase in receptor concentration until day 22 followed by a decline until parturition, and a marked increase in early lactation (32).

Prolactin binding to rat mammary gland decreased between days 30 to 100 of age in virgin glands. Binding was low during pregnancy and increased during early lactation and declined following removal of litters (43). It has been demonstrated, however, that by simply removing the ovaries and the uterus (including placentae) 24 hours prior to sacrifice, a marked increase in prolactin binding was observed, indicating that a large proportion of receptors are saturated by the high levels of circulating placental lactogen (49). PRL binding under these circumstances increases as pregnancy progresses and remains elevated during lactation. Other groups reported a peak of prolactin binding on day 2 of lactation after which receptor levels declined rapidly (9).

Up-regulation

The hormonal regulation of prolactin receptors is complex (63). Estradiol injection into male or female rats leads to an increase in hepatic prolactin binding sites (67), (97).

The fact that prolactin binding can be stimulated by estrogens, fluctuates with the estrous cycle and is reduced by ovariectomy suggests a direct physiological involvement of estradiol.

The loss of prolactin binding in rat liver following hypophysectomy implied the importance of a pituitary factor in the maintaince of these binding sites (67), (97). A direct effect of prolactin on its own receptor was first implied when we demonstrated that prolactin binding to rat liver in hypophysectomized rats given a pituitary implant under the kidney capsule began to increase approximately 3 days following the increase in serum prolactin levels (98). A direct stimulatory effect of prolactin injected in polyvinylpyrrolidone to retard absorption has more recently been reported (64), (81).

The up-regulatory effect of prolactin on prolactin receptors in rabbit mammary gland has also been demonstrated (30). Pseudopregnant rabbits injected with 100 IU oPRL showed a marked increase in prolactin receptor levels. This increase could be prevented by simultaneous administration of progesterone, suggesting that part of the progesterone block of lactation during pregnancy could be mediated by a reduction in prolactin receptor levels in the mammary gland.

Down-regulation

In contrast to the inhibitory effect of a large number of hormones on the level of their own receptor, a stimulatory effect of prolactin on its receptor in both rabbit mammary gland and rat liver has been observed (30), (98). Using 4M $MgCl_2$ to dissociate bound prolactin from its receptor (66), we investigated the short-term action of prolactin on its receptor in target tissues with the goal of evaluating if prolactin, in addition to its ability to up-regulate prolactin receptors, is, like most other hormones studied so far, capable of inducing a down-regulation of its own receptor. This in turn would lend some support to recent view (99) contending that down-regulation (and possibly up regulation as well) are ubiquitous events which might be intimately linked to the very mechanism of hormone action.

Lactating, New Zealand rabbits were injected every 12 hours over a 36-hour period with 2 mg of the dopamine agonist, CB-154, to lower circulating prolactin levels (32) after which the animals were anesthesized with 50 mg/kg of sodium pentobarbital. Three mg bovine prolactin (bPRL) were injected intravenously and 2 g biopsies of mammary gland tissue were removed at the indicated times between 0 and 30 hours after prolactin injection.

Injection of 3 mg of prolactin led to a maximal occupancy of free rabbit mammary gland prolactin receptors 15 min after the intravenous injection, corresponding to periods just following maximal serum concentrations. The highest serum levels were seen 1 min after injection with values rapidly delining thereafter. Although saturating concentrations of circulating prolactin were present 15 min after injection, 20% of the prolactin receptors remained free to bind [^{125}I]-oPRL. This could be due to an inaccessibility of the receptors to the circulating prolactin or to some dissociation occuring while membranes were isolated from the tissues.

Somewhat surprisingly, total prolactin receptor levels assayed following in vitro desaturation with 4M $MgCl_2$ declined progressively up to 6 hours after the intravenous injection of prolactin and returned to normal at 24 to 30 hours. The difference in total prolactin binding between time 0 and 6 hours was statistically significant ($p < 0.01$). A difference was observed between the pattern of occupation (free receptors) and the down-regulation reflected by total receptors. In addition, free receptors increased between 1 and 6 hours, whereas total receptors continued to decline until 6 hours (29).

A pattern similar to the time-dependent occupation of mammary gland prolactin receptors following intravenous injection of prolactin was observed with rat liver. Maximal occupation occurred at 15 min with a return to normal levels 12 hours after injection. Serum levels of bovine PRL were maximal 1 min after injection, and were still detectable 1h after injection, thus suggesting apparent dissociation of prolactin from its receptor or new receptor synthesis or processing. Total receptors were higher 1 min after PRL injection, possibly due to a protection of available binding sites, however, total receptor levels were significantly reduced at 6 hours compared to either time 0 ($p < 0.05$) or 1 min after injection ($p < 0.01$).

It has been well established that the mammary gland can be maintained in organ culture and responds well to hormones (6), (31). In addition, mammary explants can be used as an experimental model to study the steps involved in the mechanisms of hormone action (53).

Study was undertaken to verify the maintenance of PRL receptors in mammary glands in organ culture, to assess the apparent turnover of receptors and to describe the effect of large doses of prolactin on the levels of its own receptor. In the presence of insulin only, the level of PRL receptors was maintained up until 48h. The addition of cycloheximide resulted in a rapid decrease of receptors which was almost maximal at 3h. Removal of cycloheximide from the culture medium at either 6h or 24h by replacement with a medium deficient in cycloheximide resulted in a return of prolactin binding to near control levels 18-24 hours later (31).

A down-regulation of prolactin receptors in rabbit mammary gland in organ culture has also been observed. Inclusion of PRL (5 μg/ml) in the incubation medium resulted in a 80% saturation of free receptors which which was incomplete at 1h and was maximal at 24-48h. The pattern of the reduction of total prolactin receptors is different from that of free receptors with a maximal effect observed in explants cultured in the presence of prolactin for 48h.

For a number of polypeptide hormones, binding is followed by an internalization of the hormone-receptor complex (8), (17), (75), after which the labelled ligands become associated with lysosomal components in the cells (17), (41). Lysosomotropic agents such as chloroquine, methylamine or ammonium chloride have been shown to reduce clustering for α_2-macroglobulin and epidermal growth factor (EGF) on cell surface of fibroblasts (85). [^{125}I]hCG has been internalized and is associated with lysosomes is rapidly degraded to monoiodotyrosine. This process of degradation could be inhibited by lysosomotropic agents (2).

In order to examine if the down-regulation of prolactin receptors in rabbit mammary gland involved a lysosomal-mediated step, mammary explants were cultured in the presence of chloroquine (100 μM). Chloroquine, as well as the other lysosomotropic agents methylamine and ammonium chloride prevented the PRL-induced down-regulation of PRL receptors *in vitro*. Drugs which affect the cytoskeleton (colchicine and cytocalasin B) were without effect on the down-regulation of PRL receptors *in vitro* (33).

These studies suggest that prolactin receptors enter the cell following binding to the plasma membrane. However, blocking the process of down-regulation by lysosomotropic agents does not prevent the action of prolactin on mRNA production or casein synthesis in rabbit mammary gland explants (53).

HORMONAL REGULATION OF RECEPTORS IN MAMMARY TUMORS

DMBA-induced mammary tumors

Binding sites for prolactin have been identified in the particulate membrane fraction of DMBA mammary tumors (19), (29). These binding sites are rspecific for prolactin or other lactogenic hormones and have an affinity similar to that of the mammary gland. Kelly et al. (62) have previously reported that higher prolactin binding was observed in DMBA tumors which had shown the greater growth response to injected prolactin, indicating that the level of the receptor is important in determining the tissue response to prolactin. In contrast to the importance of the pituitary to the maintaince of prolactin binding sites in rat liver (67), (98), there was only a slight reduction in prolactin receptors from tumors of hypophysectomized, DMBA-treated rats (19).

Holdaway and Friesen (51) reported that it was not possible to differentiate prolactin responsive from prolactin-independent tumors by prolactin receptor determinations of biopsy samples, but that following either prolactin administration or prolactin suppression, prolactin responsive tumors had higher prolactin receptor levels. A combination of estradiol and prolactin receptor levels has also been reported to more accurately predict the responsiveness to endocrine ablation than either receptor levels alone (25).

Since estrogens are so important for the growth and maintenance of DMBA-induced mammary tumors, a logical approach, once the compounds became available, was to study analogues of the estrogen molecule or of synthesis estrogens which competed for the action of estradiol at the tumor level.

Because of the potent antiestrogenic properties of a new antiestrogenic compound, RU16117 (11α-methoxy ethinyl estradiol), we examined its effect on the development of DMBA-induced mammary tumors in the rat. In an attempt to correlate the tumor response to antiestrogen treatment with hormone receptor levels, the concentration of receptors for estradiol-17β, progesterone, and prolactin was determined in individual tumors (60).

Tumors first appeared in control rats 53 days after DMBA administration, and the incidence of tumors increased to a maximum of 94.1% at 130 days. All treatments resulted in a delayed onset of tumor appearance. After a delay of 10 days, RU16117, at a dose of 0.5 μg/day, resulted in a curve similar to that of controls, although the incidence reached only 78.6%. The important finding was that RU16117, at doses of either 8 or 24 μg/day, completely inhibited tumor development in all animals. Ovariectomy completely prevented tumor appearance until day 75, when 2 out of 14 animals (14.2% developed palpable tumors. The average number and size of tumors were also inhibited by the lower doses of RU16117.

Specific binding of [^{3}H]estradiol, [^{3}H]R5020, and [^{125}I]ovine PRL to DMBA-induced mammary tumors remained at the end of the studies showed that the antiestrogen treatment resulted in a reduction in the receptor levels for all these hormones in those tumors remaining at the end of the study.

Regression of DMBA-induced tumors by RU16117

Since antiestrogen RU16117, at relatively low doses (8 or 24 μg daily), completely prevented the development of rat mammary carcinoma when administered from the day after DMBA was administered (60), it was of interest to study the effect of this compound on the growth of DMBA tumors which were already developed and to compare the effect of such treatment with that of castration. Ovariectomy, a procedure leading to decreased levels of both estrogens and prolactin, is known to induce regression of approximately 90% of DMBA-induced tumors (101). Once again, hormone receptor levels in tumor tissue were correlated with the response to hormonal treatment (61).

In control animals, a linear increase from 3.2 ± 0.6 to 4.5 ± 0.7 tumors per rat was observed during the 4 weeks of treatment. It was also be seen that ovariectomy, a treatment well known to cause tumor regression (101) had an effect very similar to that of a daily dose of 24 μg RU16117. At the highest dose, RU16117 not only markedly decreased the number of tumors, but it also led to a marked reduction of the total tumor size. Lower doses of the antiestrogen had little or no effect on total tumor area.

In order to ascertain that the inhibitory effect of RU16117 on tumor growth was not due to any estrogenic activity of the compound in view of the slight estrogenic activity of RU16117 (36), (103), and the inhibitory effect of large doses of estradiol, the effect of increasing doses of E_2 under the experimental conditions described for RU116117 was examined. Daily injections of 0.1, 0.5, 2.5, or 12.5 μg estradiol had no significant effect on the number of tumors. Although the total tumor area decreased after castration, the two low doses of estradiol induced somewhat larger tumors, whereas the two larger doses resulted in similar or slightly smaller tumor size.

Binding of [^{125}I]oPRL to DMBA tumors was lower only in those animals injected with the highest dose of RU16117 (24 μg) and after ovariectomy. The level of progestin receptors was not markedly affected at any of the doses of E_2 or RU16117 used (61).

The studies showed that at the daily dose of 24 μg, RU16117 is as efficient as ovariectomy to inhibit tumor growth in rats bearing DMBA-induced mammary tumors. In fact, after 4 weeks of treatment, the average number of tumors per rat and tumor size are reduced to approximately 30% of control.

These findings of low levels of hormone receptors after ovariectomy or treatment with 24 μg RU16117 may indicate that tumors unresponsive to hormonal treatment are those with low levels of receptors or that ovariectomy or RU16117 treatment causes a reduction of receptor levels. A possible mechanism of action of RU16117 in the tumor tissue could involve a decrease of the hormone receptor level leading to relative unresponsiveness of the tissue to its hormonal environment.

Since we have found that RU16117 inhibits LH secretion (36), (60) and treatment with the 24 μg dose inhibits tumor growth in the presence of increased plasma prolactin levels, it is likely that RU16117 exerts its inhibitory activity through an action at both the hypothalamo-pituitary and tumor levels.

Although requiring much higher doses, other antiestrogens have been found to inhibit DMBA-induced tumor development and growth. For example, 1-[2-p-[α(p-methoxy-phenyl)-β-nitrostyril]phenoxyethyl pyrrolidine (CI-628), at a dosage of 1 mg/kg, was found to be somewhat less efficient than ovariectomy in inhibiting DMBA-induced mammary tumor growth (23). At the daily dosage of 5 mg for 40 days starting 20 days before DMBA administration, 1-[p(2-diethylaminoethoxyphenyl)]-2(p-methoxy-phenyl)-1-phenylethanol (MER-25) reduced tumor incidence to only 40% of control (72). When given every other day at a dosage of 1 mg/kg for 30 days in rats that had developed tumors, nafoxidine (U-11100 A) led to an important inhibition of tumor growth (116), (117) while, in another study, the same drug at the daily dosage of 1 mg/kg begun 2 weeks after DMBA administration almost completely prevented tumor development measured after 6 or 12 weeks (46).

The antiestrogen, tamoxifen (trans 1-(4-β-dimethylaminoethoxyphenyl)-1,2-diphenyl but-1-ene), has also been shown to be a potent inhibitor of DMBA-induced tumor growth (57), (58), (59). Injection of 5 mg twice a day for two days at the time of DMBA administration reduced tumor incidence to 10% of control (57), although injections of large doses of estradiol at this time is also associated with reduced tumor incidence (72). In all cases, tumors from tamoxifen treated rats had reduced levels of cytoplasmic estrogen receptors compared to tumors from non injected rats.

A proposed mechanism of action of tamoxifen as well as another nonsteroidal antiestrogen, U23469 (cis(3[p (1,2,3,4-tetrahydro-6-methoxy-2-phenyl-1-naphtyl)phenoxy]-1,2 propanediol) which has been shown to be effective at doses of 250 μg/day (119) resides in their interaction with the estrogen receptor. Both estradiol and the antiestrogens are able to translocate receptor proteins to the nucleus and cause an early elevation of cytopolasmic receptor levels (91). However, during the antiestrogen traetment, as much as 90% of the estrogen receptor may remain in the nucleus, while the level of progesterone receptors remains unchanged (119).

Since very little of the estrogen receptor is found in the cytoplasm, the mammary tumor becomes insensitive to its endogenous estrogens and regression of tumor growth follows.

LHRH and its agonistic analogues have potent pre- and postcoital contraceptive activity in female rats (5), (7), (18), (55) and rabbit (47). We have previously shown that treatment of adult male rats with LHRH or its agonists leads to a marked loss of testicular LH and PRL receptors accompanied by decreased testis, seminal vesicle and prostate weight, as well as lowered testosterone levels (3), (4), (76), (96). It therefore occurred to us that the antifertility effects of LHRH agonists could also be mediated by a desensitization of the ovary. We confirmed the antifertility activity of the potent LHRH agonist [D-Ala^6, des-Gly-NH_2^{10}]LHRH ethylamide. Animals injected starting on day 7 of pregnancy 4 times a day with 25 μg of the LHRH agonist showed an almost complete loss of ovarian LH receptors measured on days 10, 12 and 18 and, a 45 to 60% decline in plasma progesterone levels coincident with an almost complete resorption of fetuses (73). A similar inhibitory effect of the LHRH agonist on ovarian gonadotropin receptors was observed in cycling female rats (74).

In view of the fact that LHRH agonists have been shown to be as effective as ovariectomy or antiestrogen tratment in reducing the growth and development of DMBA-induced mammary tumors in the rat (22), (24), (35), (36), we investigated the mechanisms by which a potent LHRH agonist, [D-Ala^6, des-Gly-NH_2^{10}]LHRH ethylamide induced a regression of tumor growth.

Rats with established DMBA-induced tumors (120 days after carcinogen administration) were divided into three groups, each with approximately equal tumor number and size. One group of 17 rats served as a control, a second group of 16 rats was ovariectomized (OVX) and the final group (17 rats) received daily s.c. injections of the LHRH analogue at a dose of 1 μg/day in 1% gelatin - 0.9% NaCl for 38 days (123).

Tumor number and size of control rats increased steadily throughout the study. Ovariectomy resulted in a marked reduction in both tumor number and total mass compared to control values. When only original tumors are considered, the LHRH agonist resulted in a 38% reduction in the number of tumors present at the beginning of the study, compared to a 45% decline in the OVX group (123).

The hormonal responsiveness of the tumors was assessed by measuring receptor concentrations for estradiol, progesterone and prolactin in tumor tissue. Ovariectomy resulted in a marked reduction in the number of receptors for these three hormones. Treatment with the LHRH agonist was without significant effect on binding of [^3H]E_2 whereas [^3H]R5020 binding was reduced from 7.6 ± 0.7 to 5.5 ± 0.7 pmoles/g tissue ($p < 0.05$) and [^{125}I]oPRL binding declined from 7.2 ± 0.4 to 4.1 ± 0.4% ($p < 0.05$) (123).

The reduction in tumor growth may be partially explained by these reductions in progesterone and prolactin receptors in the tumors. However, a more direct effect of the LHRH agonist involves a desensitizing effect at the pituitary and ovarian levels. A marked decrease in ovarian LH and FSH receptor levels was accompanied by a decline in circulating estradiol and progesterone, as well as a reduction in circulating prolactin concentrations (123).

These studies confirm the antitumor effect of LHRH agonists on the growth of DMBA-induced mammary tumors. The mechanism of the inhibitory effect apears to be a "functional" castration subsequent to an ovarian desensitization. It is possible that treatment of premenopausal breast cancer patients with an LHRH analogue alone or in combination with tamoxifen could represent a useful removal of the ovaries and adrenals.

NMU-induced mammary tumors

In addition to DMBA-induced tumors, prolactin receptors as well as hormone receptors for estradiol and progesterone have been identified and characterized in nitrosomethylurea (NMU)-induced mammary tumors (120). These tumors appear to be hormonally dependent on both estrogens and prolactin (120), (121), (124), although their degree of hormonal dependence appears to differ from that of DMBA-induced mammary tumors.

In order to study the role of antiestrogens on the development of NMU-induced mammary tumors, animals were treated with NMU (5 mg/ 100 g body weight) at 50-55 days of age, with injections repeated 4 and 8 weeks after the initial injection and groups or rats were either castrated or injected with RU16117 (10 µg) or tamoxifen (50 µg). As illustrated in Fig. 1A, tumors first appeared in control and RU16117 treated rats at 71 days after the first NMU injection, however, the incidence was already higher in the control group and continued increasing gradually to a maximum of 86.4% at the end of the experiment (145 days). In the RU16117 treated rats, tumors appeared at the same time as in the control group but the incidence remained lower, reaching a maximum of 54% at the end of the experiment. A delay in the appearance of tumors was observed in the two other groups, resulting in similar patterns of incidence with a maximum of 17.4% (ovariectomized animals) and 8.7% (tamoxifen-treated animals) at the end of the experiment.

The average number of tumors per tumor-bearing rat is shown in Fig. 1B. Again the control animals showed a gradual in-

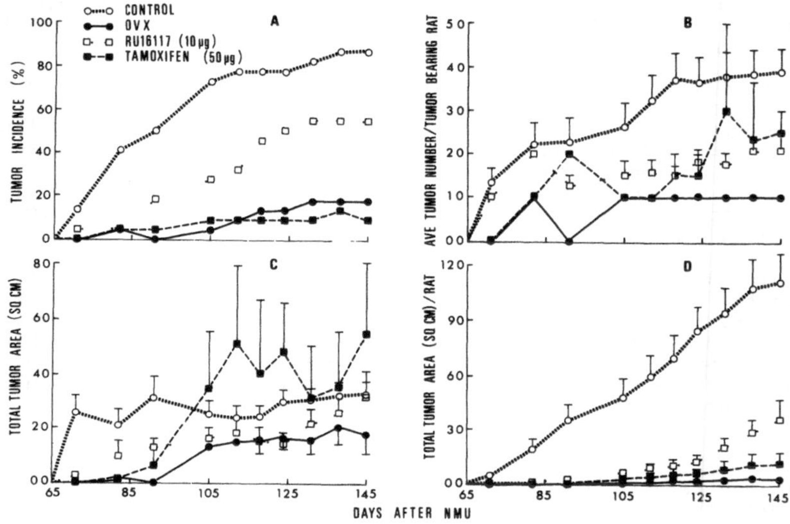

Fig. 1. Effect of ovariectomy (OVX) or treatment with RU16117 (10 μg) or tamoxifen (50 μg) on the development of NMU-induced mammary tumors. Ovariectomy was performed the day of the first NMU administration. Treatment injections began the same day and continued for 145 days. Animals were examined weekly for the presence of tumors, and, when present, tumor area (length x width) was measured. A, tumor incidence as a function of time after the first NMU injection; B, average tumor number; C, average tumor area (sq.cm); D, total tumor area (sq.cm) per animal. This value is obtained by dividing the sum of tumor areas in a group by the total number of animals in that group.

crease, reaching a plateau of 3.7 to 3.8 tumor/rat 118 days after the onset of the experiment. All treatments resulted in a reduction in tumor numbers per animal to 1, 2.1 and 2.5 for the ovariectomized, RU16117-treated and tamoxifen-treated animals, respectively. The apparent decreases in the tamoxifen-treated rats is due to the effect of 2 adjacent tumors which joined and were thereafter measured and considered as a single tumor.

Average tumor size increased rapidly in the control group and remained relatively stable for the remainder of the study (Fig. 1C) while the RU16117 treated animals and the ovariectomized animals had similar curves however delayed. There were only 2 tumor bearing rats in the tamoxifen-treated group, however, in those animals tumors increased in size sharply at 105 days and remained elevated until the study was terminated. When tumor area is represented as a function of all rats in the group as shown in Fig. 1D there is a steady increase to 11.1 ± 1.6 sq.cm/rat on day 145 in the controls. In all treated animals, the tumor size remained much smaller, being 1.2 ± 0.6 sq.cm after tamoxifen, 3.7 ± 1.1 sq.cm after RU16117 and 0.3 ± 0.1 sq.cm after ovariectomy.

The effect of antiestrogen treatment on the growth of established tumors (118 days after NMU injection is shown in Fig. 2. A steady increase in the number of tumors per rat from

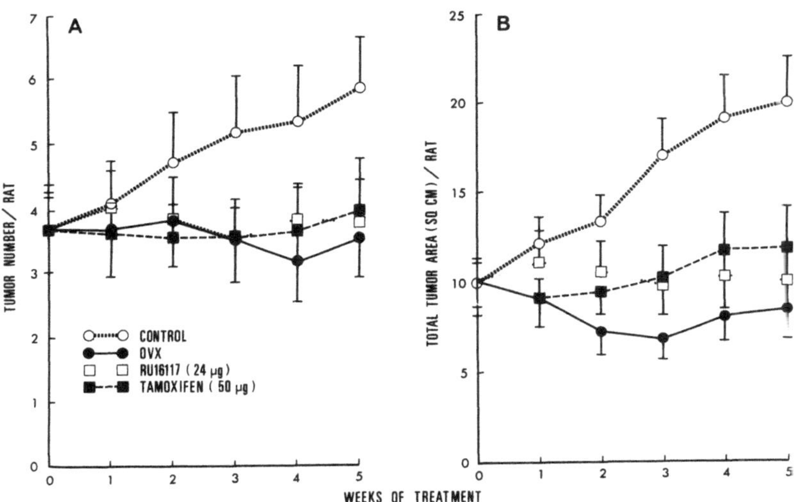

Fig. 2. Effect of 5-week treatment with RU16117 (24 µg) or tamoxifen (50 µg) or ovariectomy on the number of NMU-induced mammary tumors per rat (A) and on the total tumor area (sq.cm) per animal (B).

3.7 ± 0.7 to 5.8 ± 0.8 was observed over the 5 weeks of treatment (Fig. 2A). Ovariectomy prevented further tumor growth, but failed to induce a regression of tumor growth. The antiestrogens RU16117 and tamoxifen resulted in a similar prevention of tumor growth. The effect of these treatments on total tumor area/rat (Fig. 2B) was of a similar nature with a slight reduction in tumor size seen after 2 and 3 weeks of treatment.

When tumors present only at the outset of the experiment were included, the effect on tumor regression can be more clearly seen. Fig. 3A shows that tumor number was relatively constant in control rats and was slightly reduced by ovariectomy and more markedly depressed by RU16117. Fig. 3B shows that total tumor area/rat increased from 10.0 ± 2.2 to 15.2 ± 3.4 sq.cm in control rats. Ovariectomy was effective in inducing a regression during the first 3 weeks with a slight increase

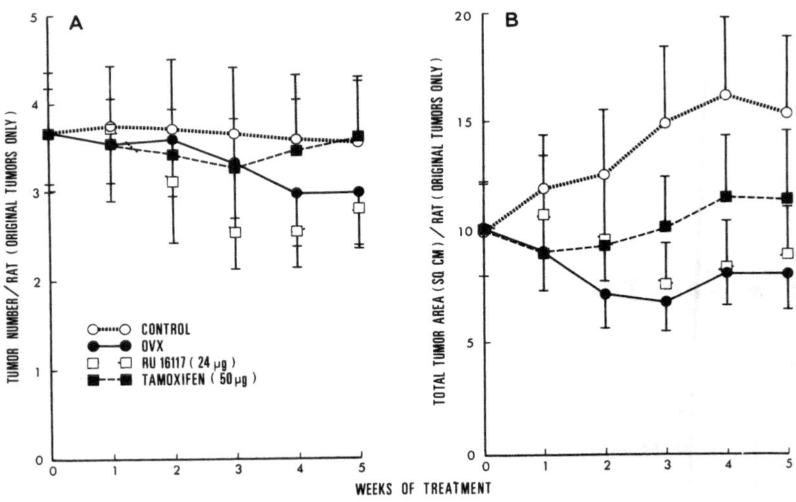

Fig. 3. Effect of 5-week treatment with RU16117 (24 μg) or tamoxifen (50 μg) or ovariectomy on the tumors only present at the beginning of the experiment. Newly appearing tumors are not considered. A, tumor number per rat; B, total tumor area (sq.cm) per animal.

in size during the fourth and fifth weeks. Both antiestrogens were at best only able to maintain tumor size, but not to induce tumor regression.

Specific binding of [^{3}H]estradiol-17β, [^{3}H]R5020 and [^{125}I]-labelled ovine PRL to NMU-induced tumors are shown in Table 1. There is a significant decrease ($p < 0.01$) of [^{3}H]estradiol receptors in both the ovariectomized and tamoxifen treated groups, however, the decreased observed in the RU16117-treated animals was not statistically significant. Binding of [^{3}H]R5020 was reduced by ovariectomy ($p < 0.05$) and tamoxifen. RU16117 treatment resulted in an increase in progesterone receptors. [^{125}I] labelled ovine PRL receptors were not affected by the antiestrogen treatment but were significantly decreased ($p < 0.05$) by ovariectomy.

NMU-induced mammary tumors have previously been shown to be dependent on the presence of ovarian hormones for growth. Ovariectomy near the time of NMU administration reduces the effectiveness of NMU to induce mammary tumors (42). Arafah et al. (1) recently reported a regression to 48% of their original size of the majority of NMU-induced mammary tumors following ovariectomy. Both cytosolic estrogen and progesterone receptor levels declined significantly but the 25% reduction in prolactin receptor levels was not significant. Our studies have shown that when larger numbers of tumors are examined, a 33% decline on prolactin receptor levels is observed, five weeks after ovariectomy, a value which is statistically significant.

In order to examine the response of NMU-induced mammary tumors to ovariectomy at various stages during tumor development, tumor-bearing animals were castrated at 2½, 3½ and 4½ months after the initial NMU injection and tumor growth was examined over a 4-week period.

Table 1. Effect of a 5-week treatment with RU16117 or tamoxifen or ovariectomy on specific binding of [^{3}H]E_2, [^{3}H]R5020 and [^{125}I]oPRL to NMU-induced mammary tumors.

Group	Number of tumors	[^{3}H] E_2 (pmol/g tissue)	[^{3}H] R5020 (pmol/g tissue)	[^{125}I]oPRL (% specific binding/300 µg protein)
Control	49	1.2±0.2	5.1±1.0	6.4±0.5
OVX	32	0.6±0.1**	0.8±0.2*	4.3±1.5*
RU16117 (24 µg)	20	0.8±0.2	11.4±3.4**	5.0±0.8
Tamoxifen (50 µg)	33	0.2±0.03**	2.5±0.5	5.9±0.7

*, $p < 0.05$ and **, $p < 0.01$ compared to control group.

As illustrated in Fig. 4, ovariectomy during the three periods of the experiment resulted in a reduction in the number of tumors compared to the control groups. Control rats showed a considerable increase in the number of tumors throughout the three periods increasing from 2.4 ± 0.5 to 5.8 ± 0.9 in the first group (140% increase) from 5.1 ± 0.8 to 6.5 ± 0.9 in the second group (27% increase), and from 4.0 ± 0.8 to 6.4 ± 0.9 in the third group (60% increase). In the OVX groups, there was a stabilization or a decrease in the number of tumors per rat from 2.3 ± 0.5 to 2.2 ± 0.5 from 5.1 ± 0.8 to 3.8 ± 0.8 (decrease of 25%) and from 3.7 ± 0.7 to 2.5 ± 0.6 (decrease of 32%) in the three periods respectively.

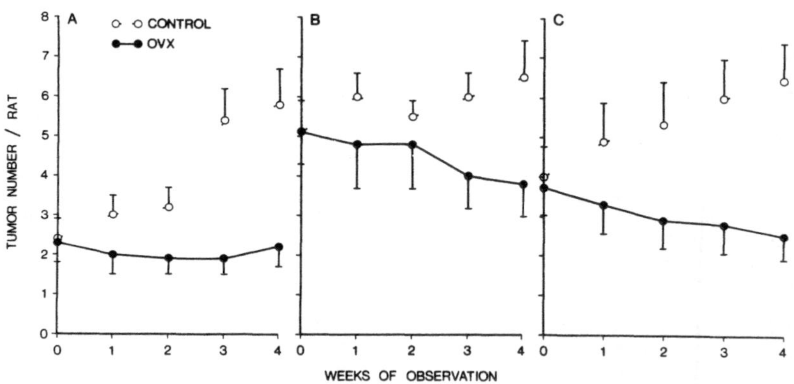

Fig. 4. Effect of ovariectomy (OVX) on the number of NMU-induced mammary tumors per rat in the first (A), second (B) and third (C) 4-week periods of observations.

The variations in tumor size per rat is shown in Fig. 5, where a somewhat similar pattern is observed. During the three periods of observation, there was a considerable increase in the average tumor area per rat in the control groups while OVX resulted in a stabilization or a regression of the size of the tumors. During the first period, the average tumor area per rat in both groups was 5.3 ± 1 cm^2. After 4 weeks of observation, control values increased to 16.6 ± 2.4 cm^2 while OVX rats had an average area of 6.4 ± 2.2 cm^2. During the second period, control tumors increased from 12.3 ± 2.5 cm^2 to 25.6 ± 4.3 cm^2 and declined to 8.0 ± 1.6 cm^2 for the OVX rats. In the third period, tumor size

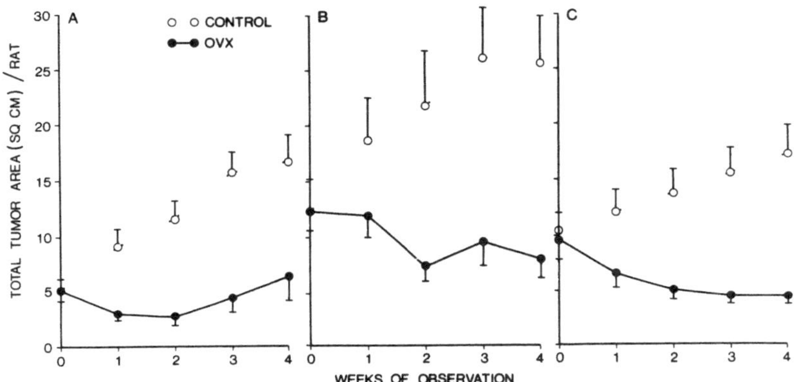

Fig. 5. Effect of ovariectomy (OVX) on the total tumor area of NMU-induced mammary tumors per rat in the first (A), second (B) and third (C) 4-week periods of observations.

changed from 10.0 ± 1.6 cm^2 to 17.2 ± 2.6 cm^2 for the controls and declined to 4.4 ± 0.7 cm^2 for the ovariectomized rats.

In order to clarify the kinds of growth responses which were seen in NMU-induced mammary tumors, the response of individual tumors were compared at various times following castration. It should be noted that approximately 50% of the tumors regressed in the first two groups, whereas 74% of the old or late appearing tumors regressed following ovariectomy.

Specific binding of [^{3}H] estradiol-17β is shown in Fig. 6A. Estradiol receptors which ranged from 2.04 ± 0.18 to 2.24 ± 0.24 pmol/g tissue in control tumors during the first two treatment periods and declined to 0.93 ± 0.14 pmol/g tissue at the last time interval studied ($p < 0.01$). Ovariectomy induced as significant ($p < 0.01$) 50% decline in E_2 receptors, regardless of the time at which OVX was performed. Fig. 6B illustrates the specific binding of [^{3}H]R5020 during the three periods of the study. The decrease of [^{3}H]R5020 receptors in the OVX groups was highly significant ($p < 0.01$) for the two first groups of rats and slightly

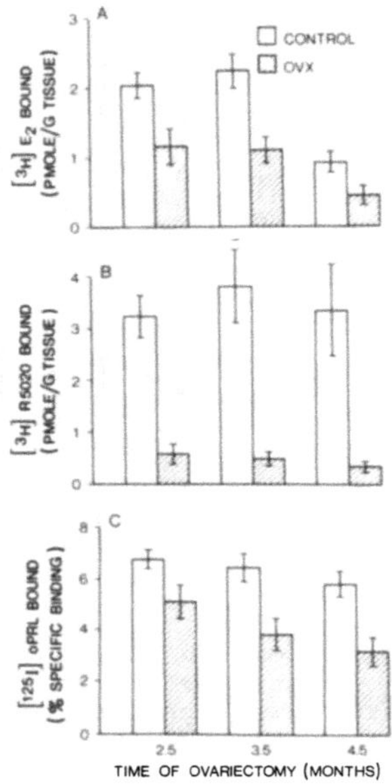

Fig. 6. Specific binding of [^{3}H]estradiol-17β (A), [^{3}H]R5020 (B) and [^{125}I]oPRL (C) on NMU-induced mammary tumors after a week period of observation starting at the indicated times, 2.5, 3.5 and 4.5 months after the first injection of NMU.

less ($p < 0.05$) for the third group. Specific binding of [^{125}I]ovine prolactin illustrated in Fig. 3C was also significantly reduced by OVX in the first ($p < 0.05$), second and third ($p < 0.01$) periods of the experiment.

It is interesting to note that there is a significant decrease in the number of estradiol receptors between the tumors of the first and second group of controls and those of the third group, either present at the beginning of the 4 weeks of observation ($p < 0.05$) or appearing during these 4 weeks ($p < 0.01$). The is also a highly significant decrease ($p < 0.01$) in receptor concentrations in old tumors used in the third group of controls compared to tumors which appeared during the same period of time, i.e. the newly appearing tumors during the first part of the experiment and the tumors already present a the beginning of the second part of the experiment.

The present data show that NMU-induced mammary tumors have similar patterns of growth in the first two months of the study (2½ to 4½ months after the first NMU injection) but are different in terms in tumor growth and estradiol-17β receptors in the last period studied. Although estrogen receptors were lower in the last treatment period studied, these tumors responded as well or better as tumors from the first or second treatment periods. It is possible that reduction in plasma prolactin concentrations observed during the last two treatment periods following OVX contributed to the increased response to ovariectomy.

Although in contrast to data for DMBA-induced tumors, these data suggest, at least for the intervals studied, that hormone responsiveness (response to ovariectomy) increases slightly with the age or time of appearance of the tumors.

Organ culture of mammary tumors

Although a great deal of information on the hormonal dependence of experimental mammary tumors has been attained by *in vivo* studies, it is important to carry out parallel studies *in vitro* to discern the mechanism by which the various hormones act. Organ culture has proven a useful tool to verify the effects of both steroid and peptide hormones on tumor growth (15), (78), (79), (92), (105). More recently, hormone receptor measurements have been carried out in both cell and organ cultures demonstrating the importance of fluctuations in hormone receptor levels for steroid and peptide hormones as an important factor in tumor growth (20), (113).

In our laboratory, we have been investigating the rate of prolactin receptor degradation and synthesis in normal mammary glands from pregnant and lactating rats, and comparing these responses to those seen in DMBA or NMU-induced mammary tumors. Although only preliminary studies have been completed thus far, it appears that prolactin can induce a down-regulation of its total receptor levels *in vitro* as occurs in the rabbit mammary glands (29), (31). Although lysosomotropic agents such as chloroquine, prevent prolactin receptor degradation in rabbits, these agents are much less effective in normal or tumour mammary tissue from rats.

Although we have been able to show a down-regulation of prolactin receptors *in vitro*, the up-regulation of prolactin receptors in vitro has yet been reported. Recently, using a continuous suspension of isolated hepatic cells, we have been able to show an up-regulation of prolactin receptors. This effect appears to be maximal at a prolactin concentrations of 50 nM. When higher concentrations are used, only a down-regulation of prolactin receptors is observed. We are currently extending these studies to normal and neoplastic mammary tissue.

PROLACTIN AND HUMAN BREAST CANCER

Evidence for role of prolactin

Although the role of prolactin in the development and promotion of experimental breast cancer in rodents is well documented, it has been much more difficult to ascertain whether prolactin is involved in mammary carcinoma in humans, even after the identification and isolation of a separate human prolactin molecule. Hypophpysectomy has been reported to induce clinical remission in a substantial number of patients with carcinoma of the breast (68), (95) although the role of prolactin in such remissions has been questioned (87).

In a retrospective study, prolactin has been implicated indirectly in human breast cancer in a report by the Boston Collaborative Drug Surveillance Program, which reported an association between regular reserpine use, which is a known stimulator of prolactin secretion, and newly diagnosed breast cancer (10). A similar correlation was found by Heinonen et al. (44) although the association was evident only for women below 50 years of age. These findings, although not conclusive, at least suggest that a causal relationship between reserpine use and breast cancer should be considered.

There is little evidence of elevated plasma prolactin levels in the etiology of human breast cancer. Basal levels have been measured in several groups of patients with established mammary carcinoma, and these studies conclude that plasma prolactin levels are not significantly different from values observed in normal women (13), (130). In a recent report, however, mastectomy has been shown to result in elevated plasma prolactin levels, both in a retrospective study as well as in an experimental study carried out over a period of several months (45). Elevated prolactin levels could of course be important in the development of subsequent metastases.

Another means of identifying whether prolactin plays a role in human breast cancer is to examine tumor response in vitro. In 1972, Salih et al. (104) described a histochemical method to determine the dehydrogenase activity of the pentose shunt of human mammary tumor biopsies in the absence and presence of ovine prolactin in the medium, thus offering a predictive tool to determine the prolactin dependency of human breast cancer. Of 50 tumors examined, 32% were prolactin dependent; for 20%, prolactin was the only hormone required. In a subsequent report, the series of patients was expanded and the percentage of prolactin-responsive tumors was similar (48). However recently, the reproducibility of this technique of measuring hormone responsiveness of human tumors in organ culture has been questioned (83).

The effect of prolactin on the growth and estrogen receptor level of a cell line of human breast cancer revealed that both bovine and human prolactin could almost double the level of estrogen receptor measured in the cells, but tha human prolactin was ten times more potent than ovine prolactin in this respect (107). Another group reported that normal human breast tissue responds, in terms of mitotic index, to either insulin or human prolactin, but not to ovine prolactin, suggesting a species specificity (28).

<u>Prolactin receptors in human breast carcinoma</u>

If prolactin does stimulate human mammary tumors, the tissue should contain prolactin receptors, as is the case for other prolactin-responsive tissues as well as for experimental mammary tumors. Holdaway and Friesen (52) have reported on the specific binding of prolactin to human breast tumors. Specific binding of greater than 1% of the added radioactivity (which the authors considered significant) occurred in 8 of 41 tumors (19.5%). For one tumor, enough material was present to perform a Scatchard plot, and an affinity constant (Ka) of 2.5 nM^{-1} was determined, which is similar to that of other prolactin receptors.

During the last two years, we have assayed prolactin receptors in 759 human breast tumors sent to our laboratory by the surrounding medical centers for steroid receptors determination. A comparison of the optimum type of labeled ligand to use in the assay of prolactin receptors in breast tumor biopsies was carried out.

Fig. 7 shows a comparison of prolactin binding sites using three different labeled ligands in human breast cancer biopsy samples. In our laboratory, we feel values greater than 0.5% of the added radioactivity represent significant specific binding of prolactin. Using [^{125}I]hPRL (Fig. 7A), 58% of the biopsies fall into this category compared to 30% with [^{125}I]oPRL (Fig. 7B) and only 12% using [^{125}I]hGH (Fig. 7C). When 1% or greater of the added radioactivity is used as the criteria for selecting prolactin-responsive

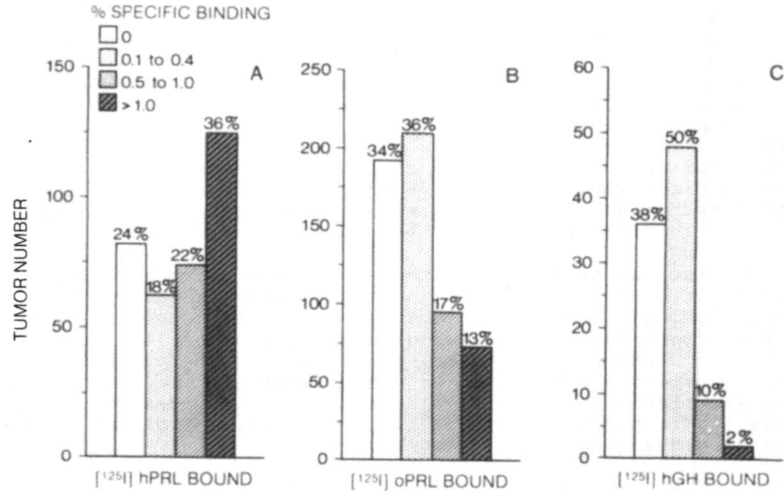

Fig. 7. Comparison of specific binding of prolactin using [^{125}I]hPRL (A, 343 tumors), [^{125}I]oPRL (B, 569 tumors) and [^{125}I]hGH, (C, 95 tumors). Binding values are arbitrarily divided into four categories (0, 0.1 to 0.4, 0.5 to 0.9 and 1% or greater of the added radioactivity specifically bound).

tumors, these values are 36, 17 and 2%, respectively for hPRL, oPRL and hGH. There are equally less tumors showing no measurable prolactin binding (0%) or borderline values (0.1 to 0.4%) when hPRL is used as the tracer.

Table 2 illustrates a specific comparison between [^{125}I]labeled ovine and human prolactin binding to 153 human breast cancer biopsies. Binding studies were carried out in parallel with freshly iodinated hormones. It is clear that the use of [^{125}I]human PRL allows the detection of almost three times as many tumors possessing prolactin receptors compared to when ovine PRL is used as tracer (29.4 vs 10.4% 10.4%) with also a two-fold increase in the tumors showing moderate binding values (0.5 to 0.9%). There was no correlation between the level of prolactin receptors and the concentration of receptors for either estradiol-17β or progesterone in these tumors.

Human breast tumors do possess membrane prolactin binding proteins in sufficient amounts to be detected when the appropriate procedure is used. Specific binding of 1% or greater of the added radioactivity has been considered positive (52). Di Carlo and Muccioli (27) using an assay similar to ours found positive values for prolactin receptors in 32.5% of their tumors which is very close to our value of 36%. Based in the present studies, importance should be placed to the use of human prolactin rather than ovine prolactin in the determination of prolactin receptors to human breast cancer biopsies (122).

These studies confirm the existence of prolactin receptors in human breast cancer biopsies. It will be important in the future to investigate the possible therapeutic implications of determining prolactin receptor levels in predicting the response of breast cancer patients to endocrine therapy.

SUMMARY AND CONCLUSIONS

The importance of prolactin in the growth and development of both normal mammary gland as well as mammary tumors has been discussed. In normal tissue, the regulation of prolactin receptors, involving both up- and down-regulation as well as modulation by steroid hormones has been discussed.

The stimulatory role of both estrogens and prolactin in the growth and development of experimental mammary tumors in rodents is clear. In a number of spontaneously developing tumors, estrogen has an important role as an inducer or carcinogen, whereas prolactin acts as a promotor of many estrogen-induced cancers. In DMBA-induced mammary tumors, optimal tumor development only occurs when the correct strain and age of rat are utilized, underlying the extremely sensitive conditions necessary to induce experimental mammary tumors.

Table 2. Comparison of specific binding to 153 human breast cancer biopsies using ovine and human prolactin as the labeled ligand.

	% specific binding				
	0	0.1/0.4	0.5/0.9	1.0/1.9	>2.0
[^{125}I]hPRL	25.5%(39)	18.3%(28)	26.8%(41)	20.3%(31)	9.1%(14) 29.4%
[^{125}I]oPRL	50.4%(77)	25.5%(39)	13.7%(21)	7.8%(12)	2.6%(4) 10.4%

The rapid acceptance of DMBA-induced mammary tumors as a model for studying hormonally-dependent human breast cancer has been based on the hormonal dependence of DMBA tumors. More recently, the importance of hormone receptors for estradiol, progesterone, and prolactin in tumor tissue, in addition to variations on circulating levels of hormones, has been recognized as an important factor in determining the tissue responsiveness of the tumor.

Several factors which inhibit tumor growth have been described, as well as proposed mechanisms for their inhibitory activity. Several of these inhibitory factors reduce the tissue sensitivity of the tumor to the stimulatory factors found in the circulation.

An alternative to the DMBA-induced mammary tumor model is the NMU-induced mammary tumors. The hormonal dependency of these tumors was studied in ovariectomized rats and intact rats injected with antiestrogens. Both treatments result in a diminution in the initiation of tumor growth. In animals with established mammary tumors, ovariectomy and antiestrogen treatment result in a prevention of further growth although none of the treatments induce marked tumor regression as occurs with DMBA-induced mammary tumors. A slight increase in the effectiveness of ovariectomy was observed in rats bearing NMU tumors as a function of the time after NMU administration. Receptors for estradiol-17β, progesterone and prolactin were significantly reduced by ovariectomy. Although NMU-induced mammary tumors may represent a better model system to study human breast cancer since they are less hormonally responsive than DMBA tumors, studies with many different model system including DMBA-induced tumors should be continued.

The role of prolactin in human breast cancer has been discussed. It is apparent that prolactin is important in normal mammary development but it is less clear if prolactin is involved as a promoter in human breast cancer. Studies in our laboratory confirm the existence of prolactin receptors in breast cancer biopsies and underline the importance of using human prolactin for the receptor determinations.

REFERENCES

1. Arafah BM, Gullino PM, Manni A, Pearson OH. Effect of ovariectomy on hormone receptors and growth of N-nitrosomethylurea-induced mammary tumors in the rat. Cancer Res 40: 4628-4630, 1980.

2. Ascoli M, Puett D. Degradation of receptor bound human chorionic gonadotropin. J Biol Chem 253: 4892-4899, 1978.

3. Auclair C, Kelly PA, Coy DH, Schally AV, Labrie F. Potent inhibitory activity of [D-Leu^6, des-Gly-NH$_2$^{10}]-LHRH ethylamide on LH/hCG and PRL testicular receptor levels in the rat. Endocrinology 101: 1890-1893, 1977.

4. Auclair C, Kelly PA, Labrie F, Coy DH, Schally AV. Inhibition of testicular luteinizing hormone receptor levels by treatment with a potent luteinizing hormone-releasing hormone agonist or human chorionic gonadotropin. Biochem Biophys Res Commun 76: 855-862, 1977.

5. Banik UK, Givner ML. Ovulation, induction and antifertility effects of an LHRH analog (AY25205) in cycling rats. J Reprod Fertil 44: 87-94, 1975.

6. Barnawell EB, A comparative study of the response of mammary tissue from several mammalian species to hormones in vitro. J Exp Zool 160: 189-206, 1965.

7. Beattie CW, Corbin A. Pre- and post-coital contraceptive activity of LHRH in the rat. Biol Reprod 16: 333-339, 1977.

8. Bergeron JJM, Posner BI, Josefsberg Z, Sikstrom R. Intracellular polypeptide hormone receptors: its demonstration of specific binding sites for insulin and human growth hormone in Golgi fractions isolated from the liver of female rats. J Biol Chem 253: 4058-4066, 1978.

9. Bohnet HG, Gomez F, Friesen HG. Prolactin and estrogen binding sites in the mammary gland of the lactating and non-lactating rat. Endocrinology 101: 1111-1121, 1977.

10. Boston Collaborative Drug Surveillance Program, Reserpine and Breast Cancer. Lancet 2: 669-671, 1974.

11. Bott LM, Muhlbock O, Ropcke G. Prolactin and the induction of mammary tumors in mice. Gen Comp Endocrinol 2: 601-603, 1962.

12. Boyns AR, Buchan R, Cole EN, Forrest APM, Griffiths K. Basal prolactin blood levels in three strains of rat with differing incidence of 7,12-dimethylbenz(a)anthracene-induced mammary tumors. Eur J Cancer 9: 169-171, 1973.

13. Boyns AR, Cole EN, Griffiths K, Roberts MM, Buchan R, Wilson RG, Forrest APM. Plasma prolactin in breast cancer. Eur J Cancer 9: 99-102, 1973.

14. Cassell E, Meites J, Welsch CW. Effects of ergocornine and ergocryptine on growth of 7,12- dimethylbenzanthracene-induced mammary tumors in rats. Cancer Res 31: 1051, 1971.

15. Chan PC, Tsuang J, Head J, Cohen LA. Effects of estradiol and prolactin on growth of rat mammary adenocarcinoma cells in monolayer cultures (39210). Proc Soc Exp Biol Med 151: 362-365, 1976.

16. Chen HJ, Bradley CJ, Meites J. Stimulation of carcinogen-induced mammary tumor growth in rats by adrenalectomy. Cancer Res. 36: 1414-1417, 1977.

17. Conn PM, Conti M, Harwood JP, Dufau ML, Catt KJ Internalization of gonadotropin-receptor complex in ovarian luteal cells. Nature 274: 598-600, 1978.

18. Corbin A, Beattie CW, Yardley J, Toell TJ. Post-coital contraceptive effects of an agonistic analogue of luteinizing-releasing hormone. Endocr Res Commun 2: 359-376, 1976.

19. Costlow ME, Buschow RA, McGuire WL. Prolactin receptors in 7,12-dimethylbenz(a)anthracene-induced mammary tumors following endocrine ablation. Cancer Res 36: 3941-3943, 1976.

20. Costlow ME, Gallagher PE, Koseki Y. Prolactin receptors in primary cultures or carcinogen-induced rat mammary tumors. Mol Cell Endocrinol 14: 81-97, 1979.

21. Cowie, A.T. Hormonal factors in mammary development and lactation. pp 3-23 in <u>Mammary Cancer and Neuroendocrine Therapy</u>, edited by BA Stoll, Butterworths, London, 1974.

22. Danguy A, Legros N, Heuson-Stiennon JA, Pasteels JL, Atassi G, Heuson JC. Effects of a gonadotropin-releasing hormone (GnRH) analogue (A43818) on 7,12-dimethylbenz(a)anthracene-induced rat mammary tumors. Histological and Endocrine Studies. Europ J Cancer 13: 1089-1094, 1977.

23. DeSombre ER, Arbogast LY. Effect of the antiestrogen CI628 on the growth of rat mammary tumors. Cancer Res 34: 1971-19761, 1974.

24. DeSombre ER, Johnson ES, White WF. Regression of rat mammary tumors affected by a gonadoliberin analog. Cancer Res 36: 3930-3933, 1976.

25. DeSombre ER, Kledzik GS, Marshall S, Meites J. Estrogen and prolactin receptor concentrations in rat mammary tumors and response to endocrine ablation. Cancer Res 36: 354-358, 1976.

26. Devinoy E, Houdebine LM, Delouis C. Role of prolactin and glucocorticoids in the expression of casein genes in rabbit mammary gland organ culture. Quantification of casein mRNA. Biochim Biophys Acta 517: 360-366, 1978.

27. Di Carlo R, Muccioli G. Prolactin receptor in human mammary carcinoma. Tumori 65: 695-702, 1979.

28. Diley WG, Kister SJ. In vitro stimulation of human breast tissue by human prolactin. J Natl Cancer Inst 55: 35-36, 1975.

29. Djiane J, Clauser H, Kelly PA. Rapid down-regulation of prolactin receptors in mammary gland and liver. Biochem Biophys Res Commun 90: 1371-1378, 1979.

30. Djiane J, Durand P. Prolactin-progesterone antagonism in self-regulation of prolactin receptors in the mammary gland. Nature 266: 641-643, 1977.

31. Djiane J, Delouis C, Kelly PA. Prolactin receptors in organ culture of rabbit mammary gland: effect of cycloheximide and prolactin. Proc Soc Exp Biol Med 162: 342-345, 1979.

32. Djiane J, Durand P, Kelly PA. Evolution of prolactin receptors in rabbit mammary gland during pregnancy and lactation. Endocrinology 100: 1348-1356, 1977.

33. Djiane J, Kelly PA, Houdebine LM. Effects of lysosomotropic agents, cytochalasin B and colchicine on the "down-regulation" of prolactin receptors in mammary explants, Mol Cell Endocrinol 18: 87-98, 1980.

34. Dubé D, Kelly PA, Pelletier G. Comparative localization of prolactin binding sites in different rat tissues by immunohistochemistry, radioautography and radioreceptor assay. Mol Cell Endocrinol 18: 109-122, 1980.

35. Dutta AS, Furr BJA, Giles MB, Valcaccia B, Walpole AL. Potent agonist and antagonist analogues of duliberin containing an azaglycine residue in position 10. Biochem Biophys Res Commun 81: 382-390, 1978.

36. Ferland L, Labrie F, Kelly PA, Raynaud JP. Inhibitory effects of RU16117, a potent estrogen antagonist, on the estrous cycle of the rat. Biol Reprod 18: 99-104, 1978.

37. Fluckiger, E. Drugs and the control of prolactin secretion, pp. 162-171 in Prolactin and Carcinogenesis, 4th Tenovous Workshop, eds AR Boyns, K Griffiths, Cardiff Wales: Alpha Omega Alpha Publishing, 1972.

38. Furth J. Experimental pituitary tumors. Recent Prog Horm Res 11: 221-255, 1975.

39. Furth J. Prolactin and carcinogenesis. pp. 137-142 in Prolactin and Carcinogenesis: 4th Tenovous Workshop, eds AR Boyns, K Griffiths, Alpha Omega Alpha, Cardiff, 1972.

40. Furth J, Clifton KH. Experimental pituitary tumors. pp 460-497 in The Pituitary Gland, eds GW Harris, BT Donovan, vol 2, Butterworths, London, 1966.

41. Gordon P, Carpentier JL, Cohen S, Orci, L. Epidermal growth factor: morphological demonstration of binding, internalization and lysosomal association in human fibroblasts. Proc Natl Acad Sci USA 75: 5025-5029, 1978.

42. Gullino PM, Pettigrew HN, Grantham FH. N-nitrosomethyl urea as mammary gland carcinogen in rats. J Natl Cancer Inst 54: 401-414, 1975.

43. Hayden TJ, Bonney RC, Forsyth IA. Ontogeny and control of prolactin receptors in the mammary gland and liver of virgin, pregnant and lactating rats. J Endocrinol 80: 259-269, 1979.

44. Heinonen OP, Shapiro S, Tuominen L, Turunen MI. Reserpine use in relation to breast cancer. Lancet 2: 675-677, 1974.

45. Herman V, Kalk WJ, de Moor, NG, Levin J. Serum prolactin after chest wall surgery: elevated levels after mastectomy. J Clin Endocrinol Metab 52: 148-151, 1981.

46. Heuson JC, Waelbroeck C, Legros N, Gallez G, Robyn C, L'Hermite M. Inhibition of DMBA-induced mammary carcinogenesis in the rat by 2-Br-α-ergocryptine (CB-154), an inhibitor of prolactin secretion and by nafoxidine (U-11,000A), an estrogen antagonist. Gynecol Invest 2: 130-137, 1971/1972.

47. Hilliard J, Pang CN, Sawyer CH. Effects of luteinizing hormone-releasing hormone in fetal survival in pregnant rabbits. Fertil Steril 27: 421-425, 1976.

48. Hobbs JR, Salih H, Flax H, Brander W. Prolactin dependence in human breast cancer. Proc Roy Soc Med 66: 866-867, 1973.

49. Holcomb HH, Costlow ME, Buschow RA, McGuire WL. Prolactin binding in rat mammary gland during pregnancy and lactation. Biochim Biophys Acta 428: 104-112, 1976.

50. Holdaway IM. Personal communication.

51. Holdaway IM, Friesen HG. Correlation between hormone binding and growth response of rat mammary tumor. Cancer Res 36: 1562, 1976.

52. Holdaway IM, Friesen HG. Hormone binding by human mammary carcinoma. Cancer Res 37: 1946-1952, 1977.

53. Houdebine LM, Djiane J. Effects of lysosomotropic agents, microfilament and microtubule disrupting drugs on the actuation of casein gene expression by prolactin in the mammary gland. Mol Cell Endocrinol 17: 1-15, 1980.

54. Huggins, C., Grand LC, Brillantes FP. Mammary cancer induced by a single feeding of polynuclear hydrocarbons and its suppression. Nature (London) 189: 204-207, 1961.

55. Humphrey RR, Windson BL, Bousley FG, Edgren RA. Antifertility effects of an analog of luteinizing hormone-releasing hormone (LHRH) in rats. Contraception 14: 625-629, 1976.

56. Johnson ES, Seely JH, White WF, DeSombre ER. Endocrine-dependent rat mammary tumor regression: use of a gonadotropin-releasing hormone analog. Science 194: 329-330, 1976.

57. Jordan VC. Effect of tamoxifen (ICI46,474) on initiation and growth of DMBA-induced rat mammary carcinomata. Eur J Cancer 12: 419-424, 1976.

58. Jordan VC, Dowse LJ. Tamoxifen as an anti-tumor agent: effect on estrogen binding. J Endocrinol 68: 297-303, 1976.

59. Jordan VC, Jaspan T. Tamoxifen as an anti-tumor agent: oestrogen binding as a predictive test for tumor response. J Endocrinol 68: 453-460, 1976.

60. Kelly PA, Asselin J, Caron MG, Labrie F, Raynaud JP. High inhibitory activity of a new antiestrogen, RU16117 (11α-methoxyethinyl estradiol), on the development of dimethylbenz(a)anthracene-induced mammary tumors. Cancer Res. 37: 76-81, 1977.

61. Kelly PA, Asselin J, Caron MG, Labrie F, Raynaud JP. Potent inhibitory effect of a new antiestrogen (RU16117) on the growth of 7,12-dimethylbenz(a)anthracene-induced rat mammary tumors. J Natl Cancer Inst 58: 623-628, 1977.

62. Kelly PA, Bradley C, Shiu RPC, Meites J, Friesen HG. Prolactin binding to rat mammary tumor tissue. Proc Soc Exp Biol Med 146: 816-819, 1974.

63. Kelly PA, Djiane J, De Léan A. Interaction of prolactin with its receptor: dissociation and down-regulation. pp. 173-188, In: Central and Peripheral Regulation of Prolactin Function, eds RM MacLeod and U. Sacpagnini, Raven Press, New York, 1980.

64. Kelly PA, Djiane J, De Léan A. Prolactin receptor dissociation and down-regulation, in Advances in Prolactin, vol 6, Progress in Reproductive Biology, eds M. L'Hermite and S. Judd, Karger, Basel, Switzerland, in press.

65. Kelly PA, Labrie F, Asselin J. The role of prolactin in tumor development. pp. 157-194 in Influences of Hormones in Tumor Development, vol. II, eds JA Kellen, R. Hilf, CRC Press Inc., Boca Raton, Florida, 1979.

66. Kelly PA, Leblanc G, Djiane J. Estimation of total prolactin binding sites after *in vitro* desaturation. Endocrinology 104: 1631-1638, 1979.

67. Kelly PA, Posner BI, Friesen HG. Effects of hypophysectomy, ovariectomy and cycloheximide on specific binding sites for lactogenic hormones in rat liver. Endocrinology 97: 1408-1515, 1975.

68. Kennedy BJ, French LA, Peyton WT. Hypophysectomy in advanced breast cancer. N Engl J Med 255: 1165-1172, 1956.

69. Kim U. Pituitary function and hormonal therapy of experimental breast cancer. Cancer Res 25:1146-1161, 1965.

70. Kim U, Furth J. Relation of mammary tumors to mammotrophs. II. Hormone responsiveness of 30-methyl-cholanthrene-induced carcinomas. Proc Soc Exp Biol Med 103: 643-645, 1960.

71. Kim U, Furth J. The role of prolactin in carcinogenesis. Vitam Horm (NY) 34: 107-136, 1976.

72. Kledzik GS, Bradley CJ, Meites J. Reduction of carcinogen-induced mammary cancer incidence in rats by early treatment with hormones or drugs. Cancer Res 34: 2953-2956, 1974.

73. Kledzik GS, Cusan L, Auclair C, Kelly PA, Labrie F. Inhibitory effect of a luteinizing hormone (LH)-releasing hormone agonist on rat ovarian LH and follicle-stimulating hormone receptor levels during pregnancy. Fertil Steril 29: 560-564, 1978.

74. Kledzik GS, Cusan L, Auclair C, Kelly PA, Labrie F. Inhibition of ovarian LH and FSH receptor levels by treatment with [D-Ala6, des-Gly-$NH_2$10]LHRH ethylamide during the estrous cycle in the rat. Fertil Steril 30: 348-353, 1978.

75. Kolata GB Polypeptide hormones: what are they doing in cells. Science 201: 895-897, 1978.

76. Labrie F, Auclair C, Cusan L, Kelly PA, Pelletier G, Ferland L. Inhibitory effect of LHRH and its agonists on testicular gonadotropin receptors and spermatogenesis in the rat. Int J Androl (Suppl 2), 303-318, 1978.

77. Lacassagne A, Duplan JF. Le mécanisme de la cancérisation de la mamelle chez la souris. Considéré d'après les résultats d'expériences au moyen de la réserpine. C R Acad Sci [D] (Paris) 249: 810-812, 1959.

78. Lee C, Oyasu R, Chen C. _In vitro_ interaction of estrogen and prolactin on hormone-dependent rat mammary tumors. Proc Soc Exp Biol Med 148: 224-226, 1975.

79. Leung BS, Sasaki GH. Prolactin and progesterone effect on specific estradiol binding in uterine and mammary tissues _in vitro_. Biochem Biophys Res Commun 55: 1180-1187, 1973.

80. Loeb L, Kirtz MM. The effects of transplants of anterior lobe of the hypophysis on the growth of the mammary gland and on the development of mammary gland carcinoma in various strains of mice. Am J Cancer 36: 56-82, 1939.

81. Manni A, Chambers MJ, Pearson OH. Prolactin induces its own receptors in rat liver. Endocrinology 103: 2168-2171, 1978.

82. Manni A, Trujilo JE, Pearson OH. Predominant role of prolactin in stimulating the growth of 7,12-dimethylbenz(a)anthracene-induced rat mammary tumors. Cancer Res 37: 1216-1219, 1977.

83. Masters JRW, Sangster K, Smith, T. II. Hormonal sensitivity of human breast tumors in vitro: pentose-shunt activity. Cancer (Philadelphia) 39: 1978-1980, 1977.

84. Matusik RJ, Rosen JM. Prolactin induction of casein mRNA in organ culture: a model system for studying peptide hormone regulation of gene expression. J Biol Chem 253: 2343-2347, 1978.

85. Maxfield FR, Willingham MC, Davies DJA, Pastan I. Amines inhibit the clustering of α_2-macroglobulin and EGF on the fiberblast cell surface. Nature 277: 661-663, 1979.

86. McCormic GM, Moon RC. Effects of pregnancy and lactation in growth of mammary tumors induced by 7,12-dimethylbenz(a)anthracene (DMBA). Br J Cancer 19: 160-166, 1965.

87. McMillin JM, Seal US, Theologides A. Prolactin dynamics following transphenoidal hypophysectomy for metastatic carcinoma of the breast. Cancer (Philadelphia) 39: 2254-2251, 1977.

88. Meites J. Relation of prolactin to mammary tumorigenesis and growth in rats. pp. 54-63 in <u>Prolactin and Carcinogenesis: 4th Tenovous Workshop,</u> eds AR Boyns and K Griffiths, Alpha Omega Alpha, Cardiff, 1972.

89. Muhlbock O, Boot LM Induction of mammary cancer in mice without the mammary tumor agent by isografts of hypophyses. Cancer Res 19: 402-412, 1959.

90. Nagasawa H. Prolactin: its role in the development of mammary tumors. Med Hypotheses 5: 1117-1121, 1979.

91. Nicholson RI, Davies P, Griffiths K. Effects of estradiol-17β and tamoxifen on nuclear estradiol-17β receptors in DMBA-induced rat mammary tumors. Eur J Cancer 13: 201-208, 1977.

92. Pasteels JL, Heuson JC, Heuson-Stiennon J, Legros N. Effects of insulin, prolactin, progesterone and estradiol on DNA synthesis in organ culture of 7,12-dimethylbenz(a)anthracene-induced rat mammary tumors. Cancer Res 36, 2162-2170, 1976.

93. Pearson OH, Llerena O, Llerena L, Molina A, Butler T. Prolactin-dependent rat mammary cancer: a model for man? Trans Assoc Am Physicians 82: 225-238, 1969.

94. Pearson OH, Murray R, Mozaffarian G, Pensky J Prolactin and experimental breast cancer. pp. 154-157 in Prolactin and Carcinogenesis: 4th Tenovous Workshop, eds AR Boyns and K Griffiths, Alpha Omega Alpha, Cardiff, 1972.

95. Pearson OH, Ray BS. Hypophysectomy in the treatment of metastatic mammary cancer. Am J Surg 99: 544-552, 1960.

96. Pelletier G, Cusan L, Auclair C, Kelly PA, Desy L, Labrie F. Inhibition of spermatogenesis in the rat by treatment with [D-Ala^{6}, des-Gly-NH_2^{10}]LHRH ethylamide. Endocrinology 103: 641-643, 1978.

97. Posner BI, Kelly PA, Friesen HG. Induction of a lactogenic receptor in rat liver: influence of estrogen and the pituitary. Proc Natl Acad Sci USA 71: 2407-2410, 1974.

98. Posner BI, Kelly PA, Friesen HG. Prolactin receptors in rat liver: possible induction by prolactin. Science 187: 57-59, 1975.

99. Posner BI, Raquidan D, Josefsberg Z, Bergeron JM. Different regulation of insulin receptors in intracellular (Golgi) and plasma membranes from livers of obese and lean mice. Proc Natl Acad Sci USA 75: 3302-3306, 1978.

100. Quadri SK, Clark JL, Meites J. Effects of LSD, pargyline and haloperidol on mammary tumor growth in rats. Proc Soc Exp Biol Med 142: 22-26, 1973.

101. Quadri SK, Kledzik GS, Meites J. Enhanced regression of DMBA-induced mammary cancers in rats by a combination of ergocornine with ovariectomy or high doses of estrogen. Cancer Res 34: 499-501, 1974.

102. Quadri SK, Meites J. Regression of spontaneous mammary tumors in rats by ergot drugs. Proc Soc Exp Biol Med 138: 999-1001, 1972.

103. Raynaud JP, Bonne C, Bouton MM, Moguilewski M, Philibert D, Azadian-Boulanger G. Screening for anti-hormones by receptor studies. J Steroid Biochem 6: 615-622, 1975.

104. Salih H, Brander W, Flax H, Hobbs JR. Prolactin dependence in human breast cancers. Lancet 2: 1103-1105, 1972.

105. Sasaki GH, Leung BS. On the mechanism of hormone action in 7,12-dimethylbenz(a)anthracene-induced mammary tumors. Cancer 35: 645-651, 1975.

106. Scatchard G. The attraction of protein from small molecules and ions. Ann NY Acad Sci 51: 660-672, 1949.

107. Shafie S, Brooks SC. Effect of prolactin on growth and the estrogen receptor level of human breast cancer cells (MCF-7). Cancer Res 37: 792-799, 1977.

108. Shiu RPC, Friesen HG. Properties of a prolactin receptor from the rabbit mammary gland. Biochem J 140: 301-311, 1974.

109. Shiu RPC, Friesen HG. Solubilization and purification of a prolactin receptor from the rabbit mammary gland. J Biol Chem 249: 7902-7911, 1974.

110. Shiu RPC, Friesen HG. Blockage of prolactin action by an antiserum to its receptors. Science 192: 259-261, 1976.

111. Shiu RPC, Friesen HG. Interaction of cell-membrane prolactin receptor with its antibody. Biochem J 157: 619-626, 1976.

112. Shiu RPC, Kelly PA, Friesen HG. Radioreceptor assay for prolactin and other lactogenic hormones. Science 180: 968-971, 1973.

113. Smith RD, Hilf R, Senior AE. Prolactin binding to dissociated cells from rat mammary tumors and mammary gland. Cancer Biochem Biophys 3: 117-121, 1979.

114. Smithline F, Sherman L, Kolodny HD. Prolactin and breast carcinoma. N Engl J Med 292: 784-792, 1975.

115. Teller MN, Stock CC, Hellman L, Mountain IM, Bowie M, Rosenberg BJ, Boyar RM, Budinger JM. Comparative effects of a series of prolactin inhibitors, 17β-estradiol and 2α-methyldihydrotestosterone propionate on growth of 7,12-dimethylbenz(a)anthracene-induced rat mammary carcinomas. Cancer Res 37: 3932-3938, 1977.

116. Terenius L. Antiestrogens and breast cancer. Eur J Cancer 7: 57-64, 1971.

117. Terenius L. Effects of antiestrogens on initiation of mammary cancer in the female rat. Eur J Cancer 7: 65-70, 1971.

118. Thompson HJ, Becci PJ, Brown CC, Moon RC. Effect of the duration of retinyl acetate feeding on inhibition of 1-methyl-1-nitrosourea-induced mammary carcinogenesis in the rat. Cancer Res 39: 3977-3980, 1979.

119. Tsai TLS, Katzenellenbogen BS. Antagonism of development and growth of 7,12-dimethylbenz(a)anthracene-induced rat mammary tumors by the antiestrogen U 23469 and effects on estrogen and progesterone receptors. Cancer Res 37: 1537-1543, 1977.

120. Turcot-Lemay L, Kelly PA. Characterization of estradiol, progesterone and prolactin receptors in nitrosomethylurea-induced mammary tumors and effect of antiestrogen treatment on the development and growth of these tumors. Cancer Res 40: 3232-3240, 1980.

121. Turcot-Lemay L, Kelly PA. Response to ovariectomy of N-nitrosomethylurea-induced mammary tumors in the rat. J Natl Cancer Inst 66: 97-102, 1981.

122. Turcot-Lemay L, Kelly PA. Prolactin receptors in human breast tumors. Submitted.

123. Turcot-Lemay L, Kelly PA. Effect of an LHRH analog on growth and hormone levels in DMBA-induced mammary tumors in the rat. Submitted.

124. Welsch CW, Brown CK, Goodrich-Smith M, Chiusano J, Moon RC Synergistic effect of chronic prolactin suppression and retinoid treatment in the prophylaxis of N-methyl-N-nitrosourea-induced mammary tumorigenesis in female Sprague-Dawley rats. Cancer Res 40: 3095-3098, 1980.

125. Welsch CW, Clemens JA, Meites J. Effects of multiple pituitary homografts or progesterone on 7,12-dimethylbenz(a)anthracene-induced mammary tumors in rats. J Natl Cancer Inst 41: 465-471, 1968.

126. Welsch CW, Jenkins TW, Meites J. Increased incidence of mammary tumors in female rat grafted with multiple pituitaries. Cancer Res 30: 1024-1029, 1970.

127. Welsch CW, Meites J. Effects of reserpine in development of 7,12-dimethylbenz(a)anthracene-induced mammary tumors in female rats. Experientia 26: 1133-1134, 1970.

128. Welsch CW, Nagasawa H. Prolactin and murine mammary tumorigenesis: a review. Cancer Res 37: 951-963, 1975.

129. Welsch CW, Nagasawa H, Meites J. Increased incidence of spontaneous mammary tumors in female rats with induced hypothalamic lesions. Cancer Res 30: 2310-2313, 1970.

130. Wilson RG, Buchan R, Roberts MM, Forrest APM, Boyns AR, Cole EN, Griffiths K. Plasma prolactin and breast cancer. Cancer (Philadelphia) 33: 1325-1327, 1974.

131. Yanai R, Nagasawa H. Inhibition of mammary tumorigenesis by ergot alkaloids and promotion of mammary tumorigenesis by pituitary isograpfs in adreno-ovariectomized mice. J Natl Cancer Inst 48: 715-719, 1972.

Chapter 3

STUDIES OF PROLACTIN RECEPTORS AND THE POSSIBLE PROLIFERATIVE ROLE OF PROLACTIN AND OTHER PITUITARY FACTORS IN HUMAN BREAST TUMOR CELLS

Robert P C Shiu

Prolactin and estrogen play key roles in influencing the growth behaviour of experimental breast tumors of rodents (7), (11), (17), (23), (43). However, the involvements of these two hormones, especially that of prolactin, in the tumorigenesis of the human breast, is still unclear (20). Whether or not trophic factors other than these two hormones are also important in growth regulation of breast cancer remains to be elucidated. Clinical investigations have indicated that pituitary hormones are important in the etiology of human breast cancer although the identity of the pituitary factors have not been elucidated. In view of the important role that prolactin plays in the tumorigenesis of rodent breast cancer, the notion that this hormone may be involved in the etiology of human breast cancer has been formulated (23). Evidence, mainly derived from clinical observations, has so far failed to establish an importance of prolactin in the breast disease of man (20). However, studies with human breast tumor biopsies maintained in organ culture using a pentose pathway histochemical effect suggest that some tumors show some form of prolactin dependency (26). Further, it has been reported that human breast biopsies maintained in organ culture (42) or transplanted in athymic nude mice (16) respond to prolactin and placental lactogen with an increase in DNA synthesis. One of the recent advances in human breast cancer research has been the development of a considerable number of cell lines derived from breast cancer specimens (4). The use of these human breast cancer cell lines maintained in tissue culture has provided new insight into the hormonal control of breast cancer in man. The proliferation of some human breast tumor cell lines in culture are affected by hormones such as insulin (1), (22) and epidermal growth factor (4).

One of the continuing interests in this laboratory is to elucidate the mechanism of action of prolactin in target cells. It is without doubt that at least four aspects of prolactin action are mediated by an initial binding of prolactin to cell surface receptor sites. These are (1) the prolactin-induced casein synthesis and amino acid transport in the mammary tissue (31), (32); (2) the prolactin-induced proliferation of Nb2 cells, a rat lymphoma cell line whose proliferation is dependent solely on prolactin (6), (35), (39); (3) the prolactin-induced luteolysis in the rat (2);

and (4) the prolactin-stimulated water transport across the human amnion (15). In view of these observations, it is rationalized that the study of prolactin receptors may gain some insight into the biological significance of prolactin in breast cancer. A number of studies have indicated that specific prolactin binding sites, which have all the characteristics of prolactin receptors, are present in some human breast cancer biopsies (8), (19), (37). Human breast cancer cells maintained in culture may, therefore, be useful for studies on prolactin binding. If these cell lines contain prolactin receptors, they may be prolactin responsive and they are potentially useful for studying the role of prolactin in human breast cancer.

A number of human breast cancer cell lines were, therefore, assayed for prolactin receptors (29). The result of such a survey is illustrated in Table 1. Twelve cell lines tested

Table 1: Prolactin Receptors in Human Breast Cell Lines

Cell Line	Number of Prolactin Receptors per Cell
Tumor Cells:	
T-47D	25,800
MCF-7	8,310
MDA-MB-157	7,663
BT-20	6,435
BT-474	5,480
MDA-MB-231	3,760
ALAB 496	3,650
SK-BR-3	3,329
Hs0578T	2,260
Levine III	1,619
Du 4475	1,094
Non-tumor Cells:	
HBL-100	1,700

Part of the results presented in this Table is reprinted, with permission, from reference No. 29.

contain varying degrees of prolactin binding activity. The number of prolactin receptor sites per cell varies among cell lines: The values range from 26,000 for T-47D to about 1000 sites for Du 4475. HBL-100, a cell line derived from human milk, also contains low levels of prolactin receptors. Hence, there is a large variation of prolactin receptor content in tumor cells derived from different patients, a finding which is similar to that of estrogen receptors in human breast cancer specimens. Furthermore, the receptor sites have very high affinity for prolactin, the dissociation constant (Kd) is about 10^{-10} M.

The hormone specificity of the prolactin receptors in the human breast cancer cells is illustrated in Fig. 1 (29). All lactogenic hormones, namely, human prolactin (hPRL), human growth hormone (hGH), and human placental lactogen (hPL) compete with ^{125}I-hPRL for the receptor sites; hPL is about 1% as potent as are hPRL and hGH. Sheep prolactin (oPRL) is almost as effective as is hPRL, consistent with its biological activity that was determined in organ culture experiments using human breast tumor biopsy specimens (12). Sheep growth hormone (oGH), which is not lactogenic, is ineffective as a competitor. Other human hormones fail to compete with ^{125}I-hPRL for the receptor sites. The same hormone specificity was reported for the prolactin binding site studied by using membrane preparations derived from human breast tumor biopsy specimens (8), (19), (37). The characteristics of the receptor sites in these human breast cancer cells are identical to that of the classical prolactin receptors (32), (33). The observation that human growth hormone shares the same receptor site for prolactin in human breast tumor cells raises the possibility that human growth hormone may have prolactin-like effects. Indeed, studies using biopsy specimens maintained in organ culture support this notion (12), (26). Assuming that prolactin has a role in the etiology of human breast cancer, attempts to induce tumor regression by the mere suppression of prolactin secretion (e.g. by bromocryptine) may not be enough. It may be essential to suppress human growth hormone secretion as well.

The binding of prolactin to some human breast cancer cell lines has also been studied morphologically by using the technique of immunocytochemistry and autoradiography (27), (34). These techniques reveal several features of prolactin binding which are not apparent from studies using the aforementioned biochemical techniques. For example, immunocytochemistry reveals that prolactin binding within a human breast cancer cell line can be heterogeneous: not all the cells are stained equally for prolactin, indicating heterogeneity of prolactin binding. We do not yet know the reasons for this observation. It is possible that the heterogeneity in prolactin binding reflects cells in different phases of the cell cycle or cells representing distinct types. Autoradiographical study using ^{125}I-hPRL reveals both surface-localized and intracellular silver grains, the latter suggesting internali-

Figure 1: Hormone specificity of binding of ^{125}I-hPRL to human breast cancer cells (T-47D). Reprinted with permission, from reference 29. hPRL, human prolactin; hPL, human placental lactogen; hGH, human growth hormone; hCG, human chorionic gonadotropin; hLH, human luteinizing hormone; oGH, ovine growth hormone; oPRL, ovine prolactin.

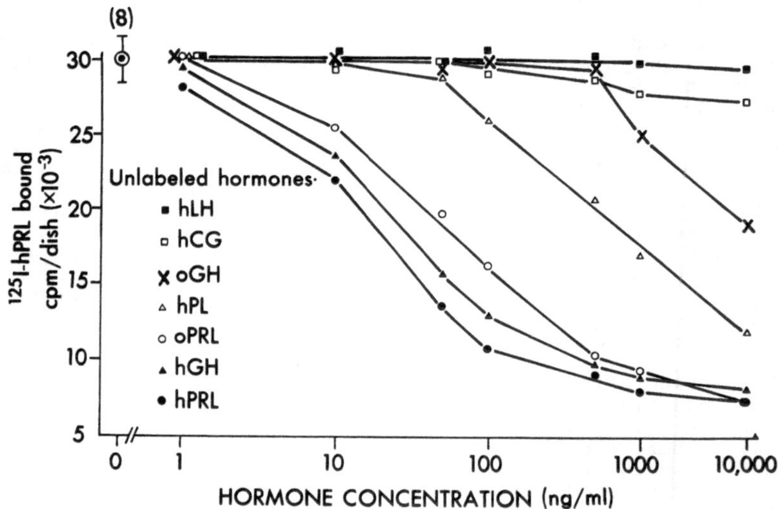

zation of prolactin by the human breast cancer cells. Our light microscopic autoradiographic study did not permit us to identify the subcellular structures that contained the internalized radioactive prolactin. The internalization of prolactin by human breast cancer cells in culture was further studied by biochemical procedures (30). It was found that receptor-bound prolactin is quickly internalized, possibly via pinocytosis, and degraded in intracellular sites (possibly the lysosomes). The internalization process can be inhibited by metabolic poisons such as 2,4-dinitrophenol and sodium azide. The internalized prolactin molecule is degraded to several small peptides which are released into the incubation media. Degradation of prolactin can be prevented by the protease inhibitor N-α-p-tosyl-L-lysine chloromethylketone, and the lysosomotropic agents ammonium chloride and chloroquine. When prolactin degradation is inhibited, specific binding and subsequent dissociation of intact prolactin is still observed, suggesting that hormone degradation is not responsible for the dissociation of prolactin. There are quantitative differences in the ability to bind and degrade prolactin among the cell lines although there is a good correlation between the number of prolactin receptor sites and prolactin degrading activity. This suggests that the prolactin molecule will be internalized and degraded only if it binds to the receptor site. It should be mentioned that intracellular prolactin has been found in normal rat and rabbit mammary epithelial cells (21), (38); prolactin internalization is not unique to human breast cancer cells in tissue culture. The physiological significance of prolactin internalization and degradation, however, remains to be elucidated, although a recent study using rabbit mammary organ cultures suggests that the internalization and degradation of prolactin is not involved in the biological action of prolactin (9).

Having established that human breast cancer cells maintained in tissue culture possess prolactin receptors, it is, therefore, essential to establish the biological significance of prolactin receptors and the biological responses that prolactin produced in these cells. There have been only limited studies on the effects of prolactin on human breast cancer cells in culture. Studies with human breast tumor biopsies maintained in organ culture suggested that some tumors responded to prolactin treatment with an increase in pentose pathway enzyme activity (26), in the production of α-lactalbumin (12), and in the uptake of ^{3}H-thymidine (42). Furthermore, it has been reported that prolactin stimulates estrogen receptor activity (28) and protein synthesis (3) in the breast tumor cell line, MCF-7. One of the important questions that remains to be answered is, "Can prolactin affect the rate of proliferation (growth) of human breast tumor cells?" We, therefore, examined whether or not prolactin and other hormones are mitogenic in several human breast cancer cell lines which contain appreciable amounts of prolactin receptors. The data of several experiments are summarized in Table 2. Purified human prolactin and growth

Table 2: Effect of Hormones and Growth Factors on Growth of Human Breast Cancer Cells In Monolayer Cultures

ADDITIONS	CELL NUMBER ($X10^{-5}$) T-47D		MCF-7	
	No Serum	1% CFCS	No Serum	1% CFCS
None	0.4±0.1	5.6±0.2	0.8±0.1	7.4±0.1
hPRL	0.4±0.1	5.5±0.6	0.8±0.2	7.2±0.3
hGH	0.5±0.1	-	0.9±0.1	-
Insulin	1.1±0.2*	10.1±0.2*	1.0±0.2	9.6±0.5*
FGF	1.6±0.4*	9.3±0.1*	0.9±0.2	7.0±0.1
EGF	0.8±0.1*	-	1.4±0.2*	-
17β-E_2	-	6.3±0.1	-	11.0±0.3*
Testo	-	5.4±0.5	-	-
Dex	-	5.7±0.4	-	4.4±0.4*
Prog	-	6.3±0.4	-	7.6±0.7
T_3	-	10.2±0.8*	-	9.6±0.4*

Cell numbers were determined seven days after the additions of hormones or growth factors. Each value represents mean of triplicate ± S.D. Astrisks indicate values which are significantly different from the control (no addition) with $P<0.05$. The final concentrations of hormones and growth factors were: hPRL, 1 μg/ml; hGH, 1 μg/ml; insulin, 10 μg/ml; FGF, 10 ng/ml; EGF, 10 ng/ml; 17β-E_2, 10^{-8} M; Testo, 10^{-8} M; Dex, 10^{-7} M; Prog, 10^{-7}M; T_3, $5x10^{-7}$ M. CFCS, charcoal-treated fetal calf serum.

hormone (at concentrations from 10 ng/ml to 1 μg/ml) fail to affect the growth rate of human breast tumor cells (T-47D and MCF-7) grown as monolayers on plastic dishes. In contrast, insulin and epidermal growth factor (EGF) stimulate the growth of both cell lines whereas pituitary-derived fibroblast growth factor (FGF) stimulates the growth of T-47D but not that of MCF-7 cells. For the steroids tested at low concentrations, 17β-estradiol is stimulatory in MCF-7 but has much less effect on T-47D cells. Progesterone and testosterone are without effect. High concentrations ($>10^{-5}$M) of all the steroids are inhibitory. The thyroid hormone, T_3, consistently stimulates the growth of both T-47D and MCF-7 cells. Furthermore, when tested in combination with several other hormones, prolactin does not produce any further stimulation over that observed for the other hormones alone (data not shown).

In view of the importance of extracellular matrix in the maintenance of cellular proliferation and differentiated functions of many cell types (5), (41), (44), we decided to examine whether or not human breast cancer cells grown in collagen matrix would become responsive to prolactin and other hormones. We (13) found that human breast cancer cells cultivated in collagen matrix exhibit altered cell shape (spherical) and grow as multilayered tumor-like clusters. They are more dependent on serum for growth as compared with cells grown as monolayers on plastic dishes. Their growth rate is slower in collagen than on plastic, and they are still responsive to a hormone combination of insulin, epidermal growth factor, estrogen and transferrin. However, prolactin and growth hormone do not affect their growth rate (Leung and Shiu, unpublished observation).

In short, we have so far been unable to demonstrate a growth regulatory role of prolactin in human breast cancer cells maintained in culture on plastic substratum or in collagen matrix. One possible explanation for these observations is that prolactin may play no role in the growth regulation of human breast tumor cells, although it affects other cellular functions, such as estrogen receptor activity and protein synthesis, as reported by others (3), (28). Therefore, further effort to examine the effect of prolactin on the expression of differentiated functions (such as the production of milk proteins) in these cells, especially when they are cultivated in extracellular matrix, is warranted. Other possible explanations for the unresponsiveness of these cells to prolactin are: (1) that permissive factors, which are absent in in vitro situations, may be needed to render the cells responsive to prolactin; (2) that prolactin may act in vivo through an intermediate pathway which is missing in our in vitro experiments; and (3) that the pituitary factor that is thought to play a role in the growth regulation of human breast cancer is something other than prolactin. The existence of a novel mammary growth factor has been suggested in a number of recent studies using rodent breast tumor cells as models (10), (24), (25).

To test some of the above possibilities, we examined whether pituitary hormones are capable of influencing the growth of the human breast cancer cells in vivo, i.e., in athymic nude mice (14). Human breast cancer cells, T-47D, that possess both prolactin and estrogen receptors were used and they were injected at a subcutaneous site in the nude mice. Pituitary hormones were supplied by subcutaneous implantation of rat pituitary glands or rat pituitary tumor cells, GH_3. These GH_3 cells secrete two known hormones: prolactin and growth hormone. Five groups of female nude mice were used; the first group (T) received a subcutaneous injection of human breast tumor cells (T-47D) only; the second group (TE) was injected with T-47D cells and estradiol valerate; the third group (TG) was injected with T-47D and rat pituitary tumor cells GH_3, one cell type on each flank; the fourth group (TEG) received T-47D cells, estradiol valerate and GH_3 cells; and the fifth group (TEP) received T-47D cells, estradiol valerate and rat pituitary transplants. The T-47D cells formed solid tumors and their growth was monitored in the five groups of nude mice (Fig. 2). The human breast cancer cells (T-47D) did not proliferate in female nude mice (T group), indicating that the hormonal milieu in these animals is not optimal for the growth of human breast cancer cells. It is interesting to note that in mice bearing GH_3 pituitary tumors (TG group), there was no apparent growth of T-47D human breast tumor despite very high concentrations of prolactin and growth hormone (437 ng/ml and 1008 ng/ml, respectively) in the blood of the animals. Thus, it seems that prolactin and growth hormone alone are not sufficient to stimulate the proliferation of T-47D tumor. On the other hand, injection of estrogen alone (TE) resulted in a very moderate growth of T-47D tumor, reaching a mean size of 63 mm^3 in 42 days. The simultaneous presence of estrogen, GH_3 pituitary tumor (i.e. TEG group), in contrast, induced rapid and sustained growth of T-47D tumors to a mean size of 528 mm^3. This value represents an eight-fold increase in volume over that of TE group, indicating that estrogen alone cannot produce maximal growth of the human breast cancer cells, T-47D. We have also observed that normal rat pituitaries implanted in estrogen-treated nude mice (TEP) also induced very rapid proliferation of T-47D tumor cells to a size comparable to that seen in the TEG group (data not shown).

It is obvious from the in vivo studies that human breast cancer cells are responsive to estrogen and pituitary hormones, even to those hormones produced from pituitary cells of a non-human species. The key question arises from these studies is, therefore, "What is (are) the pituitary factor(s) that stimulates the growth in vivo of human breast cancer cells?". Could the principle active factor be prolactin (or growth hormone) or some other unknown factors? If it were prolactin, then why does it not stimulate the

Figure 2: Growth of human breast cancer cells (T-47D) in athymic nude mice. Each point represents the mean ± standard deviation from four animals. Tumor size, in mm^3, was the product of the three dimensions. T (0), mice injected with human breast cancer cells, T-47D, only; TG (■), mice injected with T-47D and GH_3 rat pituitary tumor cells; TE (●), mice injected with T-47D cells and estradiol valerate; TEG (▲), mice injected with T-47D and GH_3 cells and estradiol valerate. Modified, with permission, from reference 14.

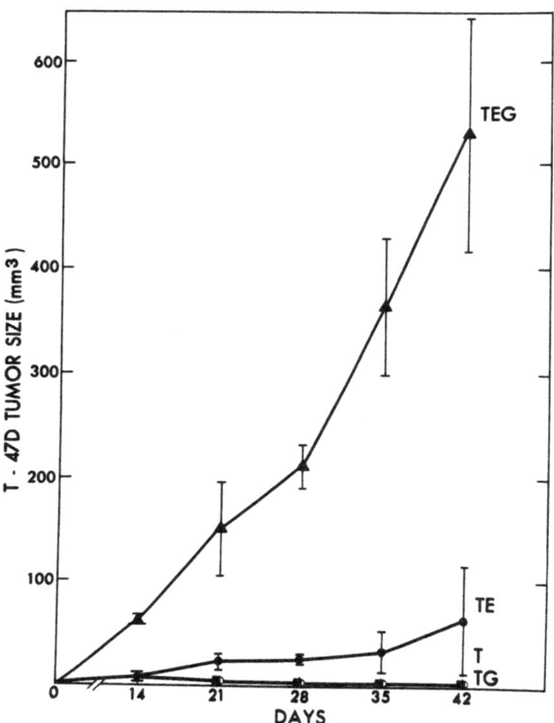

growth of the cells in vitro? In a recent review, Gospodarowicz and Tauber (5) discussed the inappropriateness of using tissue cultured cells to identify growth-promoting factors. These authors pointed out that cells cultured in vitro on plastic substratum lack the extracellular matrix, which the cells are associated with in vivo. Many properties of the cells are thus altered, and the use of tissue culture cells may lead to the identification of growth factors that are active in cell culture but are probably inactive either in organ culture or in vivo. In contrast, the use of organ culture or other in vivo models could lead to the identification of factors that are active in vivo but not in vitro. By analogy then, prolactin may still be important in the control of growth of human breast cancer in vivo, although its effect cannot be observed in vitro.

Our studies also suggest that the active pituitary principle may not be prolactin or any other "known" pituitary hormones at all. This notion is supported by several studies (18), (25) which suggest the existence of a mammary growth stimulating factor produced by the pituitary gland. This factor may be a modified form of prolactin (18) or it may not be related to prolactin at all (10). Ptashne et al (24) also reported that a factor isolated from serum promotes the proliferation of mammary epithelium; whether this serum factor originates from the pituitary is unknown. Finally, the active pituitary principle observed by us could have been induced by estrogen, a phenomenon somewhat similar to the estrogen-induced tissue growth factors described by Sirbasku (36).

The physiological factor (may it be prolactin or otherwise) that controls the growth of breast cancer has to be further characterized. The use of in vivo methodology (i.e., transplantation of human tumors into athymic nude mice) and improved tissue culture techniques (e.g., by growing human breast cancer cells in appropriately prepared extracellular matrix) would certainly improve the chances of achieving this goal. The human breast cancer cell lines that possess prolactin, estrogen and other hormone receptors should be useful models to elucidate the mechanism of action of ovarian steroids, pituitary hormones and other yet to be characterized growth factors, in the control of proliferation of human breast cancer.

BIBLIOGRAPHY

1. Barnes D, Sato G. Growth of a human mammary tumor cell line in a serum-free medium. Nature 281: 388-389, 1979.

2. Bohnet HG, Shiu RPC, Grinwich D, Friesen HG. In vivo effects of antisera to prolactin receptors in female rats. Endocrinology 102: 1657-1661, 1978.

3. Burke RE, Gaffney EV. Prolactin can stimulate general protein synthesis in human breast cancer cells (MCF-7) in long-term culture. Life Sci 23: 901-906, 1978.

4. Engel LW, Young NA. Human breast carcinoma cells in continuous culture: A review. Cancer Res 38: 4327-4339, 1978.

5. Gospodarowicz D, Tauber J-P. Growth factors and the extracellular matrix. Endocr Rev 1: 201-227, 1980.

6. Gout PW, Beer CT, Noble RL. Prolactin-stimulated growth of cell cultures established from malignant Nb rat lymphomas. Cancer Res 40: 2433-2436, 1980.

7. Holdaway IM, Friesen HG. Correlation between hormone binding and growth response of rat mammary tumor. Cancer Res 36: 1562-1567, 1976.

8. Holdaway IM, Friesen HG. Hormone binding by human mammary carcinoam. Cancer Res 37: 1946-1952, 1977.

9. Houdebine L-M, Djiane J. Effects of lysomotropic agents, and of microfilament - and microtubule-disrupting drugs on the activation of casein - gene expression by prolactin in the mammary gland. Mol Cell Endocrinol 17: 1-15, 1980.

10. Kano-Sueoka T, Cohen DM, Yamaizumi Z, Nishimura S, Mori M, Fujiki H. Phosphoethanolamine as a growth factor of a mammary carcinoma cell line of rat. Proc Natl Acad Sci USA 76: 5741-5744, 1979.

11. Kim V, Furth J. The role of prolactin in carcinogenesis. Vit Horm 34: 107-136, 1976.

12. Kleinberg DL. Human α-lactalbumin: Measurement in serum and in breast cancer organ cultures by radioimmunoassay. Science 190: 276-278, 1975.

13. Leung CKH, Shiu RPC. Growth characteristics of human breast cancer cells in collagen gel. J Cell Biol 87: 115a, 1980.

14. Leung CKH, Shiu RPC. Required presence of both estrogen and pituitary factors for the growth of human breast cancer cells in athymic nude mice. Cancer Res 41: 546-551, 1981.

15. Leontic EA, Tyson JE. Prolactin and fetal osmoregulation: water transport across isolated human amnion. Am J Physiol 232: 124-127, 1977.

16. McManus MJ, Dembroske SE, Pienkowski MM, Anderson JJ, Mann LC, Schuster JS, Vollwiler LL, Welsch CW. Successful transplantation of human benign breast tumors into the athymic nude mouse and demonstration of enhanced DNA synthesis by human placental lactogen. Cancer Res 38: 2343-2349, 1978.

17. Meites J, Lee KH, Wuttke W, Welsch CW, Nagasawa H, Quadri SK. Recent studies on functions and control of prolactin secretion in rats. Recent Prog Horm Res 28: 471-526, 1972.

18. Mittra I. A novel "cleaved prolactin" in the rat pituitary: Part II. In vivo mammary mitogenic activity of its N-terminal 16K moiety. Biochem Biophys Res Commun 95: 1760-1767, 1980.

19. Morgan L, Raggatt PR, de Souza I, Salih H, Hobbs JR. Prolactin receptors in human breast tumors. J Endocrinol 73: 17p-18p, 1977.

20. Nagasawa H. Prolactin and human breast cancer: A review. Eur J Cancer 15: 267-279. 1979.

21. Nolin JM, Witorsch RJ. Detection of endogenous immunoreactive prolactin in rat mammary epithelial cells during lactation. Endocrinology 99: 949-958, 1976.

22. Osborne CK, Bolan G, Monaco ME, Lippman ME. Hormone responsive human breast cancer in long-term tissue culture: Effect of insulin. Proc Natl Acad Sci USA 73: 4536-4540, 1976.

23. Pearson OH, Llerena O, Llerena L, Molina A, Butler T. Prolactin-dependent rat mammary cancer: A model for man? Trans Assoc Am Physicians 82: 225-238, 1969.

24. Ptashne K, Hsueh HW, Stockdale FE. Partial purification and characterization of mammary growth factor, a protein which promotes proliferation of mammary epithelium. Biochemistry 18: 3533-3539, 1979.

25. Rudland PS, Bennett DC, Warburton MJ. Hormonal control of growth and differentiation of cultured rat mammary gland epithelial cells. pp 667-700 in Hormones and Cell Culture, eds G Sato, R Ross, Cold Spring Harbour Laboratory, 1979.

26. Salih H, Flax H, Brander W, Hobbs JR. Prolactin dependence in human breast cancers. Lancet 2: 1103-1105, 1972.

27. Salih H, Cheng KW, Shiu RPC. Immunocytochemical demonstration of prolactin binding to human breast cancer cells in long term tissue culture. p 151 in Program and Abstracts, 61st Endocrine Society Meeting, 1979.

28. Shafie S, Brooks SC. Effect of prolactin on growth and the estrogen receptor level of human breast cancer cells (MCF-7). Cancer Res 37: 792-799, 1977.

29. Shiu RPC. Prolactin receptors in human breast cancer cells in long term tissue culture. Cancer Res 39: 4381-4386, 1979.

30. Shiu RPC. Processing of prolactin by human breast cancer cells in long term tissue culture. J Biol Chem 255: 4278-4281, 1980.

31. Shiu RPC, Friesen HG. Blockade of prolactin action by an antiserum to its receptors. Science 192: 259-261, 1976.

32. Shiu RPC, Friesen HG. Mechanism of action of prolactin in the control of mammary gland function. Annu Rev Physiol 42: 83-96, 1980.

33. Shiu RPC, Kelly PA, Friesen HG. Radioreceptor assay for prolactin and other lactogenic hormones. Science 180: 968-971, 1973.

34. Shiu RPC, Salih H, Paterson JA. Immunocytochemical and autoradiographical demonstration of prolactin binding to human breast cancer cells in tissue culture (submitted for publication), 1981.

35. Shiu RPC, Tanaka T, Friesen HG, Gout PW, Beer CT, Noble RL. Receptor-mediated mitogenic action of prolactin on a rat lymphoma cell line (manuscript in preparation).

36. Sirbasku DA. Estrogen induction of growth factors specific for hormone-responsive mammary, pituitary and kidney tumor cells. Proc Natl Acad Sci USA 75: 3786-3790, 1978.

37. Stagner JI, Jochimsen PR, Sherman BM. Lactogenic hormone binding to human breast cancer: Correlation with estrogen receptor. Clin Res 25: 320A, 1977.

38. Suard YML, Kraechenbuhl J-P, Aubert ML. Dispersed mammary epithelial cells: Receptors for lactogenic hormones in virgin, pregnant, and lactating rabbits. J Biol Chem 254: 10466-10475, 1979.

39. Tanaka T, Shiu RPC, Gout PW, Beer CT, Noble RL, Friesen HG. A new sensitive and specific bioassay for lactogenic hormones: Measurement of prolactin and growth hormone in human serum. J Clin Endocrinol Metab 51: 1058-1063, 1980.

40. Taylor-papadimitriou J, Shearer M, Stoker MGP. Growth requirements of human mammary epithelial cells in culture. Int J Cancer 20: 903-908, 1977.

41. Vlodarsky I, Liu GM, Gospodarowicz D. Morphological appearance, growth behaviour and migratory activity of human tumor cells maintained on extracellular matrix versus plastic. Cell 19: 607-616, 1980.

42. Welsch CW, Calaf de Iturri G, Brennan MJ. DNA synthesis of human, mouse and rat mammary carcinomas in vitro: Influence of insulin and prolactin. Cancer 38: 1272-1281, 1976.

43. Welsch CW, Nagasawa H. Prolactin and murine mammary tumorigenesis: A review. Cancer Res 37: 951-963, 1977.

44. Yang J, Richards J, Bowman P, Guzman R, Enami J, McCormick K, Hamamoto S, Pitelka D, Nandi S. Sustained growth and three-dimensional organization of primary mammary tumor epithelial cells embedded in collagen gels. Proc Natl Acad Sci USA 76: 3401-3405, 1979.

ACKNOWLEDGEMENT

The work done in the author's laboratory was supported by the Medical Research Council of Canada. The author is a Scholar of the Mecical Research Council of Canada. Some of the studies described in this chapter were done in collaboration with Dr. J. A. Paterson, Dr. H. Salih, and C.K.H. Leung. The author would also like to acknowledge Dr. E.Y. Lasfargues, Dr. M. Rich, Mr. C.V. Piczak, and Mr. J.F. Weaver for providing the cell lines used in his studies. The secretarial assistance of Miss N. Ryan is very much appreciated.

Chapter 4

MODE OF ACTION OF PROLACTIN ON NORMAL AND NEOPLASTIC MAMMARY TISSUES

James A Rıllema

Introduction

Prolactin is one of several hormones which is thought to be capable of initiating and promoting the growth of neoplastic tissues of mammary origin (10), (15), (24), (60). Accordingly, it is of critical importance to deliniate the sequel of biochemical events whereby prolactin has its actions on cellular proliferation; this knowledge will allow the use of logical approaches for creating useful methods to suppress neoplastic processes in mammary tissues. Although prolactin has a multitude of different actions in more than 80 different target tissues (17), most of the information concerning the mechanisms by which prolactin carries out its actions has been obtained using cultured normal mammary tissues. Only a limited amount of information is available concerning how prolactin has its actions on neoplastic mammary cells. Most of this chapter will therefore focus on how prolactin has its actions in normal mammary cells, but comments concerning prolactin's actions on neoplastic mammary cells will be made where appropriate. Two recent reviews (40), (55) have summarized much of the available information concerning the mechanisms of action of prolactin in mammary tissues; the present chapter will incorporate recently published information into the knowledge contained in those earlier reviews.

Prolactin receptors

Although the topic "Prolactin receptors" will be reviewed in detail in other chapters of this monograph, it is essential to make a few comments about "receptors" in order to discuss in a more intelligent fashion the subsequent actions of prolactin. Obviously, the initial interaction of prolactin with its target cells is thought to be with specific components of the plasma membrane. Accordingly, Shiu and Friesen (53), as well as other investigators (16), have demonstrated specific, dissociable binding sites for prolactin in membrane preparations from the mammary gland and other target tissues. More recently, two laboratories (9), (59) have reported a high affinity binding site for prolactin which requires a 4M magnesium ion solution to release the prolactin. That the dissociable (in the absence of magnesium) binding sites may represent physiological receptor sites for prolactin is suggested by observations from Richard's laboratory (27); he reported that the magnitude of the prolactin stimulation of ornithine decarboxylase activity varied greatly in different target tissues. But the number of dissociable prolactin-binding-sites correlates quite well with the magnitude of the prolactin responses on ornithine decarboxylase activity. Further supporting the physiological importance of the dissociable receptors is the observation (54) that an antiserum to these receptors abolishes the actions of prolactin on casein synthesis and amino acid transport. The binding sites for prolactin which are disrupted by 4M magnesium solutions may also be of physiological importance. We (42) demonstrated several years ago that it is only necessary to expose mammary tissues for a few seconds (at a reduced temperature and with low concentrations of prolactin) in order to subsequently observe actions of prolactin several hours later. These studies therefore suggest that there may be two or more types of prolactin receptors which may be responsible for carrying out different biological responses.

Internalization of prolactin

One important question concerning the actions of hormones on target cells is whether they have their actions via a plasma-membrane response, or whether they enter the target cells and have their actions. Nolin's laboratory has advocated the latter mechanism based primarily on the observation that immunoreactive prolactin can be found within a variety of prolactin target cells (18), (19). In addition, Shiu has found that prolactin is degraded by cultured neoplastic mammary cells; he has thus suggested that this may be accomplished by the proteolytic action of lysosomal enzymes (52), (55). Although the studies of Nolin and Shiu suggest that prolactin does enter its target cells, the reason why it becomes internalized is not clear. It could be that the in ternalization of prolactin is the mechanism whereby prolactin is inactivated in its target cells, i.e. it is digested by the lysosomal proteolytic enzymes. It is also possible that prolactin may have actions inside target cells. There is little evidence to support this latter possibility, however. Several years ago, Chomczynski and Topper (2) reported that lactogenic hormones stimulate the rate of [^{3}H]-uridine incorporation into RNA in isolated nucleii from rodent mammary glands. Their methods employed to isolate the nucleii, however, were such that their nuclear preparation likely contained cellular debris including plasma membranes, and it is therefore not certain if their observed effects are a result of a direct action of the lactogenic hormones on the nuclei Josefsberg et al. (7) have also reported that when [^{125}]-labeled prolactin is injected intravenously into rats, it is concentrated in the golgi apparatus of the liver. Posner et al. (26) have further identified prolactin binding proteins in the golgi apparatus as well as other cell organelles of the liver (19). What these binding sites represent is not clear. One likely possibility is that they may represent prolactin receptors being synthesized by the cells, and they will subsequently be transported to the plasma membrane. The golgi apparatus probably participates in the synthesis of the prolactin receptors since the receptors have been shown to be glycoproteins (55). In summary, it is therefore apparent that there is presently no convincing support for the idea that prolactin has biological actions directly on subcellular organelles within its target cells.

Actions of prolactin at the plasma membrane

The alternative to the hormone internalization hypothesis is that the actions of prolactin are carried out via biochemical processes which are initiated at the level of the plasma membrane. The message from the prolactin receptor complex must then be transmitted into the cell. For other hormones which work in this sort of fashion, various mechanisms involving intracellular mediators have been identified; these include altered intracellular concentrations of free calcium ions, cyclic nucleotides, prostaglandins, polyamines and sodium-potassium ions. Evidence suggests that several of these mediators may be involved in the actions of prolactin on mammary cells. In order to establish if one or more of these substances mediates the actions of prolactin, a number of experimental criteria must be established in the laboratory. These include the following:

1) One should be able to mimic the hormone effects with a proposed mediator.
2) One should be able to demonstrate an elevated tissue content of a mediator in response to the hormone.
3) One should be able to demonstrate an effect of the hormone on the enzymes that catalyze the synthesis and/or degradation of the mediator.
4) One should be able to modify or mimic the hormone effect with drugs that modulate the tissue content of the suspected mediator.

Several of these criteria have been satisfied with regard to potential mediators of prolactin's actions in normal mammary tissues. There is currently no information available concerning whether prolactin's actions in neoplastic mammary cells are carried out via intracellular mediators.

Sodium-potassium hypothesis

Falconer et al. (3), (4) have advocated the idea that certain of prolactin's actions may be carried out by an activation of membrane-associated, sodium-potassium ATPase with a consequent decreased intracellular concentration of sodium and an increased concentration of potassium. Both in vivo and in vitro, prolactin causes the appropriate changes in sodium and potassium ion concentrations in rabbit mammary tissues. In addition, μM ouabain, a specific inhibitor of sodium-potassium ATPase abolishes the effect of prolactin on fatty acid synthesis, reduces the magnitude of stimulation of protein synthesis, but has no effect on RNA synthesis in cultured rabbit mammary tissues. With cultured mammary tissues from mice in midpregnancy, the actions of prolactin on RNA synthesis (Table 1) and casein synthesis (Table 2) are still apparent when concentrations of ouabain as high as 1 mM are employed. Ouabain, by itself, inhibited in a dose-response fashion the rate of [^{3}H]-leucine incorporation into casein. The basal rate of [^{3}H]-uridine incorporation into RNA was somewhat increased by ouabain.

It is thus apparent from these studies and those of Falconer et al. that only certain actions of prolactin in cultured mammary tissues are impaired by the ATPase inhibitor, ouabain. It can be concluded then that, at best, only certain of prolactin's actions in mammary tissues may be carried out via a stimulation of membrane-associated ATPase.

Table 1. Effect of ouabain on prolactin stimulation of RNA synthesis.*

Ouabain Concentration	$[^3H]$-Uridine incorporation into RNA (dpm/μg RNA)		
	Control	Prolactin	P
0	117 ± 5**	181 ± 10	<.05
0.25 mM	160 ± 10	207 ± 10	<.05
0.50 mM	160 ± 10	210 ± 7	<.05
1.00 mM	158 ± 9	196 ± 7	<.05

*Explants from midpregnant mouse mammary glands were cultured for 2 days with Medium 199 containing insulin (2.5 μg/ml) plus hydrocortisone (1 μg/ml). Prolactin (2.5 μg/ml) and/or ouabain were then added to certain flasks and incubations were continued for 6 hours. 1 μCi/ml $[^3H]$-uridine (New England Nuclear Corp.) was added to the medium 1 hour prior to termination of the incubations. Specific activity of $[^3H]$ in RNA was then determined (28).
**Mean ± SE (7 observations).

Table 2. Effect of ouabain on prolactin stimulation of casein synthesis*.

Ouabain Concentration	$[^3H]$-Leucine incorporation into casein (dpm/mg wet tissue weight)		
	Control	Prolactin	P
0	651 ± 34**	993 ± 70	<.05
0.25 mM	607 ± 35	870 ± 32	<.05
0.50	551 ± 26	713 ± 43	<.05
1.00	344 ± 23	543 ± 32	<.05

*Explants from midpregnant mouse mammary gland were cultured for 2 days with Medium 199 containing insulin (2.5 μg/ml) plus hydrocortisone (1 μg/ml). Prolactin (2.5 μg/ml) and/or ouabain were then added to certain flasks and incubations were continued for 14 hours. 1 μCi/ml $[^3H]$-leucine (New England Nuclear Corp.) was added to the medium 1 hour prior to termination of the cultures. The incorporation of $[^3H]$ into a casein rich fraction was then determined (28).
**Mean ± SE (7 observations).

Calcium ions

We again only have limited information concerning the role of calcium ions in the actions of prolactin in mammary tissues. We have recently shown that prolactin has no actions on either RNA or casein synthesis when mammary tissues are cultured in calcium free medium (38), (40). In addition, neither high calcium ion concentrations (10 mM) nor calcium ionophores affect the rates of RNA or casein synthesis in cultured mammary tissues. It is not known if calcium ions are involved in the actions of prolactin on the proliferation of normal and/or neoplastic mammary tissues. This information may be of importance in view of the apparent involvement of calcium ions in the regulation of cell division in normal cells, but not transformed cells (61).

Polyamines, prostaglandins and cyclic nucleotides

We advocate the hypothesis that the actions of prolactin on milk protein synthesis in the mammary gland involve a complex interaction of the polyamines, prostaglandins and cyclic nucleotides (see Fig. 1). Initially, prolactin interacts with its plasma membrane receptor (R). Phospholipase A_2 (PLA_2) is then stimulated and polyunsaturated fatty acids (PUFA) including arachidonic acid (AA) are released from membrane phospholipids.

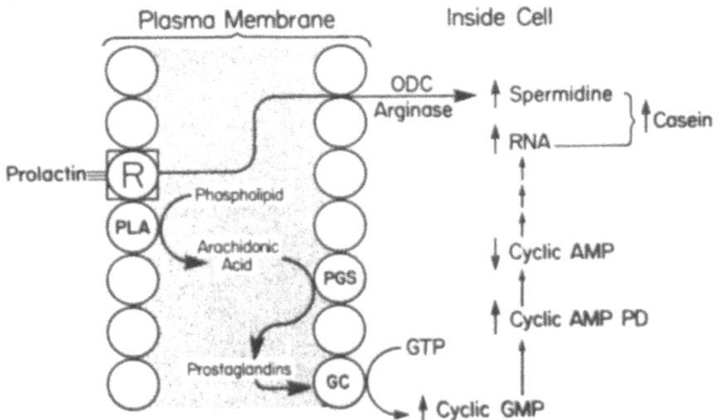

Figure 1. Proposed mechanism of action of prolactin.

The AA is then converted to the prostaglandins (PG) via the membrane-associated prostaglandin synthetase complex. The PGs may then stimulate guanylate cyclase (GC) activity and increase cyclic GMP synthesis. The cyclic GMP in turn stimulates cyclic AMP phospholiesterase and reduces the tissue content of cyclic AMP. The altered cyclic nucleotides levels may then stimulate RNA synthesis which is required for the enhanced rate of casein synthesis. The action of prolactin on casein synthesis, however, also appears to require a stimulation of polyamine synthesis.

Supporting the above hypothesis are observations from many different laboratories. The readers are referred to two earlier reviews (40), (55) which contain additional references which will not be included in this chapter.

Phospholipase A_2

Several studies suggest that the stimulation of plasma membrane associated PLA_2 may be one of the primary mechanisms by which prolactin acts on mammary cells. First of all, phospholipase A_2, when added to medium bathing mammary gland explants, mimics the actions of prolactin on RNA synthesis (41). We also observed that prolactin (NIH PS-12) stimulates phospholipase A_2 activity in broken cell preparations of mouse mammary tissues (46). In subsequent studies, however, using more purified prolactin preparations (including NIH PS-13), no stimulation of PLA_2 activity was observed. We do not presently know if the PS-12 preparation contains a contaminant which increases PLA_2 activity, or if the "purified" prolactin preparations have had varients of the prolactin molecule removed which are responsible for increasing the PLA_2 activity in the PS-12 preparation. In further studies, we have observed that inhibitors of PLA_2 activity including quinacrine (36) and p-bromphenacyl bromide (35) abolish the action of prolactin on both RNA and casein synthesis in cultured mouse mammary gland explants. These observations therefore suggest that one of prolactin's primary actions in mammary tissues may be a stimulation of membrane-associated PLA_2.

Prostaglandins (PG)

Evidence suggesting that the PGs may be involved in the actions of prolactin in mammary tissues is that indomethacin, an inhibitor of PG biosynthesis, attenuates the magnitude of the prolactin actions on RNA and casein synthesis in cultured mouse mammary tissues; indomethacin also impairs the action of PLA_2 on RNA synthesis (29), (30), (34), (41). In addition, certain of the PGs and arachidonic acid (AA, a precursor of the PGs) will duplicate the action of prolactin on RNA synthesis. The AA effect is impaired by indomethacin, thus suggesting the necessary conversion of AA to the PG's for the stimulation of RNA synthesis. In unpublished studies, we (Rillema and Mulder) have also observed that prolactin increases by more than 50 percent of the amount of radioimmunoassayable PGE_2 in the culture medium of mouse mammary gland explants. Similarly, Horobin's laboratory (6) found that prolactin stimulates PG production by more than an order of magnitude in perfused rat mesenteric beds.

Cyclic nucleotides

Most of the data in the literature suggests that cyclic AMP impairs several lactogenic processes in mammary tissues from a variety of species (11), (12), (25), (31), (51), (57). In addition, the actions of prolactin on the mammary gland may involve an elevation of cyclic GMP synthesis and a consequent reduced level of cyclic AMP (31); these actions probably occur as a consequence of prolactin's actions on PLA_2 activity and PG biosynthesis. Cyclic GMP mimics the action of prolactin on RNA synthesis in cultured mouse mammary tissues (31). It has also been found that cyclic GMP has a small, but significant stimulation of casein m RNA synthesis in cultured rat tissues (14); these experiments, however, were carried out under conditions where prolactin has no effect on casein synthesis (5), and it is therefore difficult to make meaningful conclusions from the data. In several laboratories, it has been observed that the onset of lactation following parturition is accompanied by an elevated level of cyclic GMP and a reduced level of cyclic AMP (13), (33), (48-50). It would appear that the reduced levels of cyclic AMP may be a direct result of the elevated levels of cyclic GMP since cyclic GMP, at physiological concentrations, is a powerful stimulator of cyclic AMP phosphodiesterase (56). The relationship of the altered levels of cyclic nucleotides to prostaglandin metabolism is suggested by the observation that PLA_2 and AA are potent stimulators of guanylate cyclase activity (37), (43); these effects are attenuated by the inhibition of PG biosynthesis with indomethacin.

Polyamines

Although PLA_2, AA, certain prostaglandins and cyclic GMP have prolactin-like actions on RNA synthesis in cultured mammary tissues, none of these agents affect the rate of casein synthesis. It was therefore of great interest that Russell and McVicker (47) reported spermidine levels of up to 5 mM in lactating rat mammary tissues. Moreover, it was further shown that the hormones, including prolactin, which have effects on lactogenic processes in cultured mammary tissues also have profound effects on the enzymes which catalyze the synthesis of the polyamines (1), (20-23), (32), (44). Insulin and prolactin also stimulate spermidine uptake into cultured mammary tissues (8). The importance of the polyamines for the prolactin stimulation of lactational processes is suggested by the observation that methyl-glyoxal bis guanylhydrazone, a potent inhibitor of spermidine synthesis, abolishes the prolactin stimulation of milk protein synthesis in cultured mouse tissues (21), (44). In addition, casein synthesis is enhanced when mouse mammary tissues are cultured with spermidine plus any of the agents which were shown earlier to mimic the action of prolactin on RNA synthesis. Finally, in studies to be published in the future, we (Linebaugh and Rillema) have shown that in order to demonstrate actions of prolactin on RNA, DNA and protein synthesis in normal and neoplastic mammary cells in monolayer culture, it is essential to add appropriate amounts of the polyamines to the culture medium when the cells are cultured in serum-free medium.

Actions of prolactin on the proliferation of mammary cells

Although there is some information available concerning the actions and metabolism of the cyclic nucleotides, prostaglandins, polyamines and calcium ions in mammary cells (39), there is no information about how prolactin may regulate the proliferation of normal or neoplastic mammary cells via these intracellular mediators. The observation that prolactin has a profound effect on the activity of ornithine decarboxylase in normal mammary cells is of great interest in view of the intimate relationship of the polyamines to proliferative processes. It is not currently known, however, whether prolactin has actions on polyamine metabolism in neoplastic mammary cells; nor is it known if the polyamines are involved in the proliferative processes of neoplastic mammary cells. Another recently published observation which may prove to be of great importance is the observation that phospholipase A_2 activity is elevated by more than an order of magnitude in rat mammary tumors when compared to normal rat mammary tissues (45). In view of the rate-limiting role of PLA_2 for prostaglandin biosynthesis, the high levels of PLA_2 may be an important metabolic defect in neoplastic mammary cells. Whether prolactin has an action on PLA_2 activity in neoplastic mammary cells is also not known.

One of the problems associated with trying to study the mechansim of action of prolactin in neoplastic tissues is the unavailability of an appropriate experimental model. In order to provide definitive information it is essential to work with neoplastic cells or tissue explants which are cultured under serum-free conditions. It was recently reported by Tanaka et al. (58) that lactogenic hormones stimulate the proliferation of a lymphoma cell line in suspension culture under serum-free conditions; this may prove to be an ideal model system in future studies for determining the mechanism of action of prolactin on neoplastic cells.

REFERENCES

1. Aisbitt RPG, Barry JM. Stimulation by insulin of ornithine decarboxylase activity in cultured mammary tissue. Biochim Biophys Acta 320: 610-616, 1973.
2. Chomczynski P, Topper YJ. A direct effect of prolactin and placental lactogen on mammary epithelial nuclei. Biochem Biophys Res Commun 60: 56-63, 1974.
3. Falconer IR, Forsyth IA, Wilson BM, Dils R. Inhibition of low concentrations of ouabain of prolactin-induced lactogenesis in rabbit mammary gland explants. Biochem J 172: 509-516, 1978.
4. Falconer IR, Rowe JM. Effect of prolactin on sodium and potassium concentrations in mammary alveolar tissues. Endocrinology 101: 181-186, 1977.
5. Hallowes RC, Wang DY, Lewis DJ. The lactogenic effects of prolactin and growth hormone on mammary gland explants from virgin and pregnant Sprague-Dawley rats. J Endocrinol 57: 253-264, 1973.
6. Horrobin DF, Manku MS, Karmali RA, Nassar BA, Greaves MW. Prolactin and prostaglandin synthesis. Lancet 2: 1154, 1974.
7. Josefsberg Z, Posner BI, Patel B, Bergeron JM. The uptake of prolactin into female rat liver. J Biol Chem 254: 209-214, 1979.
8. Kano K, Oka T. Polyamine transport and metabolism in mouse mammary gland. J Biol Chem 251: 2795-2800, 1976.
9. Kelly PA, LeBlanc G, Djiane J. Estimation of total prolactin-binding sites after in vitro desaturation. Endocrinology 104: 1631-1638, 1979.
10. Kim VI, Furth J. The role of prolactin in carcinogenesis. Vit Horm 34: 107-136, 1976.
11. Loizzi R. Cyclic AMP inhibition of mammary gland lactose synthesis: specificity and potentiation by 1-methyl-3-isobutylxanthine. Horm Metab Res 10: 415-419, 1978.
12. Loizzi RF, dePont JJHHM, Bonting SL. Inhibition by cyclic AMP of lactose production in lactating guinea pig mammary gland slices. Biochim Biophys Acta 392: 20-25, 1975.
13. Louis SL, Baldwin RL. Changes in the cyclic 3'-5'-adenosine monophosphate system of rat mammary gland during lactation cycle. J Dairy Sci 58: 861-869, 1975.
14. Matusik RJ, Rosen JM. Prolactin regulation of casein gene expression: possible mediators. Endocrinology 106: 252-259, 1980.
15. Nagasawa H. Prolactin and human breast cancer: a review. Eur J Cancer 15: 267-279, 1979.
16. Nagasawa H, Sakai S, Banerjee MR. Prolactin receptor. Life Sci 24: 193-208, 1979.
17. Nicoll CS. Physiological actions of prolactin. pp. 253-292 in <u>Handbook of Physiology, Section 7: Endocrinology</u>, Vol. IV, part 2, Am Physiol Soc, Bethesda, 1974.
18. Nolin JM. Intracellular prolactin in rat corpus luteum and adrenal cortex. Endocrinology 102: 402-406, 1978.
19. Nolin JM, Witorsch RJ. Detection of endogeneous immunoreactive prolactin in rat mammary epithelial cells during lactation. Endocrinology 99: 949-958, 1976.
20. Oka T, Perry JW. Arginase affects lactogenesis through its influence on the biosynthesis of spermidine. Nature (London) 250: 660-661, 1974.
21. Oka T, Perry JW. Studies on the function of glucocorticoid in mouse mammary epithelial cell differentiation in vitro. J Biol Chem 249: 7647-7652, 1974.

22. Oka T, Perry JW. Studies on the regulatory factors of ornithine decarboxylase activity during development of mouse mammary gland epithelium in vitro. J Biol Chem 251: 1738-1744, 1976.
23. Oka T, Perry JW, Kano K. Hormone regulation of spermidine synthase during the development of mouse mammary epithelium in vitro. Biochim Biophys Res Commun 79: 979-986, 1977.
24. Pearson OH, Arafak B, Manni A. Prolactin and mammary cancer. pp. 237-242 in Central and Peripheral Regulation of Prolactin Function, ed RM Macleod, U Scapagini, Raven, New York, 1980.
25. Perry JW, Oka T. Cyclic AMP as a negative regulation of hormonally induced lactogenesis in mouse mammary gland organ culture. Proc Natl Acad Sci USA 77: 2093-2097, 1980.
26. Posner BI, Josefsberg Z, Bergerch JM. Intracellular polypeptide hormone receptors: characterization and induction of lactogen receptors in the golgi apparatus of rat liver. J Biol Chem 254: 12494-12499, 1979.
27. Richards JF. Ornithine decarboxylase activity in tissues of prolactin-treated rats. Biochem Biophys Res Commun 63: 292-299, 1975.
28. Rillema JA. Early actions of prolactin on uridine metabolism in mammary gland explants. Endocrinology 92: 1673-1679, 1973.
29. Rillema JA. Possible role of prostaglandin F_2 in mediating the effect of prolactin on RNA synthesis in mammary gland explants of mice. Nature (London) 253: 466-467, 1975.
30. Rillema JA. Effects of arachidonic acid on RNA synthesis in mammary gland explants of mice. Prostaglandins 10: 307-312, 1975.
31. Rillema JA. Evidence suggesting that cyclic nucleotides may mediate metabolic effects of prolactin in the mouse mammary gland. Horm Metab Res 7: 45-49, 1975.
32. Rillema JA. Action of prolactin on ornithine decarboxylase activity in mammary gland explants from mice. Endocr Res Commun 3: 297-305, 1976.
33. Rillema JA. Cyclic AMP, adenylate cyclase and cyclic AMP phosphodiesterase in mammary glands from pregnant and lactating mice. Proc Soc Exp Biol Med 151: 748-751, 1976.
34. Rillema JA. Effects of prostaglandins on RNA and casein synthesis in mammary gland explants of mice. Endocrinology 99: 490-495, 1976.
35. Rillema JA. Inhibition of prolactin actions in mouse mammary gland explants by p-bromphenacyl bromide, a phospholipase A_2 inhibitor. Proc Soc Exp Biol Med 161: 355-357, 1979.
36. Rillema JA. Effects of Quinacrine on the prolactin regulation of metabolism in the mammary gland. Prostaglandins Med 2: 155-160, 1979.
37. Rillema JA. Activation of guanylate cyclase by arachidonic acid in mammary gland homogenates from mice. Prostaglandins 15: 857-865, 1978.
38. Rillema JA. Calcium requirement for prolactin actions on ribonucleic acid and casein synthesis in mouse mammary gland explants. Endocrinology 106: 1360-1364, 1980.
39. Rillema JA. Actions and metabolism of intracellular mediators in neoplastic mammary cells. pp. 117-147 in Breast Cancer Vol. 3, ed WL McGuire, Plenum, New York, 1979.
40. Rillema JA. Mechanism of prolactin action. Fed Proc 39: 2593-2598, 1980.
41. Rillema JA, Anderson LD. Phospholipases and the effect of prolactin on uridine incorporation into RNA in mammary gland explants of mice. Biochim Biophys Acta 429: 819-824, 1976.

42. Rillema JA, Anderson LD. Rapid interaction of prolactin with mouse mammary gland explants. Mol Cell Endocrinol 4: 131-137, 1976.
43. Rillema JA, Linebaugh BE. Effects of phospholipase A_2 and triton x-100 on guanylate cyclase activity in mammary gland homogenates from mice. Horm Metab Res 10: 331-336, 1978.
44. Rillema JA, Linebaugh BE, Mulder JA. Regulation of casein synthesis by polyamines in mammary gland explants from mice. Endocrinology 100: 529-535, 1977.
45. Rillema JA, Osmialowski EC, Linebaugh BE. Phospholipase A_2 activity in 9,10-dimethyl-1, 2-benzanthracene-induced mammary tumors of rats. Biochim Biophys Acta 617: 150-155, 1980.
46. Rillema JA, Wild EA. Prolactin activation of phospholipase activity in membrane preparations from mammary glands. Endocrinology 100: 1219-1222, 1977.
47. Russell DM, McVicker TA. Polyamine biogenesis in the rat mammary gland during pregnancy and lactation. Biochem J 130: 71-76, 1972.
48. Sapag-Hagar M, Greenbaum AL. Changes of the activities of adenyl cyclase and cAMP phosphodiesterase and of the level of 3'-5'-cyclic adenosine monophosphate in rat mammary gland during pregnancy and lactation. Biochem Biophys Res Commun 53: 982-987, 1973.
49. Sapag-Hagar M, Greenbaum AL. The role of cyclic nucleotides in the development and function of rat mammary tissues. FEBS Letters 46: 180-183, 1974.
50. Sapag-Hagar M, Greenbaum AL. Adenosine 3'-5'-monophosphate and hormone interrelationships in the mammary gland of the rat during pregnancy and lactation. Eur J Biochem 47: 303-312, 1974.
51. Sapag-Hagar M, Greenbaum AL, Lewis DJ, Hallowes RC. The effects of di-butyryl cAMP on enzymatic and metabolic changes in explants of rat mammary tissue. Biochem Biophys Res Commun 59: 261-268, 1974.
52. Shiu RPC. Prolactin receptors in human breast cancer cells in long term tissue culture. Cancer Res 39: 81-86, 1979.
53. Shiu RPC, Friesen HG. Solubilization and purification of a prolactin receptor from the rabbit mammary gland. J Biol Chem 249: 7902-7911, 1974.
54. Shiu RPC, Friesen HG. Blocade of prolactin action by an antiserum to its receptors. Science 192: 259-261, 1976.
55. Shiu RPC, Friesen HG. Mechanism of action of prolactin in the control of mammary gland function. Annu Rev Physiol 42: 83-96, 1980.
56. Smith RD, Rillema JA. Guanylate cyclase and cyclic-GMP phosphodiesterase activities in mammary glands of mice during pregnancy and lactation. Proc Soc Exp Biol Med 150: 763-765, 1975.
57. Speake B, Dils R and Mayer RJ. Interaction of insulin, prolactin and cortisol in controlling the turnover of fatty acid synthetase in rabbit mammary gland in organ culture. Biochem J 154: 359-370, 1976.
58. Tanaka T, Shiu RPC, Gout PW, Beer CT, Noble RL, Friesen HG. Rapid, sensitive and specific bioassay for lactogenic hormones using a lymphoma cell line. 62nd Annual Endocrinol Soc Abstracts 267, 1980.
59. Van der Guten AA, Waters MJ, Murthy GS, Friesen HG. Studies on the irreversible nature of prolactin binding to receptors. Endocrinology 106: 402-411, 1980.
60. Welsch CW, Nagasawa H. Prolactin and murine mammary tumorigenesis: a review. Cancer Res 37: 951-963, 1977.
61. Whitfield JF, Boyntou AL, Macmanus JP, Sikorska M, Tsang BK. The regulation of cell proliferation by calcium and cyclic AMP. Mol Cell Biochem 27: 155-179, 1979.

Chapter 5

GROWTH FACTORS FOR HORMONE-SENSITIVE TUMOR CELLS

David A Sirbasku, Frances E Leland

INTRODUCTION

The study of polypeptide growth factor interaction with cells *in vitro* and *in vivo* is a rapidly expanding new field of cell biology. Many types of cell growth factors have been identified including the steroid hormones (1), (4), (33), (65), thyroid hormones (49), (62), prostaglandins (24), (25), the classical polypeptide hormones such as insulin (53), (64), and many polypeptide and protein growth factors. Characterization of the polypeptide growth factors such as epidermal growth factor, EGF (14), (22), (51), nerve growth factor, NGF (2), (32), (68), somatomedins (48), (54), (66), fibroblast growth factor, FGF (19), (20), platelet derived growth factor, PDGF (3), (39), (40), (41), (46), and the insulin-like growth factors, IGF_1 and IGF_2 (17), (18), (45), have provided us with a detailed analysis of the biochemical properties of growth promoting proteins. These pioneering studies have led the way to two important advances in the growth control field. First, they have provided methods for purifying these activities sufficiently to allow their testing as growth regulatory agents on tissues or cell types not previously recognized as target organs. A case in point is the identification of the effects of EGF on mammary cells (5), (6), (34), (67), a growth factor which initially was believed to promote growth of only the epidermal tissues (14), (51), but is now considered important for growth of several cell types *in vivo* (11), (12), (44). The second major benefit of characterizing these new mitogens was to provide an impetus to other investigators to seek new growth regulatory polypeptides that may be involved in growth of specialized tissue *in vivo*.

Now, before entering further into the discussion of growth factors, it should be noted that in this review we will confine our comments largely to the effects of the polypeptide hormones and polypeptide growth factors on mammary tissue growth *in vivo* and *in vitro*, with only occasional reference to growth control of other tissues, or to the effects of thyroid hormones, steroid hormones and prostaglandins on mammary cells. Further, we are defining polypeptide growth factors as agents that exert their mitogenic effects at very low concentrations (10^{-11} to 10^{-9}M), well below levels considered necessary as metabolites. Growth factors are well known to interact with specific receptors either within or on the surface of the target organ cells, and that these interactions are necessary for the mitogenic response. Growth factors may be either of the type that circulate, such as EGF and somatomedins, or may be released locally at the site of action, such as proposed for FGF (19), (20), and PDGF (46).

In this review we will have the joint purposes of describing the effects of known growth factors on mammary cells in culture, as well as describing our studies that suggest that new, and as yet only partially characterized, growth factors may be involved in the estrogen-responsive growth of neoplastic and normal mammary cells.

EFFECTS OF KNOWN GROWTH FACTORS ON MAMMARY TUMOR CELL PROLIFERATION

Hormonally defined media

The fundamental observations by Hayashi and Sato (23) that GH3 rat pituitary and BHK21 hamster kidney tumor cells could be grown in serum-free media supplemented only with combinations of hormones are the forerurners of a new approach to the study of the mitogenic agents which influence mammary cell growth. In more recent reviews, Bottenstein *et al.* (8), and Barnes and Sato (6), have described the methods for culture of many different types of mammalian cells in serum-free media supplemented only with combinations of hormones and growth factors. Since the review here is mainly limited to the growth of mammary cells, it is noteworthy that this concept has been applied to the study of two types of human mammary tumor cells in culture (1), (5), and to growth of preneoplastic mouse mammary cells (34) in culture.

One of the human mammary tumor cell lines extensively studied in defined media is the MCF-7 cells orignially established in culture by Soule *et al.* (63). Barnes and Sato (5) have grown these human mammary tumor cells *in* defined media containing insulin, estradiol, EGF, prostaglandins, cold insoluble globulin, transferrin, and thyroid hormones. A different, but related, mixture has been used to grow the ZR-75-1 human mammary tumor cells in culture (1), and mouse preneoplastic nodule cells (34). In the cases of the human cells described above, variable growth effects of estrogen are reported on the MCF-7 cells in culture (5), (9), (33), (52), while the effects of physiological concentrations of estrogens on ZR-75-1 cells in culture seems somewhat more pronounced than with the MCF-7 cells (1). The clear lesson from these studies is that polypeptide hormones such as insulin, and growth factors such as EGF, are essential to the growth of the MCF-7 and ZR-75-1 cells in hormonally defined media, and that steroid hormones have, at best, variable effects.

When reviewing critically the observations just discussed, two major questions arise. First, EGF is known to be testosterone controlled in mice (10), being isolated from male submaxillary glands, but apparently not present in glands from females. Hence, the role of this growth factor in proliferation of female mammary gland tumors is difficult to understand. It may be possible that human EGF (urogastrone) is present and abundant in human females. This matter requires further study. Second, the very dramatic effect of insulin on growth of MCF-7 and ZR-75-1 cells surely points up the importance of this hormone to mammary tumor cell growth. This is further supported by work of Shafie and Hilf (53) showing that insulin is required for the estrogen-response growth of some types of rat mammary tumors *in vivo*. However, from the studies available, a question exists about whether the insulin effect on mammary tumors is that of a specific mitogen, or instead, is a requirement for growth of many types of rapidly proliferating tissues. Indeed, a generalized requirement for insulin in cell growth can be concluded from the studies reported by Sato and Reid (50), Bottenstein et al. (8), and Barnes and Sato (6), all of which show that insulin is required in the hormonally defined media used to culture cells originally derived from many non-mammary origins from several species.

Growth factor effects on cells cultured in collagen supported matrices

In recent reports by Yang et al. (67), the effect of growth factors on normal and neoplastic mammary tissue has been studied using dissociated cultures of these cells suspended in collagen gels. The exciting new methods applied in these reports have shown that dissociated normal mouse mammary gland cells respond with continuous growth to the addition of EGF, FGF, and cholera toxin to the gels containing horse and fetal calf serum supplemented media. The cholera toxin alone (at levels of less than 0.1 µg/ml) induces growth, and when the toxin is added to EGF (0.1 µg/ml) and/or FGF (0.1 µg/ml) containing media, the effects of the toxin and growth factors are synergistic. The very important advances made by these studies are that long term cultures of mouse mammary gland can be established in collagen gels, and that growth factor effects can be assessed on normal tissues without the complex problems of organ cultures, or the potential adverse effects of plating cells on plastic surface petri dishes. The effects of the cell matrix in growth experiments is currently one of the most active and controversial areas of cell biology, with many investigators feeling that an appropriate synthetic matrix is required for physiological responses of cells in culture (43), and others proposing that all growth control can be explained by basement membrane composition and interaction with cells without the necessity of growth factors at all. These issues are not yet resolved, but clearly this will be an important area in the future for any in vitro studies of the effects of matrix on mammary cell growth responses.

Effects of other growth factors on mammary origin cells

Ptashne et al. (42) have identified and partially purified a mammary cell mitogen from porcine serum. This activity is a 10,000 dalton molecular weight mitogen, and by various criteria appears similar, but not identical to somatomedins or MSA. The exact role of this activity in mammary growth in vivo awaits further study.

Another factor has been identified in bovine pituitary extracts and purified to homogeneity by Kano-Sueoka et al. (26). She has shown that this factor is phosphoethanolamine, and that a hormone-dependent clonal mammary cell line derived from an ACI rat tumor responds to this factor over the concentration range 10^{-6} to 10^{-4}M. At present, it is not clear whether this factor is a nutritional requirement for these cells, is acting as a hormone, or both. In any case, the role of phosphoethanolamine in mammary tumor cell growth has not been previously explored, and should provide interesting new insights into the components required for proliferation of mammary cells. It may be possible that phosphoethanolamine should be considered as one of the components required for optimal growth of mammary cells in hormonally defined media.

EFFECTS OF ESTROGENS ON GROWTH FACTOR ACTIVITIES FOR ESTROGEN-RESPONSIVE TUMOR CELLS

New approaches to estrogen-responsive tumor growth

During the course of the past few years, we were confronted with a paradox concerning the role of estrogens in estrogen-responsive tumor cell growth *in vivo*. We observed with three cell lines derived from different estrogen-responsive tumors of rodents that all proved to be estrogen-responsive or estrogen-dependent *in vivo*, but no direct effect of estrogens could be measured by monitoring changes in cell number *in vitro*. The cell lines used for these studies were the MTW9/PL rat mammary tumor cell line (55) that requires estrogen, prolactin, and thyroid hormones for optimal tumor formation, the GH3/C14 rat pituitary tumor cell line (61) that requires thyroid hormones and estrogens, and finally, the H-301 Syrian hamster tumor cell line (59) which requires only estrogen for tumor formation *in vivo*. We attempted many possible variations of conditions to demonstrate the direct mitogenic effects of estrogens on these cells, but were able to conclude only that estrogens do not promote complete traverse of the cell cycle resulting in a measurable increase in cell number. However, it appears possible that 1 x 10^{-9}M estradiol promotes a partial initiation of the cell cycle with MTW9/PL and GH3/C14 cells in culture (D.A. Sirbasku and J.B. Officer, unpublished data). Nevertheless, since all three of these tumor cells undergo many rounds of estrogen-dependent cell division *in vivo* to form 5g to 10g tumors in 28 to 50 days from an inoculation of 1 to 3 x 10^{6} cells, there appeared to be something missing in our understanding of the process of estrogen modulated tumor cell growth *in vivo*. Of course, one possibility was that all of the three cell lines reversibly "dedifferentiated" in culture such that they were no longer responsive to estrogens. This might happen by a reversible loss of the estrogen receptor system in the cells in culture. We have examined this possibility, but have concluded that the estrogen receptor systems of both the GH3/C14 pituitary and the MTW9/PL mammary cells are functional since estrogens have a marked effect in cellular protein synthesis in both of these lines in culture (D.A. Sirbasku and J.B. Officer, unpublished data). Thus, our laboratory sought new approaches to the problem of how estrogens promote tumor cell growth *in vivo*.

Endocrine estromedin mechanism

From the data cited above, it seemed entirely possible that estrogens could serve functions *in vivo* that have not previously been recognized, one of which might be the induction and promotion of secretion of new polypeptide growth factors from estrogen-target tissues. This mechanism is summarized in Fig. 1, and represents a mechanism we have termed the endocrine "estromedin" control. In essence, what we proposed is a search for new estrogen controlled hormones. We have designated these new growth factors with the tentative name "estromedins" or mediators of estrogen controlled growth. In order to confirm an estromedin mechanism, we considered five areas of study essential. They were as follows:

(1) Identification of tissues that produce estrogen-inducible growth factors.

(2) Demonstration of relative specificity of the growth factors for cells that form estrogen-responsive tumors *in vivo*.

(3) Biochemical characterization and purification of the growth factor.

(4) Identification of growth factors in the plasma at levels correlating with changes in estrogen concentration.

(5) Identification of specific receptors for the growth factor in target tumor cells.

The numbers in Fig. 1 correspond to these areas of study, and represent the ongoing characterization of "estromedins" that we will describe in this review.

In the first series of studies reported (56), we prepared tissue extracts from three groups of rats; normal females, ovariectomized females, and estrogen-treated, ovariectomized females, and asked whether estrogen-influenced levels of growth activity could be found in any of the tissues isolated. Our assay for these activities was done by determining MTW9/PL rat mammary, GH3/C14 rat pituitary, or H301 hamster kidney cell number increases in response to addition of increasing concentrations of extract protein to the cells in serum-free medium (56). For the purposes of this review, we will confine our description of the results to those obtained with the MTW9/PL mammary cell line, but it should be emphasized that much of what we state for the effects of the growth activities on MTW9/PL cells is true also for the GH3/C14 rat pituitary tumor cells. This is not surprising since both of these cell lines have very similar growth control patterns *in vivo* (55), (61). As shown in Fig. 2, the rat uteri from the three groups of animals showed an estrogen-inducible mammary growth factor (MGF) activity. The relative induction of this activity was 13-fold when comparing uteri from estrogen-treated, ovariectomized females to those of the animals only ovariectomized. One other tissue which demonstrated a small (i.e., 2-

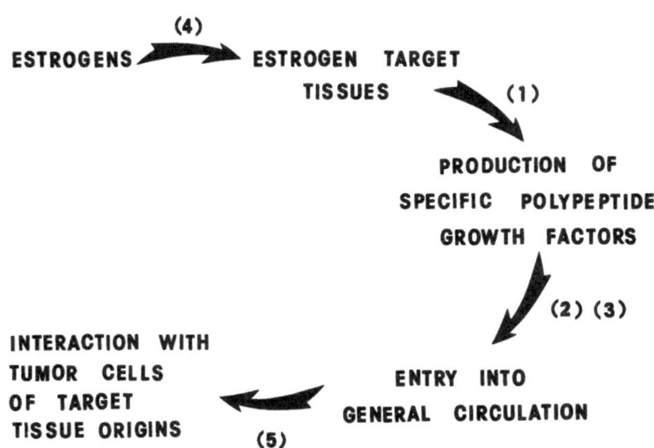

Fig. 1. Summary model of an indirect estromedin mechanism of estrogen-responsive tumor growth _in vivo_ (57).

fold), but consistent induction in activity was the kidney (Fig. 3). Comparison of the specific activities of the uterine and kidney extracts is shown in Table 1. Clearly, the uterus is a 3- to 10-fold higher specific activity source than kidney, but the total activity extracted from two kidneys is 3 to 4 times as great as extracted from one uterus, suggesting that the kidney could serve as an important source of growth factor _in vivo_.

Assays of extracts of other tissues such as liver, heart, lung, ovary, submaxillary gland, stomach, intestine, thyroid gland, and skeletal muscle showed little mitogenic activity (D.A. Sirbasku, manuscript in preparation) that could not be accounted for by proteases or the presence of small amounts of blood (serum) in the organ extracts. Brain extracts showed MTW9/PL cell growth activity which was highly variable, but in some experiments was equivalent to that seen in kidney extracts. The brain activity showed no apparent change in levels with estrogen status. the spleen showed a significant activity due to residual blood in the

TABLE 1

SUMMARY OF THE CONCENTRATIONS OF RAT UTERINE AND RAT KIDNEY EXTRACTS REQUIRED FOR ONE-HALF MAXIMAL GROWTH OF THE MTW9/PL CELLS IN CULTURE

	μg of Extract Protein Required for One-half Maximal Growth	
Animal Group	Uterine Extracts	Kidney Extracts
Normal females	75	210
Ovariectomized females	320	400
Estrogen-treated, ovariectomized females	22	260

Data taken from Sirbasku (56).

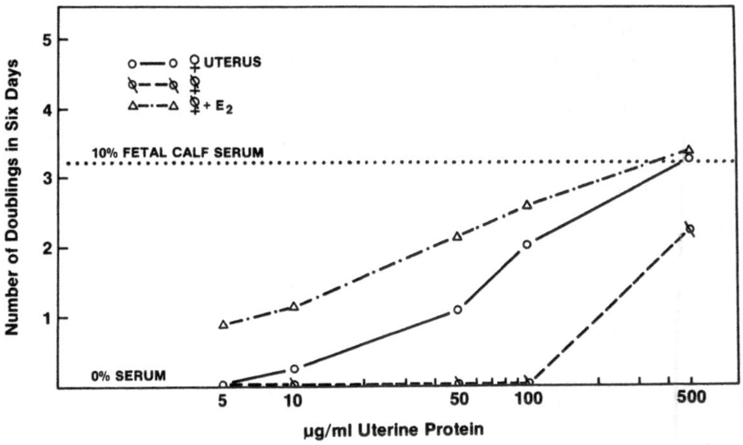

Fig. 2. Growth of the MTW9/PL rat mammary tumor cells in response to rat uterine extracts from the designated groups of animals. The extracts were added at the designated concentrations in serum-free DME, and cell numbers were determined after 6 days. Methods and data are from Sirbasku, (36).

extracts. From the data obtained from these experiments, we concluded that uterus, and probably kidney, could serve the role *in vivo* as potential sources of an estromedin activity.

In the second series of studies, we asked whether the activity from the uterus was an active mitogen for only these types of cells that form estrogen-responsive tumors, or whether this activity was a general, or nonspecific, growth factor (Table 2).

TABLE 2

CELL TYPE SPECIFICITY OF GROWTH ACTIVITY FROM RAT UTERUS

	Cell Population Doublings in Rat Uterus[a]	
Cell Lines	Ovariectomized	Estrogen-treated Ovariectomized
MTW9/PL	2.4	3.4
GH3/C14	2.6	3.8
H-301	4.2	5.1
R2C	0	0
MH_1C_1	0.1	0.3
Y1	1.2	1.4
AtT20	2.4	2.1
HAK	2.1	2.2
BHK21	2.4	2.6
Balb 3T3	1.2	0.6

[a] Data taken from Sirbasku (56).

King et al. (27) had shown previously that uterine extracts contained a growth factor for the mesenchymal origin mouse 3T6 cells. Our data, shown in Table 2, confirms this type of growth factor activity which promoted growth of the BHK21 fibroblast cells. In addition, the experiment revealed that the uterine extracts also contained growth factor activity for estrogen tumor related cells such as the MTW9/PL, GH3/C14, and H-301 lines. This activity was elevated in uterine extracts prepared from estrogen-treated animals.

Along these same lines, we investigated the ability of the uterine extracts to support the growth of two other rat mammary tumor cell lines.

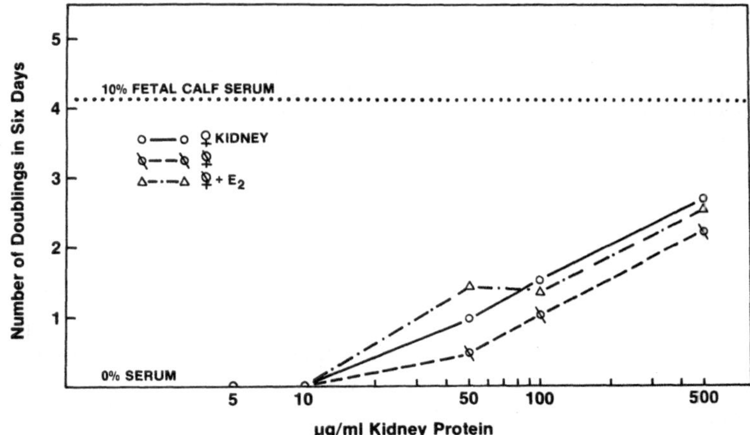

Fig. 3. Growth of MTW9/PL rat mammary tumor cells in response to rat kidney extracts from the identical three groups shown in Fig. 2. Methods are the same as in Fig. 2.

These were the RAMA-25 and RAMA-29 lines which Bennett et al. (7) have described as epithelial and myoepithelial in origin, respectively. The uterine extracts were mitogenic for both cell lines, but the RAMA-29 myoepithelial cells responded more dramatically to lower concentrations of uterine extract (58). These data suggested to us that the uterine extract may have greater specificity for some cell types in mammary tumor tissue than for others.

When rat uterine extract was tested for mitogenic activity with human origin MCF-7 mammary tumor cells, it proved to be a potent mitogen at concentrations of 50 µg/ml or less (58). The MCF-7 cell line is known to form estrogen-responsive tumors in nude mice (52). Thus, the rat uterine extracts are relatively more active with cell types that form estrogen-responsive tumors, but are not species specific in that they promote growth of human mammary tumor cells.

Beyond these studies, we have been most involved in the development of a purification scheme for the estromedins from uterine tissue. Our first concern was to establish the biochemical properties of the mitogenic activity. A series of studies was conducted, and the results are summarized in Table 3. The uterine derived activity was a heat, pH treatment and protease treatment labile, 70,000 dalton molecular weight activity which did not display either lipid or steroid hormone-like activity (60). Under all conditions tested, the activity appears to be a protein, or at least to have a required protein component.

TABLE 3

PROPERTIES OF THE MTW9/PL CELL GROWTH FACTOR ACTIVITY IN THE EXTRACTS OF RAT UTERUS

Treatment	Effect on Activity
Dialysis	Non-dialysable
80°C for 10 min.	90% inactivation
Trypsin treatment, 1 hr. at 37°C	90% inactivation
Treatment at pH 2.0 or 12.0	80% to 90% inactivation
In acetic acid for 18 hrs. at 4°C	100% inactivation
Acetone, ethanol or isopropanol (50% in aqueous solution)	50% to 60% inactivation
6M guanidine or 8M urea at 4°C for 3 hrs.	50% to 60% inactivation
Chloroform/methanol extraction	Not extractable (complete inactivation)
Charcoal extraction	No effect on activity
Ammonium sulfate precipitation	33% to 67% saturation caused precipitation

The next step in our studies was to begin a purification of the uterine derived growth factor activity. Our initial studies have shown that a four step partial purification, summarized in Fig. 4, yielded an approximate 14-fold purification of the MTW9/PL cell growth factor activity. The details of the partial purification procedure and the analysis of the proteins present in each fraction of column chromatography steps has been presented elsewhere (31).

The assays of the growth factor activity in the pooled fractions generated by this procedure are shown in Fig. 5. From these dose-responsive data we calculate the concentration of uterine extract protein which must be added to culture medium of MTW9/PL cells to achieve half-maximal growth (56). These data are then used to calculate the relative fold

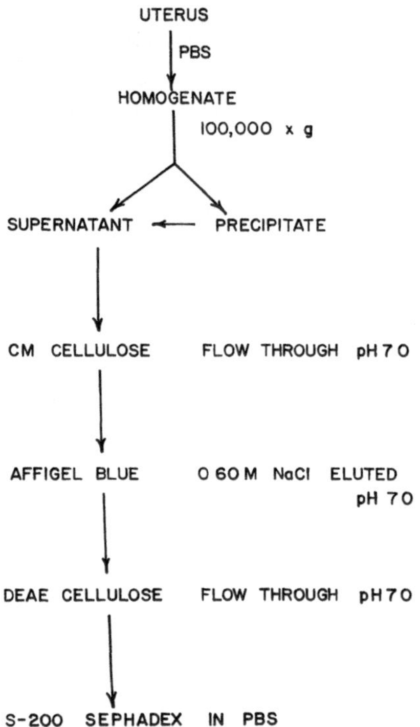

Fig. 4. Schematic diagram of the partial four step purification applied to rat uterine extracts, kidney extracts, plasma, and uterine luminal fluid.

purification (Table 4). From the information available thus far, we concluded that the growth factor activity is relatively stable during purification, and present in sufficient quantities to allow purification of reasonable amounts.

Since the major purifications of the uterine activity occurred at the Affi-Gel Blue and the DEAE cellulose steps, these have been incorporated into a more extended procedure. From the many fractionation procedures we have attempted, the tentative partial purification protocol we are presently evaluating utilized combinations of Affi-Gel Blue chromatography, DEAE cellulose chromatography, phenylsepharose hydrophobic fractionation, ultragel molecular weight separations, concanavalin A affinity chromatography, hydroxylapatite chromatography, isotachophoresis, preparative isoelectric focusing, and preparative polyacrylamide gel electrophoresis. We have been refining these various methods and will ultimately apply them sequentially to the purification of the uterine activity.

TABLE 4

PARTIAL PURIFICATION PROCEDURE FOR MAMMARY GROWTH FACTOR ACTIVITY IN RAT UTERINE TISSUE EXTRACTS, UTERINE LUMINAL FLUID, KIDNEY TISSUE EXTRACT, AND PLASMA FROM ESTROGEN-TREATED OVARIECTOMIZED RATS

Samples	Protein Concentration Required for One-half Maximal Growth Response	Relative Fold Purification
Uterine Tissue Extract	100 μg/ml	1.0
CMC column flow through	130	1.0
Affi-Gel Blue column fraction	50	2.0
DEAE column flow through	7	14.0
Uterine Luminal Fluid	< 200 μg/ml	1.0
CMC column flow through	< 200	1.0
Affi-Gel Blue column fraction	23	8.7
DEAE column flow through	0.8	250.0
Plasma	130 μg/ml	1.0
CMC column flow through	40	3.2
Affi-Gel Blue column fraction	100	1.3
DEAE column flow through	20	6.5
Kidney Tissue Extract	75 μg/ml	1.0
CMC column flow through	-	-
Affi-Gel Blue column fraction	80	1.0
DEAE column flow through	7	11.0
S-200 pooled fractions	6	12.0

In addition to the work with the uterine derived MTW9/PL growth activity, we have applied the same four step partial purification (Fig. 4) to extracts of kidneys obtained from estrogen-treated, ovariectomized rats. The assays of the various pooled column fractions from this procedure are

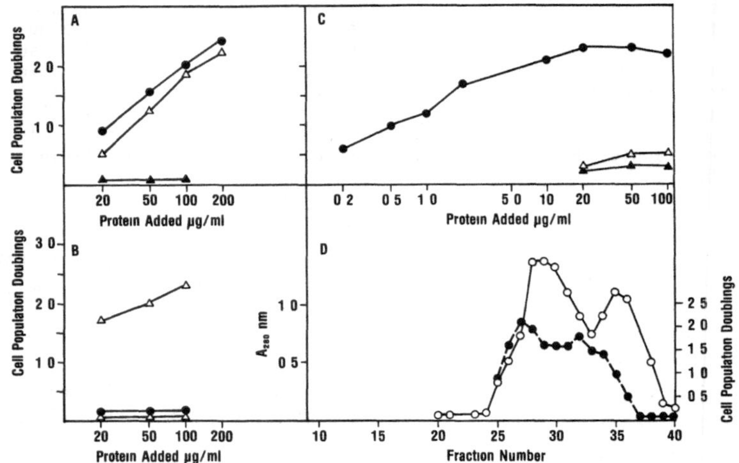

Fig. 5. Growth of MTW9/PL cells in fractions from the partial purification (Fig. 4) of uterine extracts prepared from estrogen-treated ovariectomized rats. Each fraction was assayed in the same manner as described in Fig. 6. Panel A shows the activity in crude uterine extracts (open circles), CMC flow through fraction (open triangles), and 1.0M sodium chloride eluted CMC fraction (closed triangles). Panel B shows the Affi-Gel flow through fraction (closed circles), the 0.6M sodium chloride eluted fraction (open triangles), and the 1.4M sodium chloride eluted fraction (closed triangles). Panel C shows the DEAE flow through fraction (closed circles), the 0.15M sodium chloride eluted fraction (open triangles) and the 1.0M sodium chloride eluted fractions (closed triangles). Panel D shows the 280 nm elution profile of the high molecular weight S-200 fractions (open circles) and the cell growth assays (closed circles) of these fractions.

shown in Fig. 6. The kidney derived activity was purified 11-fold by this procedure (Table 4). Comparison of data obtained in Fig. 6 and those in Fig. 5 suggest that by this limited test, the uterine and kidney derived mammary growth factor activities are very similar. The apparent molecular weights are both in the area of 70,000 daltons as estimated by the S-200

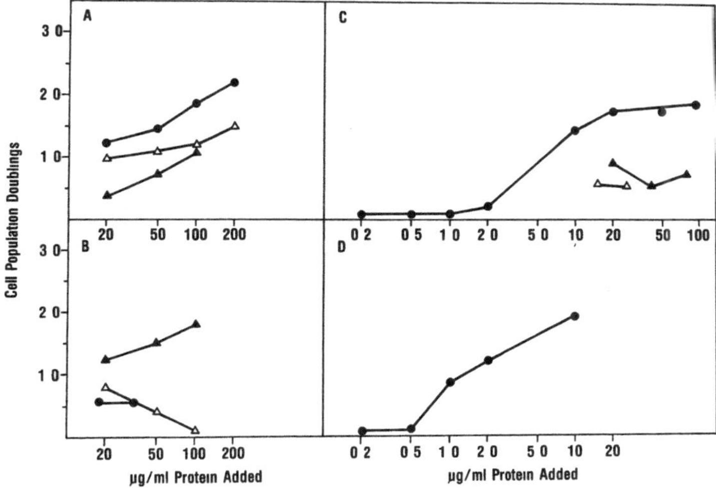

Fig. 6. Growth of MTW9/PL cells in fractions from the partial purification (Fig. 4) of kidney extracts prepared from estrogen-treated, ovariectomized rats. Each fraction was assayed in the same manner described for the rat uterine extracts in Fig. 5. Panel A shows the activity in crude kidney extracts (closed circles), CMC flow through fraction (open triangles), and the CMC fraction eluted with 1.0M sodium chloride (closed triangles). Panel B shows the assay of the Affi-Gel Blue flow through (open triangles), the 0.6M sodium chloride eluted fractions (closed triangles), and the 1.4M sodium chloride eluted fractions (closed circles). Panel C shown the assay of the DEAE flow through fractions (closed circles), the 0.15M sodium chloride eluted fractions (closed triangles) and the 1.0M sodium chloride eluted fractions (open triangles). Panel D shows the assay of the pooled S-200 column fractions at approximately 70,000 daltons molecular weight.

gel filtration. Further purification studies will be required to determine whether or not definite structural similarities exist between these activities.

It is worthwhile to note that concentrations of known growth factors which promote cell growth _in vitro_ range between 10^{-9} to 10^{-10}M. Since the molecular weight of the uterine activity is 70,000 daltons (60), this would mean that one-half maximal growth responses in culture to concentrations ranging between 7 ng to 70 ng/ml of uterine growth factor would represent pure, or nearly pure, material. From the data obtained with the partial purification procedure (Table 3), we calculate that an additional 10^2 to 10^3-fold purification will be required to obtain homogeneous uterine estromedins. This degree of purification appears well within the methods we have in hand.

However, in any purification effort, the relative abundance and costs of the starting tissue must be taken into account. We have calculated that kilogram amounts of rat uterus and rat kidney will be necessary to prepare mg quantities of estromedins for eventual amino acid sequence determination, for extensive biochemical studies of the mechanism of action, and for development of antibodies to be used for RIA methods of measurement. The average amount of uterus and kidney obtained from a 150g to 200g estrogen-treated, ovariectomized female Sprague-Dawley rat is 0.75g and 2.2g, respectively. Thus, one kilogram of fresh uterus from rat will require more than 1,300 animals, all of which must be estrogen-treated after a surgical procedure as described before (56). This represents a considerable monetary and time expenditure per kilogram of uterus.

We have sought alternative large scale sources of estromedins for both the MTW9/PL mammary tumor cells, and the GH3/C14 rat pituitary tumor cells. Our search led to the discovery that the uterus and kidneys from pregnant sheep have a high specific activity estromedin for MTW9/PL mammary cells, but little or no activity toward the GH3/C14 pituitary cells. Parenthetically, the uteri of mid-pregnant sheep have ranged in weight between 780g and 1,400g; the combined kidney weights are approximately 125g per animal. The assay of the mammary cell growth factor activity in extracts of pregnant sheep uterus and kidney are shown in Fig. 7. Calculations of the concentration of extract required for one-half maximal growth shows that uterus requires 34 μg/ml, while kidney requires 60 μg/ml. These specific activity values are greater than those seen from the same tissues of rats (see Table 4). However, it must be emphasized that one very important distinction between the rat tissue activities and those extracted from the same tissues in sheep is that the former do not support significant growth of GH3/C14 rat pituitary tumor cells in culture (Fig. 8). This means that extracts of pregnant sheep uterus are at least 15 times more active with mammary cells than pituitary cells.

In view of our general conclusion that the mammary and pituitary cell mitogens are probably one and the same in the rat extracts, we have extended our studies to ask whether the mammary and pituitary cell growth factor activities could be identified in extracts of uteri and kidneys from pregnant females of other species such as rabbit. Uteri from mid-pregnant rabbits average 60g to 70g, while those from the mature females

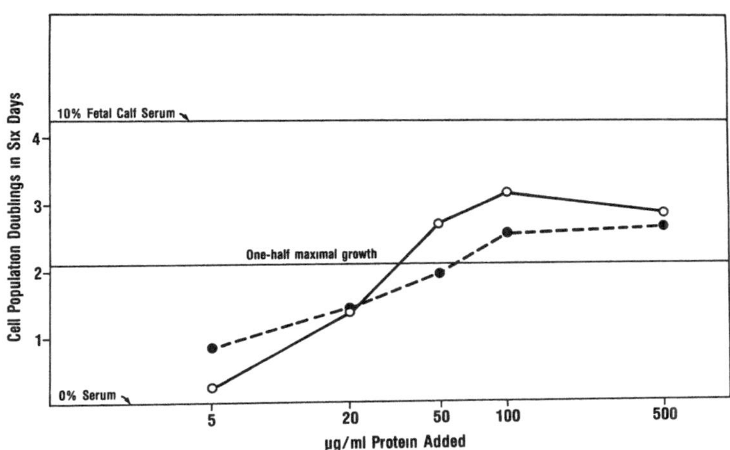

Fig. 7. Growth of MTW9/PL rat mammary tumor cells in response to extracts of kidneys (closed circles) and uteri (open circles) from mid-pregnant sheep. Methods are those from (56).

or retired breeders were approximately 20g. Kidneys from the rabbit averaged between 18g to 26g combined weight. We found that uteri from pregnant rabbits, mature females, and retired breeders all possessed a potent pituitary cell activity which was considerably greater than that found with rat (Table 5). Table 5 also shows the comparison of the one-half maximal activities for MTW9/PL cells in response to the rabbit and rat uterine and kidney extracts.

What can be summarized from these data with both cell lines, and with extracts of uterus and kidney from rat, rabbit and sheep is (i) sheep may contain only mammary cell activity in uterus and kidney extracts, and hence, is distinct from the rat and rabbit, (ii) rat contains both mammary and pituitary activity in uterine and kidney extracts, but it is not known whether both mitogens reside in one molecular species, and finally, (iii) the rabbit uteri and kidneys are a high specific activity source of both activities, and in this respect, are more like the rat than the sheep.

From these data cited above, we have commenced the purification of the MTW9/PL mammary cell mitogen from pregnant sheep uteri, and the purification of the GH3/C14 pituitary cell estromedin from pregnant rabbit uterus. Our goal in attempting both purifications is to determine whether the uterine derived mammary and the pituitary tumor growth factor are similar or different mitogens.

TABLE 5

COMPARISON OF THE MTW9/PL MAMMARY AND GH3/C14 PITUITARY CELL GROWTH FACTOR ACTIVITIES IN EXTRACTS OF UTERI AND KIDNEYS FROM RABBITS, SHEEP AND RATS

Organ Extracted	Animal Source	Cell Line	MGF or PGF Specific Activity
Uterus	Estrogen-treated ovariectomized rat	MTW9/PL	22 to 100 µg/ml
Kidney	"	"	75 to 260 "
Uterus	"	GH3/C14	130 µg/ml
Kidney	"	"	165 "
Uterus	Pregnant rabbit	MTW9/PL	39 "
	Mature rabbit	"	33 "
	Retired breeder rabbit	"	24 "
Kidney	Pregnant rabbit	"	180 "
	Mature rabbit	"	76 "
	Retired breeder rabbit	"	100 "
Uterus	Pregnant rabbit	GH3/C14	21 "
	Mature rabbit	"	12 "
	Retired breeder rabbit	"	15 "
Kidney	Pregnant rabbit	"	46 "
	Mature rabbit	"	< 500 "
	Retired breeder rabbit	"	< 500 "
Uterus	Pregnant sheep	MTW9/PL	34 "
Kidney	" "	"	130 "
Uterus	" "	GH3/C14	< 500 "
Kidney	" "	"	< 500 "

One very important study awaits the purification of the activities from the sources just described. The measurement of the levels of estromedins

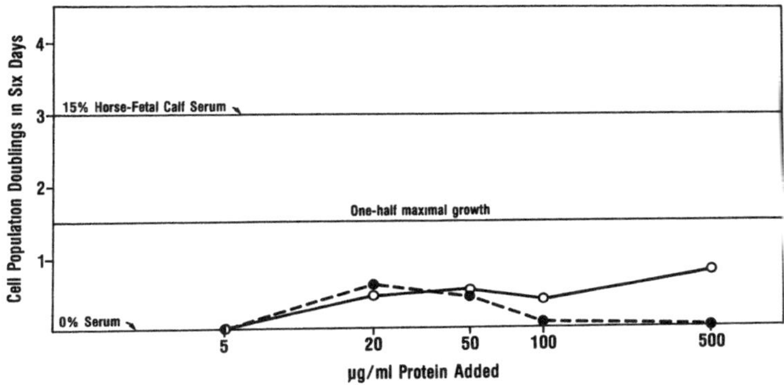

Fig. 8. Growth of the GH3/C14 rat pituitary tumor cells in response to extracts of kidneys (closed circles), and uteri (open circles) from pregnant sheep. Methods are those from (56).

in the blood is essential to the further development of this model. If estromedins are circulating hormones that act to modulate estrogen-responsive tumor growth in vivo, then their blood levels should change with the estrogen status of the host animal. We have attempted various means of demonstrating this change in growth factor content in whole serum (57) from estrogen-treated and deficient animals, but these studies have been complicated by the problem of the mitogenic effects of platelet derived growth factor in whole serum (15), (16).

Other approaches currently being used are to prepare platelet poor plasma from rats and to ask two questions. The first is whether there is one or several estromedin activities in platelet poor plasma, and the second is whether estrogen status changes these activities. The answer to the first question was obtained by submitting the plasma from estrogen-treated, ovariectomized rats to the partial purification procedure described in Fig. 4, and finding that at least two activities appear in the plasma. The second question has not been resolved satisfactorily as yet, because all of our attempts to eliminate PDGF completely from the plasma have not been successful.

At present, the best evidence that uterine derived activity may be secreted from the uterine cells in response to estrogens comes from our identification of a growth factor activity in uterine luminal fluid

(ULF) prepared from the estradiol-treated, ovariectomized rats (30), (31). The uterine horns of these animals fill with 1 to 2 ml of fluid beginning 7 days after estrogen treatment and continuing until at least day 14. This fluid has both growth promoting activity and a very potent cell growth inhibiting activity (30), (31). The cell growth inhibiting activities originate from microorganisms which probably originate in the vagina, and invade the uterus when estrogen treatment begins. Of the many organisms identified in ULF from these rats, Pseudomonas aeruginosa and Proteus mirabilis were the most common. However, others identified were: Escherichia coli, Staphylococcus epidermis, Streptococcus faecalis, Yersinea pseudotuberculosis, and α-hemolytic streptococcus. We have demonstrated that both Pseudomonas and Proteus are capable of producing exotoxins that inhibit MTW9/PL mammary and GH3/C14 pituitary cells in culture. The Pseudomonas exotoxin most likely to be present in ULF is the well known Exotoxin A described by us (30), (31), and others (35), (36) as a toxin for mammalian cells. The implications of these data were twofold when considering the assays of both uterine tissue derived activity and ULF mitogens. These inhibitors directly effect the apparent degree of induction of the mammary growth factor activity in uterine tissue. This can be seen as a decreased induction from the ten-fold or more reported with uteri from uninfected animals (56) to the four-fold or less induction of specific activity found with uteri from infected animals (30). In some experiments utilizing heavily infected uteri from estrogen treated animals, there was no induction of specific activity over uteri from animals only ovariectomized (D.A. Sirbasku and F.E. Leland, unpublished).

The same situation occurs with ULF in that some preparations show potent biological activity with MTW9/PL cells (57), while others may be inactive (30), (31). Removal of the inhibitors from either uterine extract preparations, or from ULF, was done by Affi-Gel Blue chromatography. The fraction of protein that passes through the column contains the majority of the cell growth inhibitory activity, while the fraction of protein eluted by addition of 0.6M sodium chloride to the remaining buffer contains potent mammary cell activity. The elution profile and assay of the activity in pooled fractions from Affi-Gel Blue chromatography is shown in Fig. 9.

To establish whether the uterine tissue derived growth activity is similar or different from the ULF activity, we conducted the same partial purification of the ULF activity as described for uterine tissue activity. At least a 250-fold partial purification (Table 3) of the ULF mammary cell activity was achieved by the procedure outlined in Fig. 4, and from the data presented in Table 3, it is apparent that the uterine tissue and ULF activities copurified. Of course, this represents only a partial purification of each activity, and therefore, we cannot conclude that the activities are identical. However, the data presented, along with other comparative studies presented elsewhere (30), (31), suggest

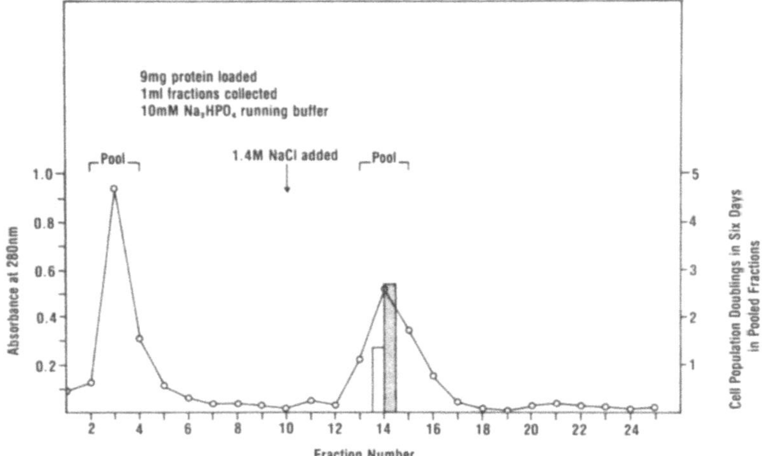

Fig. 9. Affi-Gel Blue chromatography of uterine luminal fluid (ULF) collected as described in (30), (31). ULF was dialyzed against 10 mM sodium phosphate buffer, pH 7.0, and applied to an Affi-Gel column equilibrated in the same buffer. Assay of the pooled fractions with MTW9/PL cells showed activity at 20 µg/ml (open bars) and 50 µg/ml (shaded bar) in the 1.4M sodium chloride eluted fractions, but no activity in the flow through fraction at 100 µg/ml.

that the estromedin activity of rat uterus and rat ULF have similar properties, including estimated molecular weights of 70,000 daltons (30), (31), (60). These data support the possibility that the ULF mitogen could be a secreted form of the uterine extract activity. If the activity is secreted from uterine cells, there should be a form in plasma that is similar to the activity found in ULF and uterine tissue extracts. To test this, we applied the same four step partial purification to plasma prepared from estrogen-treated, ovariectomized rats (31). The results shown in Table 4 indicate that MGF activity can be found in the same fractions as activity from either ULF or uterine tissue extracts. At least one mammary cell growth activity in plasma appears similar to that found in the uterine derived samples, although we do not know at present, whether the level of this activity is influenced by estrogens.

It must again be emphasized that the degree of purification of plasma activity is not great, and that platelet derived growth factor, which is active with MTW9/PL cells (15), (16), is not eliminated from these preparations. We recognize that there remains a need for a specific (RIA) method of measurement not dependent upon the relatively nonspecific bioassay of cell growth.

Paracrine and/or autocrine estromedin growth stimulation

Throughout the studies described above, we have asked whether the endocrine estromedin mechanism shown in Fig. 1 could be important for growth of estrogen-responsive mammary and pituitary tumor cells *in vivo*. However, another series of studies conducted recently have suggested to us that there are at least two additional mechanisms which could be involved in growth of mammary tumors *in vivo*. In these studies we have found at least two growth factor activities associated with mammary tumor cells growing *in vivo*. The MTW9/PL rat mammary cells were inoculated into W/Fu estrogen-treated castrated rats, and after tumors had formed, these were excised, washed in water and PBS, and extracts prepared as described for the rat uteri (56). The growth factor activity in MTW9/PL tumor extracts was capable of supporting very substantial growth of MTW9/PL cells in culture. As shown in Fig. 10, 50 to 100 µg of extract of MTW9/PL tumors growing in estrogen-treated castrated males, or estrogen-treated castrated females, caused greated than three MTW9/PL cell population doublings in culture. This activity appears to fractionate by Affi-Gel Blue chromatography into two distinct activities, although only a limited biochemical characterization of these activities has been done.

At present, we have concluded that one of the two activities identified in the MTW9/PL tumor extracts is similar to that found in the uterine and kidney extracts. Nevertheless, whether the activity in the tumor extracts is similar or different from that in other tissue extracts, there are at least two possible explanations for these observations, (i) the tumor concentrates this activity from the plasma, meaning that the high activity isolated could be due to growth factor associated reversibly with receptors on the tumor cells, or (ii) the MTW9/PL cells, or other cells in the tumor, are capable of producing the growth factor themselves, thereby causing growth by a "paracrine" or "autocrine" estromedin mechanism. These two mechanisms are summarized in the middle and right panels, respectively, of Fig. 11, and represent either possible alternatives to the endocrine estromedin mechanism, or mechanisms that function synergistically with an endocrine mechanism. At present we are attempting to establish whether paracrine or autocrine growth controls exist in the MTW9/PL tumor extracts, and have shown that when estrogen stimulation is removed, the MTW9/PL tumors which begin regressing within 7 days have a lower specific activity of growth factor than tumors continuing to grow in intact females (F.E. Leland and D.A. Sirbasku, manuscript in preparation).

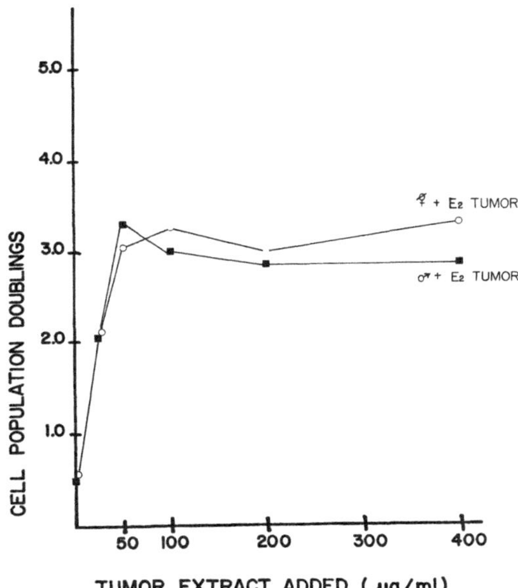

Fig. 10. Growth of MTW9/PL tumor cells in the designated concentrations of extracts of MTW9/PL tumors grown in estradiol-treated males or estradiol-treated, ovariectomized W/Fu rats.

Recent evidence from other laboratories has confirmed the presence of growth factors in human mammary tumors (47), and production of growth factors by murine mammary tumor cells (29). As yet, firm evidence for paracrine and/or autocrine control of mammary tumor growth is still lacking, but this appears to be a very promising area of future study.

PLATELET DERIVED GROWTH FACTORS

The major form of platelet derived growth factor (PDGF) has been characterized (3) as a 35,000 dalton molecular weight basic protein which, upon mercaptoethanol reduction, forms two dissimilar inactive polypeptide chains. The native activity was isolated from outdated human platelets by a series of steps involving heating platelet lysate at 100°C, carboxymethylcellulose chromatography (CMC) of the heated supernatant, and Sephadex gel filtration in 1M acetic acid which causes the growth activity to appear in the lower molecular elution volumes of the column. This activity has been shown to be an active mitogen for 3T3 mouse fibroblasts (3), (39), (40), (41), and arterial smooth muscle cells (46). Its role *in vivo* is postulated to be in wound healing and in atherosclerosis. The relationship of this factor to other platelet derived growth factors will be discussed next.

Platelet derived growth factors for mammary tumor cells

Another potential source of growth factors for both human and rat mammary tumor cells is platelets. We have shown previously (15), (16) that crude lysates of expired (3 to 5 day old) human platelets contain potent growth factors for the MTW9/PL rat mammary tumor cells in culture (Fig. 12), and for the human MCF-7 mammary tumor cells (16). The MTW9/PL cells grew at the same rate in human platelet lysates as in 5% human serum (15), (16). When growth of MTW9/PL cells was assayed in response to rat platelet lysates (Table 6), we found that these preparations stimulated cell growth as well as 5% rat serum, and that there was no significant difference between the activities of platelets prepared from male or female rats. Our observations suggested asking two questions. Is the PDGF which promotes 3T3 fibroblast cell growth (3) the same activity that promotes mammary cell growth, or could there be more than one platelet derived growth factor? Could platelet derived mammary cell growth factor function *in vivo* to promote growth of estrogen-responsive tumor cells?

TABLE 6

MITOGENIC ACTIVITY OF RAT PLATELET LYSATES AND RAT SERA

Addition	Cell Number ($\times 10^{-5}$) ± 1 s.d.	Number of Cell Population Doublings
None	0.40 ± 0.13	0
100 µg/ml female rat platelet lysate	3.27 ± 1.24	3.03
100 µg/ml male rat platelet lysate	6.92 ± 0.27	4.11
5% female rat serum	9.72 ± 0.34	4.60
5% male rat serum	5.65 ± 1.29	3.82

Data from reference (15).

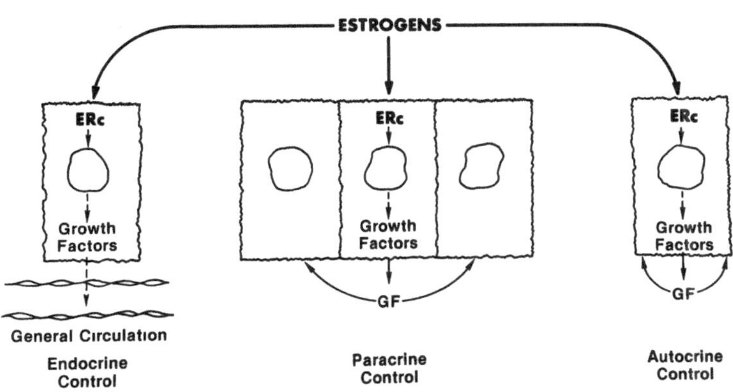

Fig. 11. Proposal of three new models in which estrogen-induced growth factors are involved in estrogen-responsive mammary tumor cell growth *in vivo*.

We approached the first of these questions by asking whether platelet lysates promoted the growth of only 3T3 cells, arterial smooth muscle cells and MTW9/PL rat mammary cells, or instead, could promote growth of a broad range of cell types. We found that many cell lines from diverse organs and species responded to growth factor(s) in crude lysates of human platelets (16). These data showed that platelet lysate, prepared as described elsewhere (15), (16), added to culture medium at 200 µg/ml supported the growth of many cell types as well, or nearly as well as 5% human serum. It thus appears that platelets were a source of significant growth factor activity, but that either multiple activities were present, or that one or a few activities were potent mitogens for many established cell lines. In order to clarify these findings further, Dr. Caroline T. Eastment of our laboratory conducted a partial two step characterization of the platelet activities for 3T3 mouse fibroblasts and MTW9/PL cells which resulted in an apparent separation of the mitogenic activities for these two cell lines. The initial step of preparation for 3T3 cell PDGF is heating the lysate at 100°C (3). The supernatant from this heating was assayed for growth activity and only 3T3 cell growth factor was found

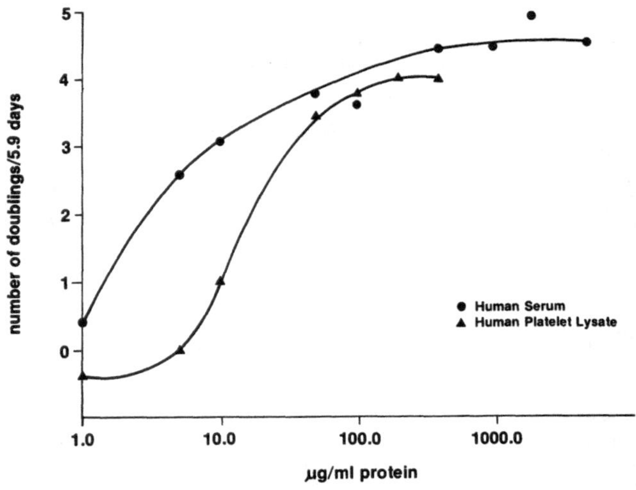

Fig. 12. Growth of MTW9/PL cells in response to increasing concentrations of protein from human serum, and from lysates of outdated human platelets.

(Fig. 13); no MTW9/PL activity was present in these extracts. However, when the heated supernatant was applied to a P-150 Bio-Gel column, separable activities for 3T3 and MTW9/PL cells were demonstrated (Fig. 14). Further characterization of this platelet derived MTW9/PL cell growth factor has not been done, but the data suggests that this area of study could provide new insights into mammary tumor growth control.

Approaching the second question stated above, we asked whether platelet derived growth factor could be released locally in the area of the growing tumors. This problem has not as yet been approached satisfactorily, but a possible working hypothesis is shown in Fig. 15, and is based on the preliminary observation by Butler et al. (9) that estrogens induce production of proteases (plasminogen activators) by MCF-7 cells in culture. If estrogens induce production of proteases by tumor cells, then these proteases could initiate platelet aggregation in the local blood supply of the tumor. The information available suggests the 3T3 PDGF is released when platelets aggregate (and release granule contents) in response to protease treatment. Thus, this type of mechanism bears fur-

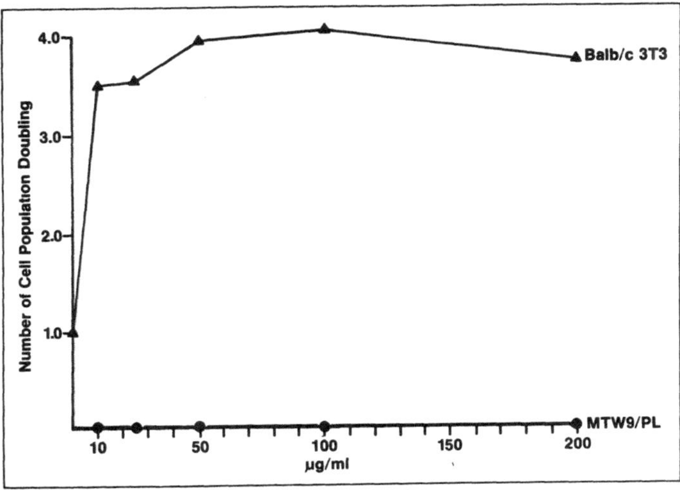

Fig. 13. Effect of heating platelet lysates to 100°C for 15 min. on growth factor activity for Balb/c 3T3 cells, and growth factor activity for MTW9/PL mammary cells. The lysate was heated as described (15), (16).

ther study under both controlled conditions *in vitro*, and with anti-platelet aggregation drugs *in vivo*.

Growth factors and growth control in normal versus malignant mammary cells

One of the very intense areas of study in growth control has been the comparison of growth factor effects and requirements of normal cells with those of their transformed counterparts. The general conclusions from the mass of these studies are that tumor cells have a reduced serum (and growth factor) requirement in culture, and no predictable pattern can be established between tumorigenesis and growth factor receptor numbers per cells.

Nevertheless, a very interesting and potentially major finding in control of normal fibroblast growth has been made by Pledger and colleagues (39), (40), (41). These investigators have proposed that normal cells resting in

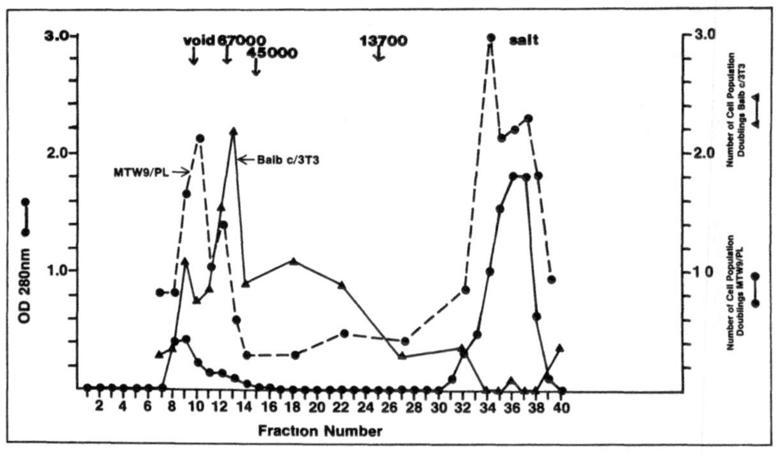

Fig. 14. P-150 gel chromatography of 100°C heated platelet lysate (Fig. 13), and assay of fractions for protein content (A280nm), MTW9/PL cell growth factor activity, and 3T3 cell growth factor activity.

the G_0 state can be stimulated by growth factors to enter the cell cycle G_1 period. The polypeptide factors that promote this transition are called "competence factors", and include PDGF and FGF. Cells in the competent state are then responsive to additional growth factors which cause the cells to pass various checkpoints in the G_1 period and enter into the S phase of the cycle. These second factors are distinct from competence factors, and because they cause movement through the cell cycle, are designated "progression factors". A summary of this model of normal cell growth is presented in Fig. 16. Points V and W represent specific G_1 cell cycle control points as reviewed by Pledger and Wharton (41). For the purposes of this review, we need only point out that these events in G_1 may be controlled by different polypeptide or protein hormones. The sum of the model proposed shows that both platelet derived factors and plasma derived factors such as somatomedins (13), are required for G_0 cells to enter into the cell cycle and arrive in S phase.

Now, if we propose a hypothetical model of normal mammary cell growth based on the concepts presented in Fig. 16, it seems entirely possible that a few to several different tyoes of growth factors may be required for entry of normal mammary cells into the cycle. These could range from

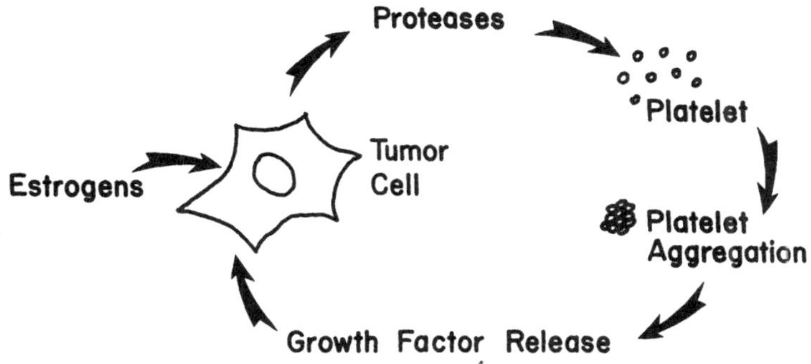

Fig. 15. Model mechanism for protease secretion and platelet aggregation and release of growth factor(s).

competence factors which could include estrogens, prolactin and growth factors, to progression factors which could be an entirely different set of activities. One of the logical possibilities that arise from the model presented in Fig. 16 is that malignant or transformed cells have gained permanent "competence", and have entered the G_1 phase of the cell cycle. This would imply that the tumor cells are not resting in G_0 state, but are always undergoing cell division, albeit, some do at only a slow rate. This has certainly proved to be the case with both MTW9/PL and MCF-7 mammary cells. Thus, the activity from uterus designated an estromedin would, most probably, be a "progression" factor rather than a "competence" factor. These matters are speculative at present, but certainly provide a new framework for considering growth control of normal versus malignant mammary cells.

PITUITARY DERIVED MAMMARY CELL GROWTH FACTORS

The most recent of our studies has been the attempt to ask whether mammary cell growth factors can be identified in extracts of rat pituitary glands, or in extracts of estrogen-dependent rat pituitary tumors. The tumors were chosen for study because they are well known to produce excessive amounts of prolactin and/or growth hormone, and may also produce excess growth factor activities. Our studies have shown that pituitaries obtained from either estradiol-treated castrated males, or estradiol-treated castrated females, have potent growth factor activity toward MTW9/PL mammary cells, but not toward GH3/C14 pituitary tumor cells (Table 7).

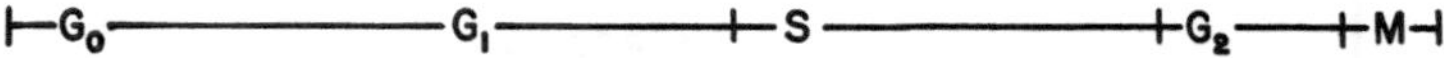

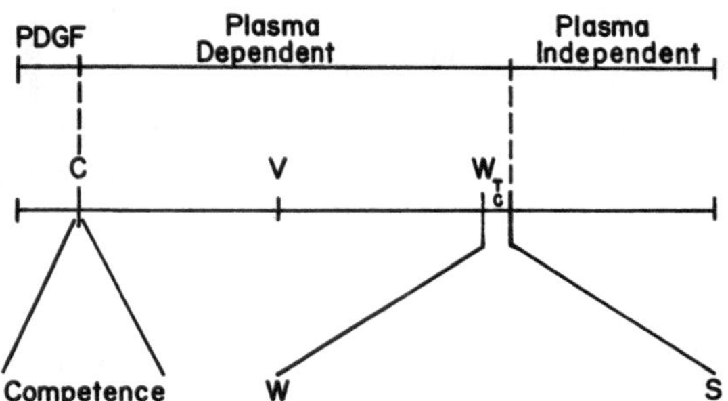

Fig. 16. Model mechanism for relationship between "competence" and "progression" factors with Balb/c 3T3 cells in culture. From Pledger and Wharton (41). The designation "c" indicates processes in the cell cycle related to competence or preparation to enter the G_1/S phases. "Progression" is plasma dependent and involves different factors than those involved in "competence".

It is possible that the activity from normal rat pituitaries is not identical to that extracted from the rat uterus since extracts of rat uterus promote growth of both kinds of cells. When mammary cell growth factor activity was sought from estrogen-dependent prolactin and growth hormone secreting GH3/C14 tumors growing in estradiol-treated, ovariectomized rats, we found that these tumors contained an MTW9/PL cell growth factor which was 2.7 times higher specific activity than that found in estrogen-primed normal pituitary glands, but again, no GH3/C14 pituitary cell activity. We have evidence that these pituitary tumor associated mammary cell activities are not the usual forms of prolactin or growth hormone, and are of much higher molecular weight than the newly described "cleaved" forms of prolactin (37), (38) which have been stated to be more mitogenic for mammary cells than the native form of prolactin. A limited, partial purification has shown these new activities extracted from pituitary tumor cells are different from others such as pituitary derived FGF and phosphoethanolamine (26). At present, a large scale characterization is planned using the estrogen-dependent GH3/C14 rat

TABLE 7

GROWTH OF MTW9/PL MAMMARY AND GH3/C14 PITUITARY CELLS IN EXTRACTS OF RAT PITUITARY GLAND AND GH3/C14 RAT PITUITARY TUMORS

Extract Source	Cell Line Tested	Concentration Producing Half-maximal Growth
Pituitary glands of estradiol-treated castrated female rats	MTW9/PL GH3/C14	46 μg/ml > 500 "
Pituitary glands of estradiol-treated castrated male rats	MTW9/PL GH3/C14	64 " > 500 "
GH3/C14 Pituitary tumors growing in female rats	MTW9/PL GH3/C14	35 " > 500 "
GH3/C14 Pituitary tumors growing in estradiol-treated castrated female rats	MTW9/PL GH3/C14	27 " > 500 "

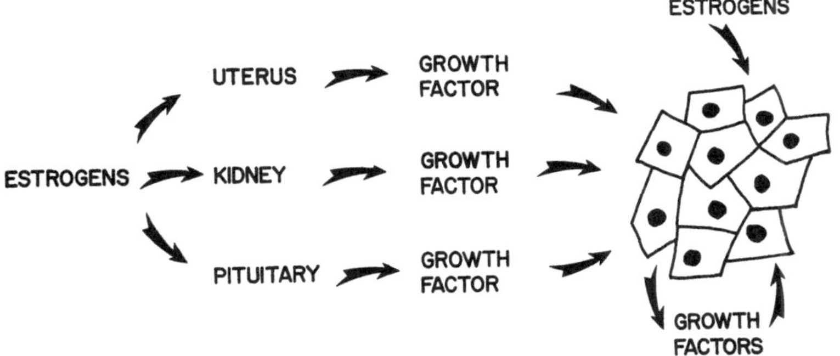

Fig. 17. Summary of the possible sources of estrogen related growth factors which may have a role in the in vivo growth of some types of mammary tumors.

pituitary tumors as sources which we hope will lead to a clear indication of whether this new activity is a mammary cell growth factor different from others already identified.

SUMMARY OF NEW APPROACHES TO GROWTH FACTOR INVOLVEMENT IN MAMMARY TUMOR GROWTH IN VIVO

In Fig. 17, we present a summary of the various new sources of mammary growth factor activities discovered by our studies of tissue extract effects on MTW9/PL and MCF-7 mammary tumor cell growth in culture. Our data suggest that at least three tissues of the rat, namely uterus, kidney and pituitary are possible sources of an endocrine type estromedin activity. Our data at present suggest that the rat uterus and rat kidney derived mammary growth factor activities are similar in properties. The pituitary derived activity remains to be better characterized, so no further conclusions can be made about this activity. Also, the MTW9/PL mammary tumors themselves may produce growth factors which are self-stimulatory (autocrine or paracrine control). Further study in this area will include attempts to determine if the MTW9/PL cells produce growth factor in culture in response to estrogen.

Beyond these studies, it is apparent from all of our work that purified growth factors are essential along with sensitive RIA methods of measurement. Nevertheless, the beginning studies presented here have encouraged us to seek new factors involved in mammary tumor growth in culture, and to attempt to evaluate their possible roles *in vivo*.

REFERENCES

1. Allegra J, Lippman ME. Growth of a human breast cancer cell line in serum-free hormone-supplemented medium. Cancer Res 38: 3823-9, 1978.
2. Andres RY, Jeng I, Bradshaw RH. Nerve growth factor receptors: identification of distinct classes in plasma membranes and nuclei of embryonic dorsal root neurons. Proc Natl Acad Sci USA 74: 2785-9, 1977.
3. Antoniades HN, Scher C, Stiles C. Purification of human platelet derived growth factor. Proc Natl Acad Sci USA 76: 1809-13, 1979.
4. Armelin HA, Armelin MCS, Farios SE, Gambarini AG, Kimura E. Effects of hydrocortisone on the growth control of a mutant derived from Swiss mouse 3T3 fibroblast. pp. 269-279 in *Hormones and Cell Culture, Cold Spring Harbor Conferences on Cell Proliferation*, eds GH Sato, R Ross. Cold Spring Harbor, New York, 1979.
5. Barnes D, Sato G. Growth of a human mammary tumor cell line in a serum-free medium. Nature 281: 388-9, 1979.
6. Barnes D, Sato G. Methods for growth of cultured cells in serum-free medium. Anal Biochem 102: 252-70, 1980.
7. Bennett DC, Peachey LA, Durbin H, Rudland PS. A possible mammary stem cell line. Cell 15: 283-298, 1978.
8. Bottenstein J, Hayashi I, Hutchings S, Masui H, Mather J, McClure DB, Ohasa S, Rizzino A, Sato G, Serrero G, Wolf R, Wu R. The growth of cells in serum-free hormone-supplemented media. Methods Enzymol 58: 94-109, 1979.

9. Butler WB, Kirkland WL, Gargola TL, Goran H, Kelsey WH. Stimulation of plasminogen activator productions in a human breast cancer cell line (MCF-7) by steroid. J Cell Biol 97 (part 2): 162a, 1980.
10. Byrny RL, Orth DN, Cohen S, Doyne ES. Epidermal growth factor: effects of androgens and adrenergic agents. Endocrinology 95: 776-82, 1974.
11. Carpenter G, Cohen S. Human epidermal growth factor and the proliferation of human fibroblasts. J Cell Physiol 88: 227-37, 1976.
12. Cattertan WZ, Escobedo MB, Sexsan WR, Gray ME, Sundell HW, Stahlman MT. Effect of epidermal growth factor on lung maturation in fetal rabbits. Pediatr Res 13: 104-108, 1979.
13. Clemmons DR, Van Wyk JJ, Pledger WJ. Sequential addition of platelet factor and plasma to Balb/c 3T3 fibroblast cultures stimulates somatomedin-c binding early in cell cycle. Proc Natl Acad Sci USA 77: 6644-48, 1980.
14. Cohen S, Carpenter G. Human epidermal growth factor: isolation and chemical and biological properties. Proc Natl Acad Sci USA 72: 1317-21, 1975.
15. Eastment CT, Sirbasku DA. Platelet derived mammary tumor growth factor. J Cell Physiol 97: 17-27, 1978.
16. Eastment CT, Sirbasku DA. Human platelet lysate contains growth factor activities for established cell lines derived from various tissues of several species. In Vitro 16: 694-705, 1980.
17. Froesch ER, Zapf E, Rinderknecht R, Humbel RE. Non-suppressible insulin-like activity (NSILA) from human serum: recent accomplishments and their physiologic implications. Metabolism 27: 1803-28, 1978.
18. Froesch ER, Zapf J, Rinderknecht E, Morell B, Schoenle E, Humbel RE. Insulin-like growth factor (IGF-NSILA) structure, function and physiology. pp. 61-77 in Hormones and Cell Culture, Cold Spring Harbor Conferences on Cell Proliferation, Vol. 6, eds GH Sato, R Ross. Cold Spring Harbor Laboratory, Cold Spring Harbor, New York, 1979.
19. Gospodarowicz D, Rudland P, Lindstrom J, Benirschke K. Fibroblast growth factor (FGF): its localization, purification, mode of action and physiological significance. Adv Metab Disor 8: 302-35, 1975.
20. Gospodarowicz D, Moran JS. Growth factors in mammalian cell culture. Annu Rev Biochem 45: 531-58, 1976.
21. Gospodarowicz D, Delgado D, Vlodavsky I. Permissive effect of the extracellular matrix on cell proliferation in vitro. Proc Natl Acad Sci USA 77: 4094-98, 1980.
22. Haigler H, Ash JF, Singer SF, Cohen S. Visualization by fluorescence of the binding and internalization of epidermal growth factor in human carcinoma cells A-431. Proc Natl Acad Sci USA 75: 3317-21, 1978.
23. Hayashi I, Sato G. Replacement of serum by hormones permits growth of cells in defined medium. Nature 259: 132-34. 1976.
24. Jimenez de Asua L, Clingan D, Rudland PS. Initiation of cell proliferation in cultured mouse fibroblasts by prostaglandin $F_2\alpha$. Proc

Natl Acad Sci USA 72: 2724-28, 1975.
25. Jimenez de Asua L, Richmond KMU, Otto AM, Kubler AM, O'Farrell MK, Rudland PS. Growth factors and hormones interact in a series of temporal steps to regulate the rate of initiation of DNA synthesis in mouse fibroblasts. pp. 403-424 in Hormones and Cell Culture, Cold Spring Harbor Conferences on Cell Proliferation, Vol 6, eds GH Sato, R Ross, Cold Spring Harbor Laboratory, Cold Spring Harbor, New York, 1979.
26. Kano-Sueoka T, Cohen DM, Yamaizumi Z, Nishimura S, Mori M, Fujiki H. Phosphoethanolamine as a growth factor of a mammary carcinoma cell line of rat. Proc Natl Acad Sci USA 76: 5741-44, 1979.
27. King RJ, Kaye AM, Shodell MJ. Copurification of an estrogen-induced protein from rat uterus and a factor able to stimulate DNA synthesis in cultured cells. Exp Cell Res 109: 1-8, 1977.
28. Kirkland WL, Sorrentino JM, Sirbasku DA. Control of cell growth: III. Direct mitogenic effect of thyroid hormones on an estrogen-dependent rat pituitary tumor cell line. J Natl Cancer Inst 56: 1159-64, 1976.
29. Knauer DJ, Iyer AP, Banerjee MR, Smith GL. Identification of somatomedin-like polypeptides produced by mammary tumors of Balb/c mice. Cancer Res 40: 4368-72, 1980.
30. Leland FE, Kohn DF, Sirbasku DA. Uterine luminal fluid growth factors: I. Promotion and inhibition of growth of estrogen-dependent tumor cell lines by factors from rat uterine luminal fluid (unpublished results).
31. Leland FE, Sirbasku DA. Uterine luminal fluid growth factors: II. Biochemical comparisons of rat uterine tissue, plasma and uterine luminal fluid growth promoting and growth inhibiting activities for estrogen-dependent tumor cells (unpublished results).
32. Levi-Montalcini R. Mechanism of action of nerve growth factor. Harvey Lect. 60: 217-59, 1966.
33. Lippman ME, Bolan G, Huff K. The effects of estrogens and antiestrogens on hormone-responsive human breast cancer in long-term tissue culture. Cancer Res 35: 4595-5601, 1976.
34. Medina D, Oborn CJ. Growth of preneoplastic mammary epithelial cells in serum-free medium. Cancer Res 40: 3982-87, 1980.
35. Middlebrook JL, Dorland RB. Serum effects on the response of mammalian cells to the exotoxins of Pseudomonas aeruginosa and Corynebacterium diphtheria. Can J Microbiol 23: 175-82, 1977.
36. Middlebrook JL, Dorland RB. Response of cultured mammalian cells to the exotoxins of Pseudomonas aeruginosa and Corynebacterium diphtheria: differential cytotoxicity. Can J Microbiol 23: 183-89, 1977.
37. Mittra I. A novel "cleaved prolactin" in the rat pituitary: part I, biosynthesis, characterization and regulatory control. Biochem Biophys Res Commun 95: 1750-59, 1980.
38. Mittra I. A novel "cleaved prolactin" in rat pituitary: part II, in vivo mammary mitogenic activity of its N-terminal 16K moiety. Biochem Biophys Res Commun 95: 1760-67, 1980.

39. Pledger W, Stiles C, Antoniades H, Scher C. Induction of DNA synthesis in Balb/c 3T3 cells by serum components: reevaluation of the commitment process. Proc Natl Acad Sci USA 74: 4481-85, 1977.
40. Pledger W, Stiles C, Antoniades H, Scher C. An ordered sequence of events is required before Balb/c 3T3 cells become committed to DNA synthesis. Proc Natl Acad Sci USA 75: 2839-43, 1978.
41. Pledger WJ, Wharton W. Regulation of early cell cycle events by serum components. pp. 165-172 in Control Mechanisms in Animal Cells, eds L Jimenez de Asua, R Levi-Montalcini, R Shields, S Iacobell-, Raven Press, New York, 1980.
42. Ptashne K, Hsueh HW, Stockdale FE. Partial purification and characterization of mammary stimulating factor, a protein which promotes proliferation of mammary epithelium. Biochemistry 18: 3533-39, 1979.
43. Rajkind M, Gatmartan A, Mackensen S, Giambrone MA, Ponce P, Reid LM. Connective tissue biomatrix: its isolation and utilization for long term cultures of normal rat hepatocytes. J Cell Biol 87: 255-63, 1980.
44. Reinwald JG, Green H. Serial cultivation of strains of human epidermal kerotinocytes: the formation of keratinizing colonies from single cells. Cell 6: 331-34, 1975.
45. Rinderknect E, Humbel RE. Primary structure of human insulin-like growth factor II. FEBS letters 89(2): 283-86, 1978.
46. Ross R, Biomset J, Kariya B, Harker L. A platelet-dependent serum factor that stimulates the proliferation of arterial smooth muscle cells in vitro. Proc Natl Acad Sci USA 71: 1207-10, 1974.
47. Rowe J, Kasper S. Partial purification and characterization of putative growth factors in extracts of human breast cancer. Endocrinology (supplement) 106: 144, 1980.
48. Salmon WD Jr, Daughaday WH. A hormonally controlled serum factor which stimulated sulfate incorporation by cartilage in vitro. J Lab Clin Med 49: 825-36, 1957.
49. Samuels HH, Tsai JS, Casanova J. Thyroid hormone action: a cell culture system responsive to physiological concentrations of thyroid hormones. Science 181: 1253-56, 1973.
50. Sato G, Reid L. Replacement of serum in cell culture by hormones. Biochem and Mode of Action of Hormones II. 20: 219-31, 1978.
51. Savage CR Jr, Cohen S. Epidermal growth factor and a new derivation. J Biol Chem 247: 7609-11, 1972.
52. Shafie SM. Estrogen and growth of breast cancer: new evidence suggests indirect action. Science 209: 701-2, 1980.
53. Shafie SM, Hilf R. Relationship between insulin and estrogen binding to growth responses in 7,12-dimethylbenz[α]anthracene induced rat mammary tumors. Cancer Res 38: 759-64, 1978.
54. Sievestsson H, Frykland L, Uthne K, Hall K, Westermark B. Isolation and chemistry of human somatomedins A and B. Adv Metab Disor 8: 47-60, 1975
55. Sirbasku DA. Hormone-responsive growth in vivo of a tissue culture

cell line established from the MT-W9A rat mammary tumor. Cancer Res 38: 1154-65, 1978.
56. Sirbasku DA. Estrogen-induction of growth factors specific for hormone-responsive mammary, pituitary and kidney tumor cells. Proc Natl Acad Sci USA 75: 3786-90, 1978.
57. Sirbasku DA, Benson RH. Estrogen-inducible growth factors that may act as mediators (estromedins) of estrogen promoted tumor cell growth. pp. 477-97 in Hormones and Cell Culture, Cold Spring Harbor Conferences on Cell Proliferation, Vol. 6, Cold Spring Harbor Laboratory, Cold Spring Harbor, New York, 1979.
58. Sirbasku DA, Benson RH. Proposal of an indirect (estromedin) mechanism of estrogen-induced mammary tumor cell growth. pp. 289-314 in Cell Biology of Breast Cancer, eds C McGrath, M Rich, Academic Press, New York, 1981.
59. Sirbasku DA, Kirkland WL. Control of cell growth: IV. Growth properties of a new cell line established from an estrogen-dependent kidney tumor of the Syrian hamster. Endocrinology 95: 1260-72, 1976.
60. Sirbasku DA, Leland FE, Benson RH. Properties of a growth factor activity present in crude extracts of rat uterus. J Cell Physiol (in press).
61. Sorrentino JM, Kirkland WL, Sirbasku DA. Control of cell growth: I. Estrogen-dependent growth in vivo of a rat pituitary tumor cell line. J Natl Cancer Inst 56: 1149-54, 1976.
62. Sorrentino JM, Kirkland WL, Sirbasku DA. Control of cell growth: II. Requirement of thyroid hormones for the in vivo estrogen-dependent growth of rat pituitary tumor cells. J Natl Cancer Inst 56: 1155-58, 1976.
63. Soule H, Vazques J, Long A, Albert S, Brennan M. A human cell line from a pleural effusion derived from a breast carcinoma. J Natl Cancer Inst 51: 1409-13, 1973.
64. Teng MH, Bartholonew JC, Bissell MJ. Insulin effect on the cell cycly: analysis of the kinetics of growth parameters in confluent chick cells. Proc Natl Acad Sci USA 73: 3173-77, 1976.
65. Thrash CR. Cunningham DD. Stimulation of division of density inhibited fibroblasts by glucocorticoid. Nature 242: 399-401, 1973.
66. Van Wyk JJ, Underwood LE, Baseman JB, Hintz RL, Clemmons DR, Marshall RN. Exploration of the insulin-like and growth promoting properties of somatomedins by membrane receptor assays. Adv Metab Disor 8: 127-50, 1975.

Chapter 6

PRIMARY AND PERMISSIVE ACTIONS OF INSULIN IN BREAST CANCER

Russell Hilf

During the past decade, more attention has been directed towards elucidation of the role of insulin as a regulatory factor in mammary cancer. This renewed interest can be attributed to a number of developments arising from research in the areas of diabetes and insulin action, such as a) development of techniques to prepare insulin with high radiospecific activity, providing a reagent for use in radioimmunoassay to measure physiological levels of insulin in blood, as well as a reagent to measure and characterize insulin receptors; b) ease of induction of diabetes with streptozotocin; c) continued improvement of *in vitro* organ and tissue culture techniques, enabling the investigator to examine hormone effects under a more "controlled" environment; and d) advances in our understanding of mechanisms of action of insulin, particularly at the membrane level. Although most of the above investigations have been applied to normal cells, such as adipocytes, hepatocytes, lymphocytes, etc., there is a need to ascertain whether such mechanisms exist in the transformed cells. Two of the well-established actions of insulin relate to regulation of glucose and amino acid entry into cells. Since it has been proposed by Holley (33) that substrate entry may be related to neoplastic cell growth, any hormone that may act as a regulator of substrate transport represents a potentially important factor in regulation of tumor growth. As such, insulin is a prime candidate for such a role and data will be presented to implicate insulin as a direct as well as a facilitative factor in regulation of mammary tumor growth.

I. DIRECT ACTIONS OF INSULIN ON EXPERIMENTAL MAMMARY TUMORS

A. Stimulation of growth: insulin-dependent tumors.

Although a few earlier reports indicated that growth of certain transplantable tumors was retarded in diabetic animals(11),(47),(48) the series of experiments reported by Heuson and his colleagues clearly demonstrated that insulin should be considered as a factor in growth of DMBA-induced mammary tumors. They (22) reported that 90% of these carcinogen-induced lesions regressed after diabetes was induced with alloxan, results that confirmed their earlier finding that insulin caused proliferation of DMBA-induced tumors in explant culture (20). In addition, they reported that estrogen treatment could not prevent tumor regression resulting from insulin removal, i.e., diabetes (23), and in hypophysectomized hosts, reactivation of tumor growth was seen when insulin was administered with prolactin whereas prolactin alone had no stimulatory effect.

To avoid the rather severe effects of alloxan, we (4) used streptozotocin to induce diabetes, which was defined as blood glucose >250mg/100ml.

urinary glucose levels >0.5gm/ml and serum insulin <10^{-10}M. Animals bearing DMBA-induced tumors, when made diabetic by the above criteria, showed the following response in tumor growth behavior subsequent to induction of diabetes: 101/190 (53.2%) lesions decreased (>20% decrease in surface area), 53/190 (27.9%) lesions continued to grow (>20% increase) and 36/190 (18.9%) were classified as static, demonstrating less than a 20% change in size. While these results are less dramatic than those reported earlier (23), body weight loss in streptozotocin-induced diabetic animals was modest compared to that reported for alloxan-treated rats. Nevertheless, the number of lesions regressing after induction of diabetes is significantly higher than would occur spontaneously in intact animals (57). If hormone-dependent cancers are analogous to hormone-dependent target tissues, e.g., uterus, replacement hormone therapy should stimulate or activate growth. Most tumors that regressed in diabetic hosts resumed growth in response to insulin treatment; in our recent report (10), 17/24 regressing lesions resumed growth, 5/24 became static and 2/24 continued to regress. On this basis, we conclude that a proportion of DMBA-induced mammary adenocarcinomas are insulin-dependent.

To examine the effects of insulin under better defined conditions, DMBA-induced neoplasms were studied by culture techniques _in vitro_. Insulin alone was found to markedly increase DNA synthesis in tumors studied by organ culture procedures (40) and Pasteels et al. (46) confirmed this by showing that 17/20 DMBA-induced tumors were classified as insulin-dependent for DNA synthesis. Likewise, similar results were reported by Welsch et al. (61) for mouse and DMBA-induced tumors of rats, as measured by enhanced incorporation of labeled thymidine into macromolecules. Curiously, when DMBA-induced tumors were grown as cell cultures, insulin alone had no effect on DNA synthesis (13). It should be noted, however, that this was also the case for insulin and normal mammary gland tissue when comparing organ explants with cell cultures.

Insulin was shown to have mitogenic activity in certain human breast cancer cells in long term tissue culture. Osborne et al. (44) reported that insulin increased the number of MCF-7 cells _in vitro_ by 50 to 100% over a range of 0.1nM to 10nM of the hormone. Similar results were reported by Rillema and Linbaugh (50) for the effect of insulin on thymidine incorporation into DNA in MCF-7 cells. At least one other human breast cancer cell line, ZR75-1, demonstrated similar results (45), although two other lines did not. Shafie showed that transplantation of MCF-7 cells to diabetic nude mice failed to yield tumors but when these diabetic mice were treated with insulin, tumors arose with 100% frequency (51). The response to insulin _in vitro_ was similar in cells derived from the solid tumors in nude mice and in cells maintained in continuous culture. Taken together, there is convincing evidence that insulin must be regarded as a growth factor in certain mammary cancers in animals and humans.

B. _Inhibition of growth: insulin-responsive tumors._

Having considered evidence that insulin stimulates growth of certain tumors, data will next be presented to demonstrate that insulin can inhibit growth of some mammary tumors. Studies from our laboratory were conducted with the R3230AC mammary adenocarcinoma, a transplantable lesion in Fischer rats that has the biochemical capacity to resemble the pregnant gland as reflected by production of a milk-like fluid containing casein, α-lactalbumin, lactose and medium-chain fatty acids in response to estrogen treatment (24),(27). Growth of this neoplasm was enhanced in diabetic rats and a dose-response inhibition of growth resulted from insulin treatment (5). This type of response to insulin appeared to be unique until recently when we examined the effects of insulin treatment on growth of DMBA-induced tumors (10). Tumors classified as insulin-indpendent, i.e., lesions continued to grow in diabetic rats, frequently demonstrated regression in response to injections of insulin. In this series, 10/28 lesions regressed, 1/25 became static and 14/25 continued to grow. Thus, two different mammary neoplasms in rodents were shown to be inhibited by insulin treatment. This resembles to some extent the paradoxical effects of estrogens, where removal or administration of the hormone may be beneficial (25). This apparent duality of action of insulin should be extended further to other models; a recent paper (35) demonstrated that proliferation of Cloudman 591 melanoma cells *in vitro* was inhibited by insulin.

C. Actions of insulin and relationship to tumor growth.

Insulin receptors and their regulation: The response of a tissue to hormonal perturbation is most likely initiated through specific receptors for the hormone. As a first approach to understanding the role of insulin as a regulatory hormone, in neoplastic tissues, specific receptors for insulin were identified and then characterized in various tumors: R3230AC mammary adenocarcinomas (14), DMBA-induced mammary tumors (54), in several human breast cancer cell lines (45) and in human tumor samples (32). Together these data demonstrate that the properties of insulin receptors in neoplastic tissues were similar to those in normal tissues, based on characteristics of saturability, affinity, specificity and curvilinearity of binding reactions as analyzed according to Scatchard. The major differences appear to be in receptor numbers, but caution is needed due to the difficulties in estimating the number of sites from curvilinear representations of Scatchard plots. It is also of interest to note that a similar conservation of properties of insulin binding has been reported for ascites forms of Zajdela hepatomas (2), transformed fibroblasts (53) and melanoma cells (6),(35). Thus, if there is a defect in the insulin regulatory action, it is most likely at a step distal to the initial hormone interaction.

An important aspect of receptor-mediated events relates to regulation of receptor number and affinity. If one assumes that response is related to the number of receptors, then an understanding of receptor regulation can offer insight into alterations in hormone-mediated events. For insulin, it has now been substantiated that the hormone itself may directly affect the number of its receptors, findings that led to the concept of down-regulation (34). This aspect of regulation was manifested for both the R3230AC and DMBA-induced tumors, since increased binding of insulin occurred in tumors in diabetic rats and insulin treatment resulted in decreased receptor number (15),(53),(54). A most interesting observation from our laboratory was the finding that estrogens exerted a negative regulation of insulin receptors (53). Insulin binding was increased in R3230AC tumors after ovariectomy and estrogen treatment reduced insulin binding; neither experimental condition altered plasma insulin levels. Similarly, DMBA-induced tumors that continued to grow after ovariectomy displayed an increase in insulin binding (54). These results demonstrate that insulin receptors can be regulated by hormonal agents and suggest that manipulation of the hormonal milieu may offer an exploitable technique for altering response. The role of sex steroids in down regulation of insulin receptors has also been noted by Bertoli et al. (1) under the physiological situation of the menstrual cycle.

Based on an earlier finding that insulin binding was increased in DMBA-induced tumors that regressed after induction of diabetes (54), we undertook studies to ascertain whether there was a relationship between the level of receptors and response to insulin (55). For these studies, we first ascertained the dependence of the lesion on insulin by its regression in the diabetic rat, removed the lesion, prepared cells from the lesion and grew the cells as primary cultures. Similar procedures were used for insulin-independent lesions, i.e., tumors continued to grow in diabetic rats. Compared to insulin-independent lesions, insulin-dependent tumors demonstrated a 2-fold higher binding capacity for insulin and this relationship was retained by the cultured cells (Table 1). To assess the relationship of binding capacity to response to insulin, cells were exposed to 5×10^{-10}M insulin and incorporation of labeled thymidine into macromolecules was measured. Compared to cells not exposed to insulin, tumors classified as independent demonstrated a modest response to insulin only at early times but were not significantly different after 8 hours. In contrast, insulin-dependent cells responded to insulin *in vitro* with significantly enhanced thymidine incorporation (Table 2). Similar results were obtained for uridine and leucine incorporation into macromolecules. We concluded that these data add further support for the role of insulin in growth regulation and that there was a relationship between insulin binding and the magnitude of response.

TABLE 1
INSULIN BINDING TO DEPENDENT AND INDEPENDENT TUMORS AND IN CELLS FROM PRIMARY CULTURE

Insulin Status	Primary Tumor	Cultured Cells
INDEPENDENT (7)	100 ± 30	100 ± 20
DEPENDENT (11)	296 ± 44	340 ± 26

Data expressed as %, wherein 100% = 14.8 ± 1.4 fmoles ^{125}I-insulin bound per 5×10^6 cells from independent lesions. Numbers in ( ) represents number of individual tumors studied.

TABLE 2

EFFECT OF INSULIN ON TIME COURSE OF THYMIDINE INCORPORATION IN DEPENDENT AND INDEPENDENT DMBA TUMOR CELLS IN PRIMARY CULTURE

HOURS	CONTROL	INDEPENDENT	DEPENDENT
2	48 ± 18	70 ± 18	164 ± 28
4	71 ± 8	115 ± 15	218 ± 19
8	100 ± 10	127 ± 12	215 ± 33
10	100 ± 9	121 ± 10	211 ± 33
16	69 ± 9	85 ± 25	198 ± 38
24	100 ± 14	113 ± 13	210 ± 16

Control consisted of an equal number of independent and dependent tumor cells with no insulin added; other cultures were exposed to 5×10^{-10}M insulin. Incorporation of ^{3}H-thymidine (5μCi) was measured at each of the times indicated and data are presented relative to incorporation in the absence of insulin. Data are mean ± SEM for 7 to 11 tumors.

Insulin, substrate transport and tumor growth: One of the most well accepted actions of insulin is its ability to regulate entry of glucose into cells, such as muscle and adipocytes. It is now becoming clear that insulin plays a regulatory role in the entry into cells of certain amino acids (12), results arising from a more discreet characterization of transport carriers with differing preferences for amino acids. Taken together with a growing knowledge that neoplastic transformation is often accompanied by enhanced entry of glucose (19), it was hypothesized by Holley (33) that neoplastic cell growth could be related to nutrient uptake. It seems logical, therefore, to question whether insulin can exert a regulatory effect on transport in neoplastic cells and further, whether other hormones act at this level of cell metabolism. Since data were presented above implicating insulin as a hormone with growth regulatory effects for certain experimental mammary tumors, it was pertinent to examine the rates of transport as they related to tumor growth behavior.

It is essential, at the outset, to ascertain the characteristics of the transport systems in the tissues to be examined and to establish procedures that are best suited for study of the selected substrates. While much of the characterizations were performed on ascites tumor cells, which have the obvious advantage of studying single cells without any intervention, information is needed on mammary tumors that grow as solid lesions. Methods to disperse solid tissues into dissociated cells invariably employ enzymatic digestions and caution is always required because of these experimental manipulations. Cells in culture also offer an experimental vehicle, but it is necessary to consider differences in transport rates that may arise attendant to growing vs. stationary cells. Thus, in order to gain an understanding of hormone action, the systems under study must be well characterized prior to perturbation by hormonal agents. Once these data are obtained and kinetically analyzed, it is then possible to attribute hormone-induced changes to alterations in carrier affinity (K_m), to the number of carriers (V_{max}), or both.

In an early report, Heuson and Legros (21) concluded that the insulin-stimulated increase in thymidine incorporation into explants of DMBA-induced tumors was not mediated by enhanced glucose uptake and utilization and concluded that growth stimulation and glucose utilization were dissociated. We examined this with a somewhat different approach (16). From a single animal made diabetic, the 3 DMBA-induced lesions present responded differently; one lesion regressed, one became static and the third continued to grow. From each tumor, cells were prepared, incubated with or without insulin (10^{-10}M), and glucose transport was measured. The data, shown in Table 3, indicate that insulin was able to stimulate glucose transport in the lesion that would be classified as insulin-dependent and was able to decrease glucose transport in the lesion classified as insulin-independent. It should also be noted that glucose transport in the absence of added insulin was related to the growth behavior of the lesion; the lowest transport was seen in the regressing lesion and the highest transport rate was seen in the growing lesion. The ability of insulin to apparently decrease glucose transport in some lesions is less surprising in light of the earlier mentioned findings of insulin treatment causing regression of some lesions *in vivo*. Since all three lesions arose from the same animal, the divergence of response would not likely be due to differences in the hormonal milieu. These results on glucose transport suggest that tumor growth behavior *in vivo* may be correlated with substrate entry.

TABLE 3
EFFECT OF INSULIN ON GLUCOSE TRANSPORT IN DMBA-INDUCED TUMORS

TUMOR GROWTH BEHAVIOR IN DIABETIC RAT	GLUCOSE TRANSPORT (pmoles/min per 10^6 cells)	
	Minus Insulin	Plus Insulin
REGRESSING	27.3	41.6
STATIC	31.2	25.8
GROWING	54.4	25.8

Carrier-mediated transport, v_1^c, was measured at 20°C with 1mM labeled 3-O-methyl glucose at 15 second intervals for 1 minute, during which time entry was linear.

A more detailed examination of glucose transport and the effects of insulin was performed with the R3230AC mammary carcinoma, which is a more uniform transplantable neoplasm. We prepared dissociated cells from the tumor and determined that the facilitated uptake of glucose was mediated by a carrier system that demonstrated saturability, substrate specificity, was inhibited by phloretin, was temperature sensitive, and gave a K_m for glucose transport 3 to 4mM (17). The effect of insulin (10^{-9}M) _in vitro_ was measured. Interestingly, glucose transport showed a decrease with time and a 2-fold increase in K_m. We next examined the time-course as related to insulin levels, ranging from 10^{-11} to 10^{-7}M, and observed that this was a dose-related response, with the greatest decreases in v_i occurring between 10^{-10} to 10^{-8}M insulin. When compared with insulin binding, it was apparent that there was a temporal relationship between hormone binding and effects on glucose transport, with the hormonal interaction preceding the response induced on transport. Thus, in at least two different mammary tumor models, DMBA-induced and R3230AC, insulin has the ability to decrease glucose transport, an action quite opposite to that seen in many normal tissues. Whether this action of insulin is peculiar to neoplastic tissues, or peculiar to these mammary neoplasms, remains to be determined.

The effects of insulin on entry of neutral amino acids has been studied in a variety of tissues. The mode of entry of neutral amino acids occurs by 3 transport carriers, the A, L, and ASC systems, which show overlapping specificities in their preferences for substrates. It is necessary, therefore, to first characterize the entry of selected substrates. This was done for the R3230AC carcinoma, using proline as a probe for the A system (28). We reported that proline transport was an active, Na^+-dependent process, was concentrative, saturable and sensitive to pH and metabolic inhibitors. Based on competition studies, we concluded that proline entry occurred by the A system, demonstrating a $K_m \sim 1$mM. The non-metabolizable amino acid analogue, α-aminoisobutyrate (AIB), has been extensively utilized as a probe for the A system, since it offers the advantage of not being influenced by subsequent metabolic events. We also examined AIB transport in R3230AC cells (29), and observed that there was more than one carrier for this probe. One system was Na-dependent, saturable, inhibited by α-methyl AIB and metabolic inhibitors, had a K_m of 1.75mM and comprised about 75% of the total AIB uptake. A second system was Na^+-independent, saturable, pH insensitive, inhibited by 2-aminobicyclo (2.2.1) heptane-2-carboxylate and had a K_m of 0.36mM for AIB. Thus, when AIB was used, entry into these tumor cells occurred by a carrier with properties of the A system as well as a carrier with properties of the L system. However, when cells from diabetic rats were studied, entry of AIB by the Na^+-dependent carrier A system was enhanced with no effect seen for entry of AIB by the Na^+-independent carrier (L-like system). This was also true for proline, but not leucine or phenylalanine, transport in cells from diabetic animals. Because of the duality of entry for AIB, we chose to use proline as the A system probe in future studies directed towards insulin action.

Since the R3230AC tumor grew faster in diabetic rats, and growth was retarded after insulin treatment, we examined the time course and dose response of insulin administration on proline and leucine transport (30). Transport of proline, which was elevated in tumors from diabetic rats, demonstrated a decrease relative to time after initiation of insulin treatment. A dose-response decrease was also observed. Leucine transport, measured on the same cell preparations, was unchanged. Curiously, when tumor cells from diabetic rats were exposed to insulin *in vitro*, we could demonstrate a stimulation of proline transport, first becoming apparent 5 hours after hormone exposure and increasing up to 9 hours. This response *in vitro* was dose-related and occurred over the physiological range. Leucine transport was unaffected. Interestingly, the effects of insulin *in vitro* were not manifested on tumor cells obtained from intact rats, and the response was blunted when studied in tumors from diabetic rats that had been treated with insulin *in vivo*. We proposed that these paradoxical effects of insulin *in vivo* versus *in vitro* may be due to the presence of other hormonal factors *in vivo*, which modulate the effects of insulin. Such differences between hormone actions *in vivo* and *in vitro* need to be resolved as well as extended to other tumor models.

II. FACILITATIVE EFFECTS OF INSULIN ON MAMMARY TUMORS

There have been many studies directed towards understanding the regulation of hormone receptors, particularly estrogen receptors (ER). It is now clear that the levels of ER can be modulated by hormones other than estrogens, themselves. Earlier studies implicated prolactin (39), (52), (59) progesterone (38) and thyroid hormone (43) as playing a role in regulation of ER.

In an earlier report, we (9) observed that ER levels were reduced in DMBA-induced tumors that regressed or became static after induction of diabetes, whereas tumors that continued to grow in diabetic rats contained approximately the same estrogen binding capacity as that seen in growing tumors from intact rats. We also found that in tumors from lergotrile-treated rats, an agent that effectively reduced prolactin secretion, the levels of ER were reduced even though many of these lesions continued to grow. Because of these findings, we wished to ascertain the effects of insulin administration on subsequent tumor growth and ER levels in diabetic rats bearing DMBA-induced neoplasms (10). The results pertaining to tumor growth responses were presented earlier (see I, A). Tumors regressing or becoming static after induction of diabetes had ER levels that were 20.3% and 21.6%, respectively, of those in growing tumors from intact rats (controls; average was 39fmoles/mg cytosol protein). Tumors that continued to grow in diabetic animals had somewhat lower ER levels (61.4% of control). When insulin was administered to tumor-bearing diabetic rats, tumors that had been regressing and then resumed growth contained ER levels that actually exceeded controls (average of 53fmoles/mg cytosol protein). Tumors that were growing in diabetic rats that continued to grow after insulin treatment did not demonstrate a difference in ER levels attributable to insulin administration. However, tumors that were growing in diabetic rats that regressed in response to administration of insulin demonstrated ER levels that were equal to the controls. Likewise, when growing tumors became static after insulin treatment, the ER levels were elevated to those seen in controls. The estimated K_d for the ER was comparable in all groups, ranging from 0.5 to 2.0 x 10^{-9}M. We concluded that cessation of tumor growth after induction of diabetes resulted in a reduction in ER and resumption of growth in response to insulin treatment was accompanied by an increase in ER levels that were equal to or greater than those in control (growing tumors in intact rats) animals. A most interesting observation was the increase in ER levels that occurred in tumors that regressed in response to insulin treatment, suggesting that the insulin-induced response in ER was independent of the tumor growth response. We proposed that insulin may play a role in regulation of ER (see Table 4).

TABLE 4
MODULATION OF ESTROGEN RECEPTOR LEVELS IN DMBA-INDUCED TUMORS BY DIABETES AND INSULIN TREATMENT

TUMOR GROWTH BEHAVIOR		ESTROGEN RECEPTOR LEVELS
DIABETIC	INSULIN TREATMENT	(fmoles/mg cytosol protein)
—	CONTROL (INTACT ANIMAL)	39.4 ± 3.8
GROWTH	-	24.2 ± 2.9
REGRESSION	-	8.5 ± 0.7
STATIC	-	8.0 ± 0.4
REGRESSION	GROWTH	52.8 ± 9.9
STATIC	GROWTH	58
STATIC	STATIC	10
GROWTH	REGRESSION	39.9 ± 6.0
GROWTH	STATIC	48
GROWTH	GROWTH	27.5 ± 10.5

Data presented as mean ± SEM from 4 to 18 tumors.

Due to the heterogeneity of DMBA-induced tumors, it is possible that the above results could be explained by changes in cell populations. Assuming at least two populations, one with high ER and a second with low or no ER, regression of lesions after diabetes could yield low ER-containing tumors if the cell population with high ER was diminished but was stimulated following insulin treatment and resumption of growth. For the tumors regressing after insulin treatment, it would be necessary to propose that the low ER-containing cells were preferentially diminished, leaving the high ER-containing cells in the regressing lesions. Obviously, additional experiments are required to provide further insight. It is interesting, however, that we observed a considerable reduction in ER levels in R3230AC tumors growing in diabetic rats, levels that were restored upon treatment with insulin (53). Further, we observed a modest increase in ER levels in R3230AC tumor cells in primary culture when exposed to insulin *in vitro*. Support for a role of insulin as a regulatory factor in estrogen responsiveness has come from Kirchick et al. (36) who found that the diabetic rat had a reduced sensitivity to estradiol, as reflected by a loss of pituitary LH surge, and from the work of Gentry et al. (8), who noted that nuclear uptake of labeled estradiol in the hypothalamus and pituitary was reduced in diabetic rats. Still another possibility is based on the findings of Smith et al. (56), who noted that prolactin binding was reduced in DMBA-induced tumors from diabetic rats; such an effect could impair the proposed stimulatory role of prolactin on ER. Regardless of the mechanisms, should insulin prove to have a regulatory role for ER, its use as a potentiator of estrogen therapy could be considered.

III. ESTROGEN-INSULIN INTERACTIONS

We have noted that estrogens may interfere with the action of insulin by decreasing insulin binding. Another possible site of action of estrogens is at the level of membrane transport, an action regulated by insulin. Our attention was initially drawn to this aspect by the work on glucose transport, in which facilitated carrier-mediated entry is known to be inhibitable by phloretin, which is weakly estrogenic. LeFevre (37) had extended this apparent relationship to other synthetic estrogens and reported that diethylstilbestrol was a potent inhibitor of glucose transport. We performed studies with R3230AC tumor cells in culture (7) to determine the effects of steroidal estrogens on glucose transport. These data demonstrated that estradiol-17β, estrone and estriol were capable of inhibiting carrier-mediated glucose transport, with estradiol-17β demonstrating the highest potency among the three steroids. In the same system, diethylstilbestrol was equal to or slightly more potent than phloretin as an inhibitor of glucose transport.

During our study of amino acid transport, we observed that estradiol was able to partially antagonize the stimulatory effects of insulin *in vitro*. We reported that ovariectomy resulted in enhanced proline transport, which was reduced after treatment with estrogens (31). The time course of this effect was somewhat similar to that seen earlier for insulin treatment. However, there was some question as to the specificity of the estrogen-induced response *in vivo*, since estrogen treatment appeared to cause a reduction in leucine transport as well as the inhibition of proline transport. To resolve this, we examined the effects of several estrogens *in vitro* on proline and leucine transport in dissociated R3230AC tumor cells (26). The ability of estradiol-17β to inhibit proline transport was both time- and dose-dependent. Kinetic analysis indicated that estradiol-17β acted as a non-competitive inhibitor, with an estimated K_i of ∿2μM. Diethylstilbestrol was similar in potency as estradiol-17β, but estrone, estriol and estradiol-17α were not as effective as inhibitors, with the estimated K_i in the range of 6 to 8μM. No effect on leucine transport was observed in the presence of 1μM levels of these estrogens, indicating the effect was specific for the A system. These effects, together with those on glucose transport, suggest that at pharmacological levels, estrogens may inhibit cell growth by interfering with substrate transport. This could offer a partial explanation for the therapeutic action of estrogens in treatment of breast cancer. Pertinent to this suggestion are the reports of inhibition of growth of estrogens of a human pituitary cell line (62) and the human breast cancer cell line, MCF-7 (60), observations that were seen at estradiol concentrations around 2μM. Caution is necessary, however, regarding the specificity of this response in neoplastic as well as normal tissues.

IV. INSULIN AND HUMAN BREAST CANCER

We have reviewed the literature on this subject (18) and cannot at this time offer many conclusions. This is due to discordance in the conclusions from the older epidemiological studies with those conducted more recently. There are reports (41),(42), using matched-pairs analysis, that suggest a higher incidence of diabetes in breast cancer patients compared to patients with benign breast disease. It would be most informative if studies of breast cancer incidence were examined in patients with juvenile onset diabetes vs. diabetes arising in the adult population. The fact that abnormal glucose tolerance was seen in many advanced disease breast cancer patients (3) is certainly indicative of an altered metabolism and insulin milieu, but its relationship to disease course is not known. In one interesting report, Rhomberg (49) observed that a higher percentage of diabetic breast cancer patients responded favorably to hormone therapy than seen in the non-diabetic cancer patients. Such a finding warrants a re-examination of diabetic patients treated by various therapeutic regimens to ascertain if this sub-group has a different response rate.

V. CONCLUSIONS

The multihormonal nature of breast cancer implies that a full understanding of the disease process requires elucidation of the role of numerous hormones, singly and as they interrelate to one another. There are now sufficient data from animal models to implicate a role for insulin; directly, as its actions to enhance substrate entry, protein and DNA synthesis would lead to enhanced cell growth and replication, and indirectly, as it may facilitate the actions of other hormones, such as by regulating receptor levels. Antagonism of the insulin stimulatory actions could account, at least in part, for the apparent efficacy of certain hormones, such as estrogens. The observation that pharmacological doses of insulin may inhibit tumor growth is interesting, may be somewhat reminiscent of the duality of actions known for estrogens, and requires that a mechanistic basis be found for such a paradoxical observation. The role of insulin in the human disease is not resolved and warrants attention.

Acknowledgement

The research presented from the author's laboratory was supported by USPHS Grant CA16660. The continued support of the University of Rochester Cancer Center (CA11198) and its Animal Tumor Research Facility is gratefully noted. I am most appreciative of the dedicated efforts of former and current students, fellows and technicians who have participated in this research. Typing of this manuscript was done by A. Stevenson.

REFERENCES

1. Bertoli A, DePirro R, Fusco A, Greco AV, Magnatta R, Lauro R. Differences in insulin receptors between men and menstruating women and influences of sex hormones on insulin binding during the menstrual cycle. J Clin Endocrinol Metab 50: 246-250, 1980.
2. Capeau J, Picard J, Caron M. Insulin receptors in Zajdela rat ascites hepatoma cells and their sensitivity to certain enzymes and lectins. Cancer Res 38: 3930-3937, 1978.
3. Carter AC, Lefkon BW, Farlin M, Feldman EB. Metabolic parameters in women with metastatic breast cancer. J Clin Endocrinol Metab 40: 260-264, 1975.
4. Cohen ND, Hilf R. Influence of insulin on growth and metabolism of 7, 12-dimethylbenz(a)anthracene-induced mammary tumors. Cancer Res 34: 3245-3252, 1974.
5. Cohen ND, Hilf R. Influence of insulin on estrogen-induced responses in the R3230AC mammary carcinoma. Cancer Res 35: 560-567, 1975.
6. Coppock DL, Covey LR, Straus DR. Growth response to insulin in mouse melanoma cells and fibroblast x melanoma hybrids. J Cell Physiol 105: 81-92, 1980.
7. Gay RJ, Hilf R. Paradoxical effects of 17β-estradiol on glucose transport in primary cell cultures of a rat mammary tumor. Biochem Biophys Res Comm 92: 1180-1188, 1980.
8. Gentry RT, Wade GN, Blauskin JD. Binding of [^{3}H]estradiol by brain cell nuclei and female rat sexual behavior: inhibition by experimental diabetes. Brain Res 135: 135-146, 1977.
9. Gibson SL, Hilf R. Influence of hormonal alteration of host on estrogen binding capacity in 7,12-dimethylbenz(a)anthracene-induced mammary tumors. Cancer Res 36: 3736-3741, 1976.
10. Gibson SL, Hilf R. Regulation of estrogen-binding capacity by insulin in 7,12-dimethylbenz(a)anthracene-induced mammary tumors in rats. Cancer Res 40: 2343-2348, 1980.
11. Goranson ES, Tilser GJ. Studies on the relationship of alloxan-diabetes and tumour growth. Cancer Res 15: 626-631, 1955.
12. Guidotti GG, Borghetti AF, Gazzola GC. The regulation of amino acid transport in animal cells. Biochim Biophys Acta 515: 329-366, 1978.
13. Hallowes RC, Rudland PS, Hawkins RA, Lewis DJ, Bennett D, Durbin H. Comparison of the effects of hormones on DNA synthesis in cell cultures of nonneoplastic and neoplastic mammary epithelium from rats. Cancer Res 37: 2492-2504, 1977.
14. Harmon JT, Hilf R. Identification and characterization of the insulin receptors in the R3230AC mammary adenocarcinoma of the rat. Cancer Res

36: 3993-4000, 1976.
15. Harmon JT, Hilf R. Insulin binding and glucose transport in the R3230AC mammary adenocarcinoma. J Supramol Structure 4: 223-240, 1976.
16. Harmon JT, Hilf R. Effect of insulin on glucose transport in DMBA-induced mammary tumors. Eur J Cancer 12: 933-934, 1976.
17. Harmon JT, Hilf R. Effect of insulin to decrease glucose transport in dissociated cells from the R3230AC mammary adenocarcinoma of diabetic rats. Biochim Biophys Acta 433: 114-125, 1976.
18. Harmon JT, Hilf R. Insulin and Mammary Cancer. pp 111-128, Vol. II in Influences of Hormones in Tumor Development, eds JA Kellen, R Hilf CRC Press, Boca Raton, Florida, 1979.
19. Hatanaka, M. Transport of sugars in tumor cell membranes. Biochim Biophys Acta 355: 77-104, 1974.
20. Heuson JC, Coune A, Heimann R. Cell proliferation induced by insulin in organ culture of the rat mammary carcinoma. Exp Cell Res 45: 351-360, 1967.
21. Heuson JC, Legros N. Study of the growth-promoting effect of insulin in relation to carbohydrate metabolism in organ culture of rat mammary carcinoma. Eur J Cancer 4: 1-7, 1968.
22. Heuson JC, Legros N. Effect of insulin and of alloxan diabetes on growth of the rat mammary carcinoma in Vivo. Eur J Cancer 6: 349-351, 1970.
23. Heuson, JC, Legros, N, Heimann, R. Influence of insulin administration of growth of the 7,12-dimethylbenz(a)anthracene-induced mammary carcinoma in intact, oophorectomized and hypophysectomized rats. Cancer Res 32: 233-238, 1972.
24. Hilf R. Milk-like fluid in a mammary adenocarcinoma: biochemical characterization. Science 155: 826-827, 1967.
25. Hilf R. Dose-time relationships in the effect of estrogens on mammary cancer. pp 11-16 in Reviews on Endocrine-related Cancer, ed BA Stoll, Imperial Chemical Industries, Ltd, Cheshire, England, 1979.
26. Hilf R, Helton DL. Inhibition of proline transport in R3230AC mammary carcinomas by estrogens in Vitro. Submitted for publication.
27. Hilf R, Michel I, Bell, C. Biochemical and morphological responses of normal and neoplastic mammary tissue to hormonal treatment. Recent Prog Horm Res 23: 229-295, 1967.
28. Hissin PJ, Hilf R. Characteristics of proline transport into R3230AC mammary tumor cells. Biochim Biophys Acta 508: 401-412, 1978.
29. Hissin PJ, Hilf R. α-Aminoisobutyrate transport into cells from the R3230AC Mammary adenocarcinoma. Evidence for a sodium-dependent and -independent carrier-mediated entry and effects of diabetes. Biochem J 176: 205-215, 1978.
30. Hissin PJ, Hilf R. Effects of insulin in Vivo and in Vitro on amino acid transport into cells from the R3230AC mammary adenocarcinoma and their relationship to tumor growth. Cancer Res 38: 3646-3655, 1978.
31. Hissin PJ, Hilf R. Effects of estrogens to alter amino acid transport in R3230AC mammary carcinomas and its relationship to insulin action. Cancer Res 39: 3381-3387, 1979.
32. Holdaway IM, Friesen HG. Hormone binding of human mammary carcinoma. Cancer Res 37: 1946-1952, 1977.

33. Holley RW. A unifying hypothesis concerning the nature of malignant growth. Proc Natl Acad Sci USA 69: 2840-2841, 1972.
34. Kahn CR. The role of insulin receptors and receptor antibodies in states of altered insulin action. Proc Soc Exptl Biol Med 162: 13-21, 1979.
35. Kahn R, Murray M, Pavelik J. Inhibition of proliferation of Cloudman 591 melanoma cells by insulin and characterization of some insulin resistant variants. J Cell Physiol 103: 109 119, 1980.
36. Kirchick HJ, Keyes PL, Frye BE. Etiology of anovulation in the immature alloxan-diabetic rat treated with pregnant mare's serum gonadotrophin: absence of the preovulatory luteinizing hormone surge. Endocrinology 102: 1867-1873, 1978.
37. LeFevre PG. Molecular structural factors in competitive inhibition of sugar transport. Science 130: 104-105, 1959.
38. Leung BS. Hormonal dependency of experimental breast cancer. pp 219-261 in Hormones, Receptors and Breast Cancer, ed WL McGuire, Raven Press, New York, 1978.
39. Leung BS, Sasaki GH. On the mechanism of prolactin and estrogen action in 7,12-dimethylbenz(a)anthracene-induced mammary carcinoma in rat. II. In vivo tumor responses and estrogen receptor. Endocrinology 97: 564-572, 1975.
40. Lewis DJ, Hallowes RC. Correlation between the effects of hormones on the synthesis of DNA in explants from induced rat mammary tumours and the growth of the tumours. J Endocrinol 62: 225-240, 1974.
41. Muck BR, Trotnow S, Egger H, Hommel G. Cancer of the breast, diabetes and pathological glucose tolerance. Arch Gynaekol 220: 73-81, 1975.
42. Muck BR, Trotnow S, Egger H, Hommel G. Altered carbohydrate metabolism in breast cancer and benign breast affections. Arch Gynaekol 221: 83-91, 1976.
43. Muldoon TG. Mouse mammary tissue estrogen receptors: ontogeny and molecular heterogeneity. pp 225-247 in Ontogeny of Receptors and Reproductive Hormone Action, eds TH Hamilton, JH Clark, WA Sadler, Raven Press, New York, 1979.
44. Osborne CK, Bolan ME, Lippman ME. Hormone responsive human breast cancer in long-term tissue culture: effect of insulin. Proc Natl Acad Sci USA 73: 4536-4540, 1976.
45. Osborne CK, Monaco ME, Lippman ME, Kahn CR. Correlations among insulin binding, degradation and biologic activity in human breast cancer cells in long term tissue culture. Cancer Res 38: 94-102, 1978.
46. Pasteels JL, Heuson JC, Heuson-Stiennon J, Legros N. Effects of insulin, prolactin, progesterone, and estradiol on DNA synthesis in organ culture of 7,12-dimethylbenz(a)anthracene-induced rat mammary tumors. Cancer Res 36: 2162-2170, 1976.
47. Pavelic K. Slijepcevic M, Pavelic J, Ivic J, Andy-Jurkovic S, Pavelic ZP, Boranic M. Growth and treatment of Ehrlich tumor in mice with alloxan-induced diabetes. Cancer Res 39: 1807-1813, 1979.
48. Puckett CL, Shingleton WW. The effect of induced diabetes on experimental tumor growth in mice. Cancer Res 32: 789-790, 1972.
49. Rhomberg W. Metastasierendes Mammakarzinom und Diabetes mellituseine prognostich gunstige Krankheits kombination. Dtsch Med Wochenschr 100:

2422-2427, 1975.
50. Rillema JA, Linebaugh BE. Characteristics of the insulin stimulation of DNA, RNA and protein metabolism in cultured human mammary carcinoma cells. Biochim Biophys Acta 475: 74-80, 1977.
51. Shafie SM. Estrogen and the growth of breast cancer: new evidence suggests indirect action. Science 209: 701-702, 1980.
52. Shafie SM, Brooks SC. Effect of prolactin on growth and the estrogen receptor level of human breast cancer cells (MCF-7). Cancer Res 37: 792-799, 1977.
53. Shafie SM, Gibson SL, Hilf R. Effect of insulin and estrogen on hormone binding in the R3230AC mammary adenocarcinoma. Cancer Res 37: 4641-4649, 1977.
54. Shafie SM, Hilf R. Relationship between insulin and estrogen binding to growth response in 7,12-dimethylbenz(a)anthracene-induced rat mammary tumors. Cancer Res 38: 759-764, 1978.
55. Shafie SM, Hilf R. Insulin receptor levels and magnitude of insulin-induced responses in 7,12-dimethylbenz(a)anthracene-induced mammary tumors in rats. Cancer Res 41: in press, 1981.
56. Smith RD, Hilf R, Senior AE. Prolactin binding to 7,12-dimethylbenz-(a)anthracene-induced mammary tumors and liver in diabetic rats. Cancer Res 37: 4070-4074, 1977.
57. Teller MN, Stock CC, Stohr G, Marker PC, Kaufman RJ, Escher GJ, Bowie M. Biological characteristics and chemotherapy of 7,12-dimethylbenz-(a)anthracene-induced tumors in rats. Cancer Res 26: 245-252, 1966.
58. Thomopoulos P, Roth J, Lovelace E, Pastan I. Insulin receptors in normal and transformed fibroblasts: relationship to growth and transformation. Cell 8: 417-423, 1976.
59. Vignon F, Rochefort H. Regulation of estrogen receptors in ovarian-dependent rat mammary tumors. I. Effects of castration and prolactin. Endocrinology 98: 722-729, 1976.
60. Weichselbaum RR, Little JB, Nove S, Hellman S, Piro AJ. Lack of selective killing by steroids in normal and malignant cells. J Cell Physiol 103: 429-433, 1980.
61. Welsch CN, deIturri GC, Brennan MJ. DNA synthesis of human, mouse and rat mammary carcinomas _in vitro_. Cancer 38: 1272-1281, 1976.
62. Wyche JH, Noteboom WD. Growth regulation of cultured human pituitary cells by steroidal and nonsteroidal compounds in defined medium. Endocrinology 104: 1765-1773, 1979.

Chapter 7

EFFECT OF THYROID HORMONES ON MAMMARY TUMOR INDUCTION AND GROWTH

Barbara K Vonderhaar

INTRODUCTION

Normal development (i.e., growth and differentiation) of the mammary gland is a complex process subject to the influence of many hormones including insulin, growth hormone, steroids, prolactin and thyroid hormones (100). In turn, each of these hormones has also been implicated in mammary tumorigenesis and development (48), (49), (63), (64), (82), (113), (114). Because of these multiple hormonal interactions as well as the ubiquitous role that thyroid hormones play in the body's overall metabolism, it is not at all surprising that there is confusion as to the role thyroid hormones may play in establishing and maintaining breast cancer. It has been established that altered thyroid status can affect the growth and maintenance of a variety of tumors in different organs (5), (53), (66), (67), suggesting an indirect or systemic mode of action. Whether the role of thyroid hormones in mammary tumorigenesis, if any, is solely indirect, or is mediated directly on the mammary tissue as well, remains to be clarified. Indeed, recent studies (10), (41), (91), (104), (105), (106) have clearly established a direct action of thyroid hormones on the development of the normal mammary gland. But whether an alteration in thyroid status affects mammary tumor risk as well as development and growth is not entirely clear.

EPIDEMIOLOGIC AND CLINICAL STUDIES

In humans, attempts to correlate breast cancer incidence with alterations in thyroid function have resulted in a variety of conflicting reports. The majority of epidemiologic and clinical evidence suggests that asymptomatic hypothyroidism, either secondary to iodine deficiency or to primary disease of the thyroid gland, may predispose to the development of breast cancer (70), (74). In areas of high incidence of endemic goiter in Australia, Belgium, Denmark, England, Holland, Mexico, Poland, Soviet Union, Switzerland, Thailand, USA and Wales increased mortality from breast cancer has been observed (21), (22), (70), (74). In contrast, in areas where endemic goiter is uncommon, such as Ceylon, Chile, Iceland, Japan and Venezuela, breast cancer mortality is low (9), (22), (70), (74). Endemic goiter may be due to increased thyroid stimulating hormone (TSH) secretion in response to the subclinical hypothyroidism which results from iodine deficiency (70). Thus Mittra and Hayward (70) compared the mean basal level of plasma TSH in 50 British women with early breast cancer and 50 women with advanced breast cancer with the levels detected in a group of 50 age-matched women who were in the hospital for a variety of conditions unrelated to the breast. They reported TSH levels 2 to 3 times higher in both breast cancer groups compared to controls. These investigators also reported (70), (71) that at 20 and 60 minutes after administration of thyrotropin releasing hormone (TRH) a significantly higher mean TSH response was obtained in the breast cancer groups. From this study the authors concluded that decreased thyroid function in breast cancer patients is primarily of thyroid and not of hypothalamic or pituitary origin and that increased susceptibility to mammary cancer is associated with the hypothyroid state. Consistent with this hypothesis, Itoh and Maruchi (42) observed a 5- to 6-fold increase in breast cancer incidence in Japanese women with Hashimoto's thyroiditis compared to the general population of Japan. Similar results were reported by Lender et al. (56) who found an increased incidence of both autoimmune thyroid disorders and mammary dysplasias in a group of diabetic women. However, others who studied circulating thyroid antibodies, thought to be indicative of Hashimoto's thyroiditis and Graves' disease, found no evidence that these autoimmune diseases are associated with an increased risk of breast cancer for British, American or Japanese women (72), (77).

Despite these conflicting reports, but supported by some experimental observations in rats (68), Mittra et al. (71) were prompted to suggest that a "suboptimal level of circulating thyroid hormones may abnormally sensitize mammary epithelial cells to prolactin stimulation, leading to dysplasia and eventual neoplasia." Experimental evidence to support this hypothesis in humans has been scant and contradictory. In addition to the reports cited above, several investigators (83), (85) have also found mean plasma TSH levels elevated in breast cancer patients compared to controls which appeared to worsen with progression of the disease. However, Adami (1) has reported that there was no significant change in thyroid function in women followed for up to 2 years after diagnosis of breast cancer as well as no differences between patients who developed recurring disease and those who did not. In addition, several other investigators (2), (60), (61) found no differences in mean TSH or thyroxine levels in women with breast cancer or benign breast disease compared to controls, or between British (high incidence group) and Japanese (low incidence group) women (52). And finally, in a carefully performed study reported by Aldinger et al. (3), the altered TSH and prolactin response to TRH in breast cancer patients was not found to be directly related to the presence of breast cancer, but rather was associated with a general pituitary dysfunction in the disease.

In direct contrast to the above observations is the report of Wanebo (110) which indicated that breast cancer patients have a higher incidence rate of hyperthyroidism. In addition, a controversial report (29), (39), (55), (59), (78), (87), (99), (103) by Kapdi and Wolfe (46) raised the question of increased breast cancer risk for women on thyroid therapy. They found that the incidence of breast cancer was twice as high in women taking thyroid hormones compared to matched women not on such medication. While it appeared that the odds of getting breast cancer associated with thyroid medication did not increase with age (59), their data clearly showed significantly more women in all age groups given thyroid supplements for more than 15 years developed the disease (99), (103). As emphasized by Kapdi and Wolfe (46), many of the women taking the thyroid hormones had been placed on the medication because of earlier hypothyroidism. Therefore, it is not clear whether the high breast cancer incidence is due to the thyroid supplements or the earlier hypothyroidism for which they were being treated. Moreover, the long latent period believed to occur between induction of human breast cancer and clinical presentation of the disease makes such interpretation difficult. While association of thyroid dysfunction with breast cancer does not necessarily prove a cause and effect relationship (109), it is quite reasonable to suggest that thyroid dysfunction and associated endocrine and metabolic imbalances at a critical period of mammary gland development are of primary importance in predisposing an individual to eventual development of breast cancer (101).

ANIMAL STUDIES

Mammary tumorigenesis

In an attempt to clarify the role of thyroid hormone imbalance in breast cancer development and growth, animal models must be employed. An association of altered thyroid function and mammary development and tumorigenesis has been studied primarily in rats and mice although several other species (20), (25), (30), (34), (41), (112) have also been examined.

Growth in culture of both mouse (40) and rat (92) as well as human (4) (11) cells derived from mammary tumors has been shown to increase with the addition of thyroid hormones to the culture medium. In addition, several studies using transplanted cells from established mammary tumor lines in both rats (13), (92) and mice (89), (90) have shown that physiological levels of thyroid hormones are necessary for establishing and growing the tumors *in vivo* and that hypothyroidism appears to retard tumor growth once established (89), (90), (92), thus increasing animal survival (89), (90). While these data suggest that established mammary tumors are dependent on thyroid hormones for growth, the published reports on the role of altered thyroid status in the *in vivo* induction of the mammary tumors in rodents, as in humans, is not clear. This lack of clarity arises, among other reasons, because these studies differ with regard to the manner in which altered thyroid status is achieved (i.e., hypothyroidism induced by iodine deficiency, ^{131}I treatment, thyroidectomy or treatment with goitrogens; hyperthyroidism induced by either injection or ingestion of T_3, T_4 or thyroid powder). The method of tumor induction frequently varies, with some studies examining "spontaneous" tumors in the mouse while others, both in mice and rats, utilizing chemical carcinogens such as 3-methylcholanthrene (3-MC), 7,12-dimethylbenz(α)anthracene (DMBA) or nitrosomethylurea (NMU). The time of initiation of the altered thyroid state in relation to the administration of a carcinogen likewise is not consistent. These latter two points are especially important as thyroid status is known to affect metabolism of some chemical carcinogens (7) and some of these agents, such as 3-MC (80) or NMU (50), increase the incidence of hypothyroidism in certain inbred strains of rats. In addition to the above difficulties, many authors have either not reported or not minimized the effects of altered thyroid status on the serum levels of other hormones, especially prolactin and estrogens, both of which play key roles in mammary tumorigenesis (63), (64), (82), (114). Nor have they always provided information on body weights and food and water consumption throughout the experiment. In some studies the number of animals was either not given or was too small to allow for meaningful interpretation of the data. Most striking in the rat studies, but not in those of mice, is the lack of any definition of the morphology of the mammary gland itself at the onset of the experiment or as a result of the alteration of thyroid status.

Thus, using rats as the model system, apparently similar experiments frequently gave different results. Several reports indicated that hypothyroidism induced either by ^{131}I treatment (17), (31), (32), iodine-deficient diets (17), (21), (23), propylthiouracil (PTU) treatment (21), (23), or thyroidectomy (33) resulted in increased incidence of DMBA-induced mammary tumors. Davidson (17) used ^{131}I treatment or iodine-deficient diets begun 4 weeks prior to DMBA treatment. These treatments resulted in 90% and 64% tumor incidence, respectively, compared to a 43% TI in controls. Although the authors state that these numbers are significant, the number of animals in the study was not given. They also concluded that the "increased incidence of breast cancer in rats treated with ^{131}I may be a consequence of radiation injury of breast tissue rather than the associated hypothyroidism" since the mammary gland (21), (98) and some mammary tumors (58) are known to concentrate iodide. Grice et al. (31) initially reported that ^{131}I treatment resulted in a 67% TI vs. a 42% TI for controls although neither the number of animals nor the timing of DMBA treatment relative to the onset of hypothyroidism was given. Subsequently they reported (32) no significant difference in TI for ^{131}I-treated rats, ^{131}I-treated animals given T_4 and controls.

Eskin and co-workers (21), (23) induced hypothyroidism by use of either low iodine diet or PTU 3 days before DMBA treatment. While there were very few animals in each group, all groups eventually had a 100% TI. The animals with impaired thyroid function, however, developed their tumors at a significantly faster rate. By contrast, when hypothyroidism was induced 3 days after administration of DMBA, there was no acceleration of tumor development, leading Eskin (21) to conclude that the effect of induced hypothyroidism may be on the "initiation" phase of tumorigenesis. Shellabarger (88) obtained completely opposite results. For this study hypothyroidism was induced by PTU given before and/or after DMBA. In the control group 11 of 22 animals developed tumors. When PTU was given for 15 days prior to DMBA, 17 of 22 developed tumors. The author states that this number is not significantly different from the control. When PTU treatment was begun at the time of DMBA administration and continued throughout the experiment, significantly fewer rats (3 of 22) developed tumors. When the PTU treatment was initiated 15 days prior to the carcinogen treatment and continued throughout the experiment, no animals developed tumors (0 of 22). These data prompted Shellabarger to suggest that "hypothyroidism does not interfere with the initiation phase of DMBA carcinogenesis but rather hypothyroidism inhibits the growth of mammary adenocarcinomas subsequent to their initiation." This concept is in agreement with the observations of Newman and Moon (81) in which animals given PTU 10 days prior to 3-MC treatment and then maintained in the hypothyroid state had significantly fewer tumors (67% TI) than did 3-MC-treated euthyroid animals (100% TI) or hypothyroid animals restored to the euthyroid state after 3-MC treatment (94% TI). However, in a subsequent report by Cave et al. (13) rats were injected 3 times with the carcinogen NMU over an 8-week period and 2 days after the last dose were made either mildly hypothyroid with PTU, hyperthyroid by ingestion of T_4 or maintained in the euthyroid state. When the animals were killed 3 months after the initial NMU dose, no differences in TI were seen among the 3 groups.

Eskin's studies using iodine-deficient diets to induce hypothyroidism resulted in animals whose growth rate throughout the experiment was similar to controls (21). However, the control animals were fed standard lab chow while the iodine-deficient group were on a specially formulated diet. In a similarly designed experiment reported by Cave et al. (14) using NMU-induced tumors, rats on an iodine-deficient diet had no greater tumor incidence or growth than did animals receiving an iodine-supplemented form of the same diet.

The work of Gruenstein et al. (33) points out another difficulty in selecting proper controls for studies on altered thyroid status. Rats were thyroidectomized 7 days prior to DMBA or 3-MC treatment. No significant difference in TI was observed between control (31%) and thyroidectomized (35%) animals treated with DMBA, while 3-MC-treated thyroidectomized animals showed only a 12% TI vs. a 74% TI in the control group. However, pair fed animals in both carcinogen studies showed even lower TI than the thyroidectomized animals (5% for DMBA and 0% for 3-MC), pointing out that dietary restrictions alone can strongly influence results. Severely impaired weight gains, dramatic loss of weight and restricted food intake similarly influence the interpretation of the studies of Jull and Huggins (45), Kellen (47) and Jabara and Maritz (43) which also indicate that hypothyroidism decreases mammary tumor incidence. Baker and Yaffe (6) also reported decreased TI in thyroidectomized animals treated with 3-MC. While they reported impaired food intake by the thyroidectomized animals, they also stated that there was no significant difference in tumor induction or survival time between euthyroid rats fed ad libitum or rats pair fed with the thyroidectomized animals. Both Helfenstein (37) and Cameron et al. (12) also reported that PTU (37) or thyroidectomy and/or ^{131}I-induced (12) hypothyroidism significantly reduced the incidence of DMBA-induced mammary tumors. In neither of these studies was information given on body weights of the animals.

Similar problems have arisen in studies attempting to assess the effects of hyperthyroidism in mammary tumorigenesis. Baker and Yaffe (6) reported that rats fed thyroid powder beginning one week before 3-MC treatment had a 36% TI vs. a 92% TI in control animals. These observations are consistent with the studies of Jull and Huggins (45) indicating that a low daily dose (0.5 mg) of T_4 did not change TI compared to control rats but that larger doses (1 mg/day) significantly reduced the tumor incidence. In neither experiment was food intake found to be a significant factor. Gruenstein et al. (33) also reported that treatment with thyroxine significantly reduced TI in 3-MC-treated rats while he found no significant difference in TI in control vs. T_4-treated animals given DMBA. By contrast, St. Gerard et al. (97) reported that T_3 administration begun 29 days prior to or simultaneous with 3-MC treatment and then continued throughout the experiment resulted in a significantly more rapid onset of tumors.

Perhaps the most definitive and best controlled experiments attempting to clarify the effects of altered thyroid status on induction and growth of mammary tumors in rats is that of Goodman et al. (28) using DMBA. In these studies moderate hypothyroidism was induced by PTU and in most cases the effects on body weight were minimized. When moderate hypothyroidism was induced prior to DMBA treatment and continued for 4 days after the carcinogen, the subsequent TI was not significantly different (89 of 116) from controls (81 of 115), thus suggesting that mild hypothyroidism does not affect mammary tumor induction. However, when PTU treatment was begun 4 days after DMBA treatment, significantly fewer animals developed tumors in the hypothyroid group (64 of 121) compared to the euthyroid controls (82 of 119). The observation prompted Goodman to conclude that "hypothyroidism does not enhance and may suppress promotion or growth of DMBA-induced cancer." Mild hypothyroidism, either PTU induced or resulting from iodine deficiency, did not affect the tumor latent period, histological appearance or estrogen dependence. When a severe hypothyroidism, which resulted in significantly lower body weights, was induced by PTU, only 7% of the animals subsequently developed tumors compared to 63% of the controls. Rats given the same PTU treatment but supplemented with T_3 and T_4 had body weights similar to controls and a 78% TI.

All studies on mammary tumorigenesis in the mouse are consistent with the observations of Goodman in the rat. Morris et al. (76) showed that ingestion of thiouracil (TU) by BALB/c mice infected with the mammary tumor virus (MMTV) by foster nursing on C3H dams resulted in a 20% decrease in body weight but no difference in survival. The hypothyroid animals did have relatively normal estrous cycles. However, no mammary tumors arose in 62 mice that ingested TU while 48% of 62 control animals developed tumors. The appearance of hyperplastic alveolar nodules (HAN) believed to be precursors of mouse mammary tumors (18) correlated with this observation as only 2 of the 62 hypothyroid animals compared to 25 of 62 controls had HAN. When young C3H mice which carry the endogenous MMTV were placed on TU at 9-10 weeks of age, their body weights were significantly different from those of controls by 8 months of age and their estrous cycles became very irregular (20). Only 19% of these 52 severely hypothyroid animals developed mammary tumors after 1 1/2 years while 92% of the 53 controls had tumors. HAN were reduced in number and size, thus confirming the observations of Vasquez-Lopez (102). A significant difference in body weight was not observed when fully developed 11-month-old C3H mice were placed on a TU-containing diet (75). While all of these animals did eventually develop tumors, the appearance of the tumors was significantly delayed compared to controls.

A similar delay in the onset of appearance of "spontaneous" mammary tumors was observed in mildly hypothyroid primiparous mice (108). Mature lactating mice were made either hypothyroid (by ingestion of TU), hyperthyroid (by ingestion of T_4) or maintained as euthyroid at the time that the pups were removed. The animals were maintained in the various thyroid states for one year during which time tumor development was examined. The involuted mammary glands of all three groups were morphologically indistinguishable from each other 10 weeks after removal of the pups even though significant changes in serum T_3 and T_4 levels were observed at this time. These changes were not accompanied by significant alterations in serum PRL levels and the animals maintained normal estrous cycles. However, at the end of one year over 96% of the euthyroid and hyperthyroid animals developed tumors while only 72% of hypothyroid animals had tumors. The mean latent days for the hyperthyroid and euthyroid groups were 237 and 242 days, respectively, while 50% tumor incidence was not reached until 290 days in the hypothyroid group. The reduction in TI in hypothyroid animals correlated with the appearance of HAN. At 12 weeks post-lactation 14 of 20 hypothyroid animals had HAN compared to 20 of 20 euthyroid mice. The average number of HAN was 8.8 for hypothyroid and 14.9 for euthyroid.

Marked decreases in plasma levels of T_3 and T_4 without changes in the estrous cycle, ovarian structure, prolactin levels, body weights, anterior pituitary weight and adrenals were achieved by Nagasawa <u>et al</u>. (79) by giving mice potassium thiocyanate (KSCN) in their drinking water. In the high mammary tumor incidence SHN strain of mice, administration of KSCN resulted in the dose-related inhibition of the number of HAN as well as incidence of mammary tumors. The incidence and number of pregnancy-dependent mammary tumors in GR/A mice were also significantly suppressed by KSCN with no apparent influence on reproduction or the levels of prolactin and growth hormone. Thus it is becoming clear that under conditions where altered thyroid status has minimal effects on the growth of the animals and does not dramatically alter the levels of other hormones, particularly prolactin and the ovarian steroids, effects on mammary tumorigenesis occur. In the mouse and probably in the rat as well, hypothyroidism can result in reduced mammary tumor incidence. In the mouse such reduced TI occurs even with mild hypothyroidism. In the rat, while mild hypothyroidism may have little or no effect (28), severe hypothyroidism can lead to decreased TI, suggesting a greater sensitivity of mouse mammary glands to thyroid hormones.

Normal mammary gland development

By understanding the role of thyroid hormones in normal development of the mammary gland considerable insight can be gained into the mechanism by which they affect mammary tumorigenesis. It is clear that thyroid hormones are not absolutely essential for ductal growth in the mouse but alveolar development requires normal thyroid function. Conflicting reports in the literature make the situation in the rat unclear.

Using C3H mice or BALB/c mice foster nursed on C3H dams, Morris and coworkers (19), (76) clearly showed that the initiation of severe hypothyroidism by TU treatment begun at an early age resulted in a drastic arrest in mammary gland development. Lateral budding of mammary ducts was greatly reduced and no alveoli were observed even after one year.

The hypothyroidism thus induced resulted in TU-treated animals which weighed on the average 20% less than controls and had highly irregular and infrequent estrous cycles. This prompted Dubnik et al. (19) to suggest that the effects on mammary development were due to "creation of a hormonal imbalance initiated by the inability of the thyroid gland to secrete thyroxine under the influence of thiouracil; followed by a compensatory oversecretion of thyrotrophin by the pituitary gland and a concomitant undersecretion of other trophic hormones." This concept was supported by the work of Flux (24) who reported increased mammary duct growth in ovariectomized animals treated with TSH and growth hormone. Thus an indirect or systemic action of thyroid hormones may explain their observations. However, the work of Vonderhaar and Greco (107) also showed a lack of alveolar development with lateral ductal branching in C3H mice made mildly hypothyroid at weaning. Animals made hyperthyroid showed a greater degree of ductal branching and extensive alveolar development compared to euthyroid controls of a similar age. Under these conditions of mild alteration of thyroid status, animals had normal estrous cycles, body weights were not significantly different from controls and circulating levels of prolactin were not altered. Very similar results were obtained by Nagasawa et al. (79) using chronic treatment with KSCN to induce very mild hypothyroidism in SHN mice. These latter reports suggest that at least in the mouse, while altered thyroid status may indeed affect levels of other mammotropic hormones, the thyroid hormones themselves may also play a principal and direct role in mammary gland development.

In the rat it is less clear if thyroid hormones play a direct as well as indirect or systemic role in mammary gland development. In addition, confusion exists as to whether thyroid hormones have a negative or positive influence. In 1941 Leonard and Reece (57) reported that the mammary glands of young female rats, examined 54 days after thyroidectomy, on the whole showed some increased thickening and extension of the ductal system and in most cases greater development of lateral and end buds as well as alveoli than did those of the controls. In addition, they found that thyroidectomy favored a better mammary development in either castrated or estrogen (E_2)-injected castrated rats when compared with the appropriate controls. The injection of thyroxine (T_4) after thyroidectomy countered these effects. However, Smithcors (95) was unable to repeat these results when rats were made hypothyroid by injections of the goitrogen thiouracil (TU). He reported that even in castrated female rats, TU-treatment failed to alter mammary gland development. Using male rats as a model, Smithcors and Leonard (96) reported decreased ductal extension and increased development of the lobulo-alveolar system after thyroidectomy. This effect was intensified when thyroidectomy was coupled with castration and E_2-treatment. These data suggested that the hypothyroid state increases the sensitivity of the mammary glands of rats to estrogens (57) at least in terms of alveolar development.

The effects of altered thyroid status in relation to prolactin (PRL), as well as to the ovarian steroids, were explored by several investigators. Meites and Kragt (65) reported that PRL-induced alveolar development in the mammary glands of immature hypophysectomized rats receiving a pituitary transplant under the kidney capsule was abolished when the animals were simultaneously treated with T_4. An antagonism between PRL and T_4, similar to that between E_2 and T_4, was reported by Mittra (68), (69). He found that in E_2-primed rats, thyroidectomy induced a marked stimulation of mammary alveolar development which was suppressed by replacement doses of thyroxine. In addition, he reported that when E_2-treated thyroidectomized rats were given 2-bromo-α-ergocryptine (CB154) to reduce PRL secretion, mammary gland development was suppressed compared to E_2-treated thyroidectomized controls. He also reported that elevation of PRL levels by perphenazine injections resulted in enhanced alveolar development in E_2-treated animals which was further increased by thyroidectomy. These data led Mittra (68) to suggest that in the absence of thyroid hormones, in addition to increased sensitivity of the gland to E_2 (57), the mammotropic effect of a normal level of endogenous PRL is markedly increased and that further stimulation occurs when the PRL level is raised by pharmacological means.

However, apparently contradictory reports have also been published by several authors. Schmidt and Moger (86) and Kumaresan and Turner (54) reported that thyroxine treatment throughout pregnancy, when PRL levels are elevated, had a stimulatory effect on mammary gland growth. Jacobsohn (44) reported that while mild hyperthyroidism induced by T_4 treatment alone in hypophysectomized rats had no effect on mammary gland development, simultaneous injection of T_4 and E_2 to hypophysectomized animals did increase end bud development and total area of epithelial growth. These observations were supported by the studies of Moon and Turner (73) who suggested that "thyroid hormone may be a limiting factor in mammary gland growth when estrogen and progesterone secretions are adequate, but when the thyroid secretion rate is optimal, estrogen and progesterone secretion may limit growth." Thus alterations in the levels of thyroid hormones themselves (either up or down) without changes in other hormones may directly affect the <u>sensitivity</u> of the mammary gland to these hormones. This appears to be especially true in the mouse whose mammary glands appear to be more responsive to changes in thyroid hormone levels than are the glands of rats. However, when the manipulation of thyroid status is accompanied by a change in levels of other hormones, then the <u>balance</u> between thyroid hormones and the mammotropic agents such as PRL and the ovarian steroids becomes overriding.

This concept of hormonal balance was tested directly by Singh and Bern (91) who examined the influence of changes in the ratio of PRL to T_4 on growth of the mouse mammary gland in organ culture. Using whole glands from estrogen-progesterone-primed immature mice, both positive and negative effects of thyroid hormones on lobulo-alveolar development could be demonstrated. In the presence of optimal concentrations of insulin and aldosterone and 5 μg PRL per ml, T_4 at low concentrations had no effect while higher concentrations (2-5 μg/ml) resulted in less lobulo-alveolar development than in the same medium without T_4. However, when cultures were maintained in media containing suboptimal (3 μg/ml) or low (1 μg/ml) amounts of PRL, lower levels of T_4 (0.01-0.5 μg/ml) enhanced PRL-induced development whereas greater amounts (1-5 μg/ml) inhibited growth. Using a similar culture system, Warner (111) found that in the absence of PRL and ovarian steroids, thyroxine at 5 μg/ml could not promote lobulo-alveolar development. When PRL only was omitted but E_2 and progesterone were present, intermediate levels of growth were obtained in the presence of T_4. Maximal differentiation was obtained in media containing T_4, PRL, E_2 and progesterone in addition to insulin, growth hormone and aldosterone.

POSSIBLE MECHANISMS

The systemic effects of thyroid hormones on mammary gland development may be exerted through alterations in circulating levels of mammotropic hormones. Thyroid hormones are known to affect the metabolism, secretion and clearance rates of estrogens in serum as well as play a role in determining what proportion of the total steroid concentration circulating in the blood is protein-bound (38), (51). In addition, severe hypothyroidism frequently results in elevated serum PRL levels. However, in rats, Cave *et al.* (14), (15) have clearly shown that this increase does not represent an alteration in pituitary PRL synthesis, but rather decreased clearance of the hormone from the serum.

The mechanism by which thyroid hormones directly act on mammary tissue is also becoming clear. Studies using mouse mammary tissue in organ culture have shown that physiological concentrations of T_3 added to serum-free medium resulted in increased sensitivity of the tissue to E_2 (10) and to PRL (8), (105). At physiological concentrations of PRL, T_3 is essential for E_2-stimulation of both lactose synthetase activity and casein synthesis in mid-pregnancy mammary explants (10). In the absence of T_3 no effect of E_2 on differentiation is demonstrable. T_3 also increases the responsiveness of mouse mammary glands to PRL, resulting in increased lactose synthetase activity *in vitro* (8), (105). When explants from glands of adult virgin mice were cultured in the presence of optimal levels of insulin and hydrocortisone and various concentrations of PRL, lactose synthetase activity in tissues from hyperthyroid animals was induced at PRL concentrations as low as 0.01 μg per ml. Euthyroid tissue required at least 0.05 μg per ml while induced activity was not observed in hypothyroid tissue until PRL concentrations were at least 0.1 μg per ml. In the presence of 10^{-9} M L-T_3, all tissues responded to PRL concentrations as low as 0.01 μg per ml (8). Similar cultures of mid-pregnancy mammary glands resulted in consistent induction of lactose synthetase activity at 10^{-3} μg PRL per ml in the absence of thyroid hormones. Only 10^{-4} μg per ml were required when T_3 was also present in the culture medium.

One explanation for these results *in vitro* is that thyroid hormones modulate either the number of or affinity characteristics of the E_2 and PRL receptors. Although the concentration of cytoplasmic estrogen receptors in uterus, hypothalamus and anterior pituitary is modulated by alterations in thyroid status (16), the retention of E_2-receptor complexes by uterine nuclei is not affected (26). A recent report by Reimer *et al.* (84) has attempted to correlate estrogen receptor status of human breast cancers with the patients' TSH levels. They found that the frequency of detectable TSH is significantly greater in patients with estrogen receptor positive breast cancer than in their receptor negative counterparts (87% vs. 57%). Several laboratories have reported that the level of PRL binding in several target tissues in rats varies with alterations in the circulating levels of thyroid hormones (27), (35), (62), (94). In both rats (35) and mice (8), the level of PRL binding to mammary gland membranes is also exquisitely sensitive to _in vivo_ alterations in thyroid hormone levels. Thyroid hormones are also able to induce PRL receptor activity _in vitro_. When mammary gland explants from mid-pregnant mice were cultured overnight in the presence of insulin, hydrocortisone and 10^{-9} M L-T_3, a 60-80% increase in PRL binding to membranes was seen compared to similarly prepared membrane from explants cultured in the presence of insulin and hydrocortisone alone (8). Whether such regulation of PRL receptors exists in hormonally responsive mammary tumors is not known. One report (94) has shown that PRL binding to membranes of DMBA-induced tumors in rats made mildly hypo- or hyperthyroid was not significantly different from the level of binding to tumors from euthyroid rats. However, the authors did not make it clear that the particular tumors studied were indeed PRL dependent, and the failure to see a difference could be due to the fact that thyroid status alterations were begun after the DMBA tumors were well established. No such studies have yet been reported using human tissue or human breast cancer cell lines. The recent demonstration of the presence of thyroid hormone receptors in human breast cells (11) (93), similar to those reported in normal rat breast tissue (36), offers the possibility that such a mechanism of receptor modulation operates in the human tissue as well.

REFERENCES

1. Adami HO, Hansen J, Rimsten A, Wide L. Thyroid function in breast cancer patients before and up to two years after mastectomy. Upsala J Med Sci 84: 228-234, 1979.
2. Adami HO, Rimsten A, Thoren L, Vegelius J, Wide L. Thyroid disease and function in breast cancer patients and non-hospitalized controls evaluated by determination of TSH, T_3, rT_3 and T_4 levels in serum. Acta Chir Scand 144: 89-97, 1978.
3. Aldinger KA, Schultz PN, Blumenschein GR, Samaan NA. Thyroid-stimulating hormone and prolactin levels in breast cancer. Arch Intern Med 138: 1638-1641, 1978.
4. Allegra JC, Lippman ME. Growth of a human breast cancer cell line in serum-free hormone-supplemented medium. Cancer Res 38: 3823-3829, 1978.
5. Aoki N, Wakisaka G, Nagata I. Effects of thyroxine on T-cell counts and tumor cell rejection in mice. Acta Endocrinol 81: 104-109, 1976.
6. Baker DG, Yaffe AH. The influence of thyroid stimulation on the incidence of 3-methylcholanthrene-induced tumors. Cancer Res 35: 528-530, 1975.
7. Bather R, Franks WR. Further studies on the role of thyroxine in chemical carcinogenesis. Cancer Res 12: 247-248, 1952.
8. Bhattacharya A, Vonderhaar BK. Thyroid hormone regulation of prolactin binding to mouse mammary glands. Biochem Biophys Res Commun 88: 1405-1411, 1979.

9. Bogardus GM, Finley JW. Breast cancer and thyroid disease. Surgery 49: 461-468, 1961.
10. Bolander FF Jr, Topper YJ. Stimulation of lactose synthetase activity and casein synthesis in mouse mammary explants by estradiol. Endocrinology 106: 490-495, 1980.
11. Burke RE, McGuire WL. Nuclear thyroid hormone receptors in a human breast cancer cell line. Cancer Res 38: 3769-3773, 1978.
12. Cameron H, Owen J, Thomas CG Jr. Further studies on the effects of hypothyroidism on the incidence of DMBA induced breast cancer in Sprague-Dawley rats. Proc Am Assoc Cancer Res 11: 14, 1970.
13. Cave WT Jr, Dunn JT, MacLeod RM. Effects of altered thyroid states on mammary tumor growth and pituitary gland function in rats. J Natl Cancer Inst 59: 993-999, 1977.
14. Cave WT Jr, Dunn JT, MacLeod RM. Effects of iodine deficiency and high-fat diet on N-nitrosomethylurea-induced mammary cancers in rats. Cancer Res 39: 729-734, 1979.
15. Cave WT Jr, Paul MA. Effects of altered thyroid function on plasma prolactin clearance. Endocrinology 107: 85-91, 1980.
16. Cidlowski JA, Muldoon TG. Modulation by thyroid hormones of cytoplasmic estrogen receptor concentrations in reproductive tissues of the rat. Endocrinology 97: 59-67, 1975.
17. Davidson A, Owen J, Thomas CG Jr. Further studies on the role of altered thyroid function on experimentally induced breast cancer in Sprague-Dawley rats. Proc Am Assoc Cancer Res 10: 17, 1969.
18. DeOme KB, Faulkin LJ, Bern HA, Blair PB. Development of mammary tumors from hyperplastic alveolar nodules transplanted into gland-free mammary fat pads of female C3H mice. Cancer Res 19: 515-520, 1959.
19. Dubnik CS, Morris HP, Dalton AJ. Inhibition of mammary-gland development and mammary-tumor formation in female C3H mice following ingestion of thiouracil. J Natl Cancer Inst 10: 815-841, 1950.
20. El Etreby MF. Thyroid function in the dog and its possible relationship to mammary tumorigenesis. Pharmac Ther 5: 403-405, 1979.
21. Eskin BA. Iodine metabolism and breast cancer. Trans NY Acad Sci 32: 911-947, 1970.
22. Eskin BA. Iodine and mammary cancer. pp 293-304 in <u>Inorganic and Nutritional Aspects of Cancer</u>, ed GN Schrauzer, Plenum Press, New York, 1977.
23. Eskin BA, Murphey SA, Dunn MR. Induction of breast cancer in altered thyroid states. Nature 218: 1162, 1968.
24. Flux DS. The growth-stimulating effect of growth hormone and L-thyroxine on the mammary glands and uterus of the mouse. J Endocrinol 15: 266-272, 1957.
25. Frank DW, Kirton KT, Murchison TE, Quinlan WJ, Coleman ME, Gilbertson TJ, Feenstra ES, Kimball FA. Mammary tumors and serum hormones in the bitch treated with medroxyprogesterone acetate or progesterone for four years. Fertil and Steril 31: 340-346, 1979.
26. Gardner RM, Kirkland JL, Ireland JS, Stancel GM. Regulation of the uterine response to estrogen by thyroid hormone. Endocrinology 103: 1164-1172, 1978.

27. Gelato M, Marshall S, Boudreau M, Bruni J, Campbell GA, Meites J. Effects of thyroid and ovaries on prolactin binding activity in rat liver. Endocrinology 96: 1292-1296, 1975.
28. Goodman AD, Hoekstra SJ, Marsh PS. Effects of hypothyroidism on the induction and growth of mammary cancer induced by 7,12-dimethylbenz(a)anthracene in the rat. Cancer Res 40: 2336-2342, 1980.
29. Gorman CA, Becker DV, Greenspan FS, Levy RP, Oppenheimer JH, Rivlin RS, Robbins J, VanderLaan WP. Breast cancer and thyroid therapy. JAMA 237: 1459-1460, 1977.
30. Gorski J. Endocrine factors in genetic improvement of milk production. J Dairy Sci 62: 814-817, 1979.
31. Grice OD, Faircloth S, Thomas CG Jr. The effect of hypothyroidism on induced cancer of the breast. Proc Am Assoc Cancer Res 7: 26, 1966.
32. Grice OD, Faircloth S, Thomas CG Jr. The effect of hypothyroidism on induced cancer of the breast---further observations. Proc Am Assoc Cancer Res 8: 23, 1967.
33. Gruenstein H, Meranze DR, Acuff M, Shimkin MB. The role of the thyroid in hydrocarbon-induced mammary carcinogenesis in rats. Cancer Res 28: 471-474, 1968.
34. Hart IC, Morant SV. Role of prolactin, growth hormone, insulin and thyroxine in steroid-induced lactation in goats. J Endocrinol 84: 343-351, 1980.
35. Hayden TJ, Bonney RC, Forsyth IA. Ontogeny and control of prolactin receptors in the mammary gland and liver of virgin, pregnant and lactating rats. J Endocrinol 80: 259-269, 1979.
36. Hayden TJ, Forsyth IA. Thyroid hormone binding in rat mammary gland. J Endocrinol 75: 38P-39P, 1977.
37. Helfenstein JE, Young S, Currie AR. Effect of thiouracil on the development of mammary tumors in rats induced with 9,10-dimethyl-1,2-benzanthracene. Nature 196: 1108, 1962.
38. Hembree WC, VandeWiele RL. Female reproductive system. pp 757-772 in The Thyroid: a Fundamental and Clinical Text, eds SC Werner, SH Ingbar, Harper and Row, Publishers, Inc, Hagerstown Maryland, 1978.
39. Hodges RE. Thyroid supplements and breast cancer. JAMA 236: 2743, 1976.
40. Hosick HL, Nandi S. Preliminary survey of hormonal influences on multicellular architecture in primary cultures of mammary carcinoma cells. J Natl Cancer Inst 52: 897-902, 1974.
41. Houdebine LM, DeLouis C, Devinoy E. Post-transcriptional stimulation of casein synthesis by thyroid hormone. Biochimie 60: 809-812, 1978.
42. Itoh K, Maruchi N. Breast cancer in patients with Hashimoto's thyroiditis. Lancet 1: 1119-1121, 1975.
43. Jabara AG, Maritz JS. Effects of hypothyroidism and progesterone on mammary tumours induced by dimethylbenz(a)anthracene in Sprague-Dawley rats. Br J Cancer 28: 161-172, 1973.
44. Jacobsohn D. Effects of thyroxine on growth of mammary glands, whole body, heart and liver in hypophysectomized rats treated with insulin, cortisone and ovarian steroids. Acta Endocrinol (Kbh) 35: 107-134, 1960.

45. Jull JW, Huggins C. Influence of hyperthyroidism and of thyroidectomy on induced mammary cancer. Nature 188: 73, 1960.
46. Kapdi CC, Wolfe JN. Breast cancer: Relationship to thyroid supplements for hypothyroidism. JAMA 236: 1124-1127, 1976.
47. Kellen JA. Effect of hypothyroidism on induction of mammary tumors in rats by 7,12-dimethylbenz(a)anthracene. J Natl Cancer Inst 48: 1901-1904, 1972.
48. Kelsey JL. A review of the epidemiology of human breast cancer. Epidemiologic Reviews 1: 74-109, 1979.
49. Ketcham AS, Sindelar WF. Risk factors in breast cancer. Prog Clin Cancer 6: 99-114, 1975.
50. Kieffer JD, Vickery AL Jr, Ridgway EC, Mover H, Kern K, Maloof F. Induction of breast cancer by nitrosomethylurea in rats of the Buffalo strain: frequent association with thyroid disease. Endocrinology 107: 1218-1225, 1980.
51. Kirschner MA. The role of hormones in the etiology of human breast cancer. Cancer 39: 2716-2726, 1977.
52. Kumaoka S, Takatani O, Abe O, Utsunomiya J, Wang DY, Bulbrook RD, Hayward JL, Greenwood FC. Plasma prolactin, thyroid-stimulating hormone, follicle-stimulating hormone and luteinizing hormone in normal British and Japanese women. Eur J Cancer 12: 767-774, 1976.
53. Kumar MS, Chiang T, Deodhar SD. Enhancing effect of thyroxine on tumor growth and metastases in syngeneic mouse tumor systems. Cancer Res 39: 3515-3518, 1979.
54. Kumaresan P, Turner CW. Effect of various hormones on mammary gland growth of pregnant rats. Endocrinology 78: 396-399, 1966.
55. Lender M, Hardt N, Paloyan E, Lawrence AM. Thyroid supplements and breast cancer. JAMA 236: 2743, 1976.
56. Lender M, Lawrence AM, Paloyan E. Diabetes, autoimmune thyroid disease, and breast cancer. Lancet 1: 1110, 1977.
57. Leonard SL, Reece RP. The relation of the thyroid to mammary gland growth in the rat. Endocrinology 28: 65-69, 1941.
58. Lyttle CR, Thorpe SM, DeSombre ER, Daehnfeldt JL. Peroxidase activity and iodide uptake in hormone-responsive and hormone-independent GR mouse mammary tumors. J Natl Cancer Inst 62: 1031-1034, 1979.
59. MacCornack FA. Thyroid hormone and breast cancer. JAMA 238: 1147, 1977.
60. MacFarlane IA, Robinson EL, Bush H, Durnings P, Howat JMT, Beardwell CG, Shalet SM. Thyroid function in patients with benign and malignant breast disease. Br J Cancer 41: 478-480, 1980.
61. Malarkey WB, Schroeder LL, Stevens VC, James AG, Lanese RR. Twenty-four-hour preoperative endocrine profiles in women with benign and malignant breast disease. Cancer Res 37: 4655-4659, 1977.
62. Marshall S, Bruni JF, Meites J. Effects of hypophysectomy, thyroidectomy, and thyroxine on specific prolactin receptor sites in kidneys and adrenals of male rats. Endocrinology 104: 390-395, 1979.
63. McGuire WL, Chamness GG, Costlow ME. Hormone dependence in breast cancer. Metabolism 23: 75-100, 1974.

64. Meites J. Relation of prolactin and estrogen to mammary tumorigenesis in the rat. J Natl Cancer Inst 48: 1217-1224, 1972.
65. Meites J, Kragt CL. Effects of a pituitary homotransplant and thyroxine on body and mammary growth in immature hypophysectomized rats. Endocrinology 75: 565-570, 1964.
66. Mishkin S, Morris HP, Yalovsky MA, Murthy PVN. Increased survival of rats bearing Morris hepatoma 7800 after induction of hypothyroidism. Cancer Res 39: 2371-2375, 1979.
67. Mishkin S, Morris HP, Yalovsky MA, Murthy PVN. Inhibition of the growth of Morris hepatoma # 44 in rats after induction of hypothyroidism: evidence that Morris hepatomas are thyroid dependent. Gastroenterology 77: 547-555, 1979.
68. Mittra I. Mammotropic effect of prolactin enhanced by thyroidectomy. Nature 248: 525-526, 1974.
69. Mittra I. Potency of thyroid hormone analogues in suppressing prolactin-mediated mammary growth in thyroidectomized rats. Experientia 31: 1218-1221, 1975.
70. Mittra I, Hayward JL. Hypothalamic-pituitary-thyroid axis in breast cancer. Lancet 1: 885-889, 1974.
71. Mittra I, Hayward JL, McNeilly AS. Hypothalamic-pituitary-prolactin axis in breast cancer. Lancet 1: 889-891, 1974.
72. Mittra I, Perrin J, Kumaoka S. Thyroid and other autoantibodies in British and Japanese women: an epidemiological study of breast cancer. Br Med J 1: 257-259, 1976.
73. Moon RC, Tuner CW. Thyroid hormone and mammary gland growth in the rat. Proc Soc Exp Biol Med 103: 149-151, 1960.
74. Moossa AR, Evans DA, Brewer AC. Thyroid status and breast cancer. Ann R Coll Surg Engl 53: 178-188, 1973.
75. Morris HP, Dubnik CS, Dalton AJ. Effect of prolonged ingestion of thiourea on mammary glands and the appearance of mammary tumors in adult C3H mice. J Natl Cancer Inst 7: 159-169, 1946.
76. Morris HP, Green CD, Dalton AJ. The effect of ingestion of thiouracil on strain C mice. J Natl Cancer Inst 11: 805-815, 1950.
77. Munoz JM, Gorman CA, Elveback LR, Wentz JR. Incidence of malignant neoplasms of all types in patients with Graves' disease. Arch Intern Med 138: 944-947, 1978.
78. Mustacchi P, Greenspan F. Thyroid supplementation for hypothyroidism. An iatrogenic cause of breast cancer? JAMA 237: 1446-1447, 1977.
79. Nagasawa H, Yanai R, Nakajima Y, Namiki H, Kikuyama S, Shiota K. Inhibitory effects of potassium thiocyanate on normal and neoplastic mammary development in female mice. Eur J Cancer 16: 473-480, 1980.
80. Newman WC, Moon RC. Effect of 3-methylcholanthrene on thyroid function in Sprague-Dawley rats. Cancer Res 26: 1938-1942, 1966.
81. Newman WC, Moon RC. Chemically induced mammary cancer in rats with altered thyroid function. Cancer Res 28: 864-868, 1968.
82. Pearson OH, Llerena O, Llerena L. Prolactin-dependent rat mammary cancer: a model for man? Trans Assoc Am Physicians 82: 225-238, 1969.
83. Perry M, Goldie DJ, Self M. Thyroid function in patients with breast cancer. Ann R Col Surg of Engl 60: 290-293, 1978.

84. Reimer R, Hardesty I, Kumar M, Sheeler L, Greenstreet R, Livingston R. Thyroid stimulating hormone levels correlate with estrogen receptor (ER) status of human breast cancer. Proc Am Assoc Cancer Res 21: 52, 1980.
85. Rose DP, Davis TE. Plasma triiodothyronine concentrations in breast cancer. Cancer 43: 1434-1438, 1979.
86. Schmidt GH, Moger WH. Effect of thyroactive materials upon mammary gland growth and lactation in rats. Endocrinology 81: 14-18, 1967.
87. Shapiro S, Slone D, Kaufman DW, Rosenberg L, Miettinen OS, Stolley PD, Knapp RC, Leavitt T Jr, Watring WG, Rosenshein NB, Schottenfeld D. Use of thyroid supplements in relation to the risk of breast cancer. JAMA 244: 1685-1687, 1980.
88. Shellabarger CJ. Hypothyroidism and DMBA rat mammary carcinogenesis. Proc Am Assoc Cancer Res 10: 79, 1969.
89. Shoemaker JP, Bradley RL, Hoffman RV. Increased survival and inhibition of mammary tumors in hypothyroid mice. J Surg Res 21: 151-154, 1976.
90. Shoemaker JP, Dagher RK. Remissions of mammary adenocarcinoma in hypothyroid mice given 5-fluorouracil and chloroquine phosphate. J Natl Cancer Inst 62: 1575-1578, 1979.
91. Singh DV, Bern HA. Interaction between prolactin and thyroxine in mouse mammary gland lobulo-alveolar development _in vitro_. J Endocrinol 45: 579-583, 1969.
92. Sirbasku DA. Hormone-responsive growth _in vivo_ of a tissue culture cell line established from the MT-W9A rat mammary tumor. Cancer Res 38: 1154-1165, 1978.
93. Smallridge RC, Latham KR. Nuclear thyroid hormone receptors in human breast tumors. Clin Res 28: 421a, 1980.
94. Smith RD, Hilf R, Senior AE. The effect of altered thyroid state on prolactin binding to livers and 7,12-dimethylbenz(a)anthracene-induced mammary tumors in rats. Proc Soc Exp Biol Med 158: 517-520, 1978.
95. Smithcors JF. Effects of thiouracil on the mammary gland. Proc Soc Exp Biol Med 59: 197-200, 1945.
96. Smithcors JF, Leonard SL. Relation of thyroid to mammary gland structure in the rat with special reference to the male. Endocrinology 31: 454-460, 1942.
97. St Gerard S, Gardner B, Patti J, Husain V, Shouten J, Alfonso AE. Effect of triiodothyronine and reserpine on induction and growth of mammary tumors in rats by 3-methylcholanthrene. J Surg Oncol 14: 213-218, 1980.
98. Strum JM. Site of iodination in rat mammary gland. Anat Rec 192: 235-244, 1978.
99. Taylor WF, Hayles AB. Thyroid hormone and breast cancer. JAMA 238: 1147-1148, 1977.
100. Topper YJ, Freeman CS. Multiple hormone interactions in the developmental biology of the mammary gland. Physiol Rev 60: 1049-1106, 1980.
101. VanderLaan WP, Larson BA. The thyroid, prolactin and breast cancer. Arch Intern Med 138: 1611, 1978.
102. Vazquez-Lopez E. The effects of thiourea on the development of spontaneous tumors in mice. Br J Cancer 3: 401-414, 1949.

103. Venezian EC. Thyroid hormone and breast cancer. JAMA 238: 1147, 1977.
104. Vonderhaar BK. A role of thyroid hormones in differentiation of mouse mammary gland *in vitro*. Biochem Biophys Res Commun 67: 1219-1225, 1975.
105. Vonderhaar BK. Studies on the mechanism by which thyroid hormones enhance u-lactalbumin activity in explants from mouse mammary glands. Endocrinology 100: 1423-1431, 1977.
106. Vonderhaar BK. Lactose synthetase activity in mouse mammary glands is controlled by thyroid hormones. J Cell Biol 82: 675-681, 1979.
107. Vonderhaar BK, Greco AE. Lobulo-alveolar development of mouse mammary glands is regulated by thyroid hormones. Endocrinology 104: 409-418, 1979.
108. Vonderhaar BK, Greco AE. Effect of altered thyroid status on development of spontaneous mammary tumors in primiparous C3H mice. Submitted for publication.
109. Vorherr H. Thyroid disease in relation to breast cancer. Klin Wochenschr 56: 1139-1145, 1978.
110. Wanebo HJ, Benua RS, Rawson RW. Neoplastic disease and thyrotoxicosis. Cancer 19: 1523-1526, 1966.
111. Warner MR. Effect of perinatal oestrogen on the pretreatment required for mouse mammary lobular formation *in vitro*. J Endocrinol 77: 1-10, 1978.
112. Warner MR. Mammary pathology. pp 210-228 in *Aging in Non-human Primates*, ed DM Bowden, VonNostrand-Rheinhold, New York, 1979.
113. Welsch CW. Prolactin and the development and progression of early neoplastic mammary gland lesions. Cancer Res 38: 4054-4058, 1978.
114. Welsch CW, Nagasawa H. Prolactin and murine mammary tumorigenesis: a review. Cancer Res 37: 951-963, 1977.

Chapter 8

MODE OF CYCLIC AMP ACTION IN GROWTH CONTROL

Yoon Sang Cho-Chung

INTRODUCTION

It is now well recognized that cyclic adenosine 3',5'-monophosphate (cyclic AMP), a nucleotide present in a wide variety of organisms, is a major regulator of numerous cellular activities (71), (93), (113). The intracellular accumulation of cyclic AMP, either endogenously generated or exogenously supplied, inhibits the growth of normal and transformed cells *in vivo* and *in vitro* [see review (16)]. There is also evidence that an inverse correlation exists between the level of cellular cyclic AMP and the rate of cell growth. Unrestrained growth, a characteristic of neoplastic cells, however, is not always associated with diminished levels of cyclic AMP. Several studies have shown wide ranges of cyclic AMP levels in proliferating tissues of animals and humans (16). Moreover, an increase in cellular cyclic AMP has been produced in tumors following treatment with $N^6,O^{2'}$-dibutyryl cyclic AMP (dibutyryl cyclic AMP) although tumor regression occurs only in tumors that are responsive to dibutyryl cyclic AMP (14). In our investigations on the mechanism of dibutyryl cyclic AMP-responsiveness, we utilized rat mammary tumor models that were either "responsive" or "unresponsive" to dibutyryl cyclic AMP treatment.

The objective of this chapter is to discuss the mechanism of cyclic AMP-mediated growth regulation of mammary tumors *in vivo*. Our findings also concern the involvement of cyclic nucleotides in the functional development of the mammary gland and in the expression of neoplastic transformation and reversion.

NORMAL AND NEOPLASTIC GROWTH OF THE MAMMARY GLAND

Intracellular content of cyclic nucleotides

Sapag-Hagar and Greenbaum (102) reported that the content of cyclic AMP in rat mammary gland shows a diphasic pattern and is related to the growth, development and differentiation of the tissue. The level of cyclic AMP in the gland rose continuously to the end of pregnancy, then fell progressively to its lowest value by the 16th day of lactation. The transition at the time of parturition coincided with a considerable increase in the metabolic activity of the gland consequent to the onset of lactation. A reverse pattern was observed with cyclic guanosine 3',5'-monophosphate (cyclic GMP), the second cyclic nucleotide found in a variety of organisms (2), (50), (62) during the various stages of the gestation cycle. In studies (103) with rat mammary gland explants in culture, cyclic AMP was found to inhibit the increase of enzymes associated with lipogenesis and to depress the synthesis of DNA, RNA and fatty acids. More recently, cyclic AMP was identified as a negative control factor for the induction of milk protein synthesis in mouse mammary gland organ culture (94). These observations suggest that the functional development of the mammary gland is, indeed, related to the cyclic nucleotide concentration.

Several investigators have examined cellular cyclic AMP levels in mammary tumors and obtained different results. Minton *et al.* (86) and Guerinot *et al.* (52) found high cyclic AMP levels in human breast carcinomas and intermediate levels in benign breast tumors, as compared to normal breast tissues, whereas Oertel *et al.* (88) reported cyclic AMP levels to be 70% lower in human breast tumors than in adjacent normal mammary tissues: these cyclic AMP levels were expressed on the basis of wet tissue weight. Eppenberger and associates (74) measured both cyclic AMP and cyclic GMP in normal, dysplastic and neoplastic human breast tissues and found that the levels expressed on the basis of the wet tissue weight were higher in neoplastic tissues than in normal adjacent tissues; however, if the results were expressed on a per cell basis, the levels of both cyclic AMP and cyclic GMP were significantly lower in the neoplastic tissues.

Cohen and Chan (41) found higher cyclic AMP levels in 7,12-dimethylbenz-(α)anthracene (DMBA)-induced rat mammary carcinomas (60) than in mammary glands from non-pregnant rats, but lower cyclic AMP levels in cultured mammary adenocarcinoma cells than in their normal mammary epithelial counterpart. They concluded that the low levels of cyclic AMP found in normal mammary gland *in vivo* might be due to the larger amount of fat cells present.

The studies on cyclic nucleotide levels in mammary tissues are difficult to interpret but the disparity of results may be due in part to differences in sample preparation or the method of nucleotide measurement or because of the heterogeneity of tissue samples.

On the basis of the observations reported, it is apparent that the involvement of cyclic nucleotides in tumor growth is complex and cannot be explained by a simple relationship between the intracellular concentration of cyclic nucleotides and the rate of cell proliferation.

Hormone-cyclic nucleotide interrelation

The development and involution of the mammary gland occur in response to changes in serum levels of hormones from various endocrine organs. Of these hormones, estrogen, prolactin and progesterone are important for the development of the gland. For the functional differentiation of mammary epithelium, however, studies (115) of mouse mammary gland in organ culture have shown that insulin, prolactin and glucocorticoid are required.

The growth regulatory function of hormones has also been demonstrated in some mammary carcinomas. Estrogen is believed to be essential for the growth of hormone-dependent mammary tumors. This assumption stems from observations that deprivation or antagonism of estrogen produces regression of certain mammary carcinomas in both experimental animals and humans (3), (12), (54), (59), (77), (104), (106). Prolactin, on the other hand, cannot sustain growth of rat mammary tumors by itself but plays a combined regulatory role with estrogen in the growth of mammary tumor cells _in vitro_ and _in vivo_ (13), (45), (46), (78).

Estrogen, like other steroid hormones, acts by binding to a specific binding protein in the cytoplasm; the complex formed is then activated and translocated into the nucleus where it triggers the biological responses (63), (89). Hormone-dependent mammary tumors contain the specific estrogen-binding protein (estrogen receptor) (69), (76), (85) just as estrogen-responsive normal tissues (68), (79), (119). Thus the presence of an appreciable concentration of cytoplasmic estrogen receptor can be an indicator of hormone-dependency of mammary tumors and, indeed, the measurement of the receptor is now used extensively as an assay to identify patients likely to respond to endocrine therapy. However, the prediction of hormone-dependency by the estrogen receptor assay is far from satisfactory since about one-half of the tumors containing estrogen receptor do not regress after ovariectomy (84). It is conceivable, therefore, that the estrogen receptor may interact with other cellular regulator(s) in growth control.

The first indication that a relationship exists between estrogen and cyclic AMP in mammary tumor regression was provided by the observation that both hormone removal (ovariectomy) and dibutyryl cyclic AMP treatment produce new synthesis of acid RNase within a few hours from the initiation of treatment (14), (33), (34), (35). In regressing DMBA tumors, an increase in the cyclic AMP level follows ovariectomy (22), (23), (83), high dose estrogen or tamoxifen administration (9), dibutyryl cyclic AMP treatment (7), streptozotocin-induced diabetes (83), (107) and inhibition of prolactin secretion (83). In rat uterus, the cyclic AMP level decreases while the cyclic GMP level increases when a low dose estrogen injection is given following ovariectomy or during proestrus when the plasma estrogen level is maximal (73). These results indicate that cyclic AMP levels are low in estrogen-target tissues that are under a physiological concentration of estrogen and high under supra- or sub-physiological concentrations of estrogen. Thus there appears to be a counter-relationship between cyclic AMP and estrogen in target tissues.

How might cyclic AMP and estrogen interact? Involvement of the specific cytoplasmic binding proteins for cyclic AMP and estrogen has been shown: 1) in hormone-dependent mammary tumors during growth and regression induced by hormonal manipulations or dibutyryl cyclic AMP treatment (7), (9), (22), (23), (107), 2) in several rat target tissues during *in vivo* administration of steroid hormones following hormone withdrawal (80), and 3) during induction of ornithine aminotransferase in rat kidneys following cyclic AMP injections *in vivo* (120). The antagonistic action between cyclic AMP-binding protein and estrogen receptor in mammary tumor regression is discussed later.

MECHANISM OF MAMMARY TUMOR REGRESSION

Exogenous cyclic nucleotides

Gericke and Chandra (49) first and Keller (65) later reported growth inhibition of a mouse lymphosarcoma and Walker 256 (W256) rat mammary carcinoma, respectively, by treatment with cyclic AMP, dibutyryl cyclic AMP, theophylline, epinephrine and isoproterenol. Our studies showed that cyclic AMP derivatives exhibit a growth inhibitory effect on a variety of established rat mammary tumors (14), (35). Dibutyryl cyclic AMP, 8-thiomethyl cyclic AMP and 8-bromo cyclic AMP (8 mg/day/200 g rat s.c.) arrested the growth of hormone-dependent DMBA and MTW9 (66) mammary carcinomas. Growth inhibition was reversible upon cessation of the treatment. The same dibutyryl cyclic AMP treatment also produced growth arrest in about 30% of W256, a hormone-independent mammary carcinoma. Some W256 carcinomas regressed completely within two weeks from the start of dibutyryl cyclic AMP treatment and did not reappear until 10 months after the treatment was terminated. A response similar to that of W256 carcinomas was also shown with hormone-responsive nitrosomethylurea (NMU)-induced (53) and R3230AC (58) mammary tumors. These results show that inhibition of tumor growth by exogenous cyclic nucleotides varies with the tumor cell population.

Cyclic AMP receptor proteins

The action of cyclic AMP on mammalian tissues appears to be mediated by the interaction of cyclic AMP with its "receptor" protein (a high affinity binding protein), the regulatory subunit of cyclic AMP-dependent protein kinase (72), (75). This enzyme has been purified from various tissues of several animal species and consists of two catalytic (C) and two regulatory (R) subunits, the latter interacting with cyclic AMP. When cyclic AMP binds to R, the holoenzyme (RC) dissociates, freeing C from R, thus activating the enzyme. The catalytically active C then phosphorylates specific proteins.

Daniel _et al_. (44) were the first to find a correlation between deficiency of cyclic AMP receptor protein and resistance of S49 lymphosarcoma cells to the cytolytic effect of dibutyryl cyclic AMP. Subsequently, Coffino and associates (39), (40) reported on a variety of parallel defects in both cyclic AMP-binding and cyclic AMP-dependent protein kinase activities that they observed in several hundred independently selected mutants of S49 lymphoma cells resistant to dibutyryl cyclic AMP. They also found a correlation between a charge alteration of the regulatory subunit of cyclic AMP-dependent protein kinase and the resistance of the mutant S49 cells to dibutyryl cyclic AMP (112). In the studies of Simantov and Sachs (109), clones of neuroblastoma cells resistant to the cytotoxic effects of dibutyryl cyclic AMP were shown to be associated with an abnormal property of cyclic AMP receptor protein, i.e., an increased temperature sensitivity and a resultant decrease in cyclic AMP-dependent protein kinase.

An interesting finding of Tisdale and Phillips (114) was a correlation between an alteration of cyclic AMP-dependent protein kinase and resistance to the cytotoxic effects of both dibutyryl cyclic AMP and an alkylating agent in a W256 mammary carcinoma cell line.

The mechanism by which dibutyryl cyclic AMP exerts its effect was studied (27), (28), (30) in two cell populations selected from W256, one regressing (responsive) and the other growing (unresponsive) under dibutyryl cyclic AMP treatment. The difference between the two cell populations was found to reside in the physicochemical properties of their cyclic AMP receptor proteins, i.e., affinity for cyclic AMP, heat stability, electrophoretic mobility and sedimentation profile in sucrose density gradient. A striking correlation between the heat stability of cyclic AMP receptor protein and dibutyryl cyclic AMP-induced regression has also been found in other types of mammary tumors and hepatomas (24).

If alteration of cyclic AMP receptor proteins could account for the "unresponsiveness" of neoplastic cells to cyclic AMP-mediated growth regulation, then a comparison of the responses of the receptor proteins of dibutyryl cyclic AMP-responsive and -unresponsive cells should help to explain the role of this protein in growth control. The results of our experiments showed that following dibutyryl cyclic AMP treatment _in vivo_, or incubation of tumor slices with cyclic AMP _in vitro_, cyclic binding and protein kinase activities increase in the _nuclei_ of responsive but not of unresponsive W256 tumor (27), (28). We further demonstrated that in a cell-free system the cytoplasmic cyclic AMP receptor protein-cyclic AMP complex from the responsive tumor binds to isolated nuclei from both responsive and unresponsive tumors, whereas the complex from the unresponsive tumor does not bind to either nuclei (27). Thus the nuclear accumulation of cyclic AMP receptor protein may be a critical step in cyclic AMP-mediated growth control and the presence of the cyclic AMP receptor protein complex in the cytoplasm may be a determinant of this event.

Several species of cyclic AMP receptor proteins have been identified in normal tissues. Purified cyclic AMP-dependent protein kinase type I from rabbit skeletal muscle has a regulatory subunit with a molecular weight of 48,000 (61), whereas cyclic AMP-dependent protein kinase type II from bovine heart has a regulatory subunit with 56,000 daltons (42), (99). The proteolytic fragments of these regulatory subunits with 39,000 and 17,000 daltons have also been identified (42), (118).

We examined the molecular species of cyclic AMP receptor proteins involved in the regression of hormone-dependent DMBA-induced tumors by the use of the photoaffinity label, 8-azido-[^{32}P]cyclic AMP (95). Growing DMBA-induced tumors contained two major cyclic AMP receptor proteins, with apparent molecular weights of 39,000 and 56,000, in the cytosol but not in the nuclei (20), (29). Following ovariectomy, the 56,000-dalton protein increased appreciably in the cytosol of regressing tumors, whereas the 39,000-dalton protein showed no change; moreover, only the 56,000-dalton protein appeared in the nuclei of regressing tumors (20). An increase of the 56,000-dalton receptor protein has also been found in DMBA tumors regressing after dibutyryl cyclic AMP treatment (19), injection of tamoxifen or pharmacologic doses of estrogen (5), (9) and in DMBA tumor slices incubated with cyclic AMP in the presence of benzamidine and arginine _in vitro_ (20), (21). In contrast, autonomously growing mammary tumors [about 12% of DMBA-induced tumors that fail to regress after ovariectomy or dibutyryl cyclic AMP treatment (7), (22)] incorporated 8-azido-[^{32}P]cyclic AMP into the cytosol protein of 56,000 daltons but showed no increase of this receptor in either the cytosol or nuclei (20).

It seems reasonable to assume that the inability of the 56,000-dalton cyclic AMP receptor protein of hormone-independent DMBA tumors to penetrate the nucleus is due to a structural alteration of the protein. In fact, on two-dimensional gel electrophoresis, the 56,000-dalton receptor of the hormone-independent tumor migrates as a doublet with a shift to a more acidic charge than that of the receptor of the hormone-dependent tumor (20). This charge alteration of the cyclic AMP receptor protein did not affect the cyclic AMP-binding affinity but correlated with the decreased self-phosphorylation of the receptor molecule (20). Self-phosphorylation [phosphorylation of the regulatory subunit of protein kinase by its own catalytic subunit (48)] has been shown to be a characteristic of protein kinase type II from various tissues (81), (101), (116). It has also been shown that the decreased self-phosphorylation of cyclic AMP receptor protein results in a decreased ability of the receptor protein to interact with the catalytic subunit of protein kinase (42). Indeed, the majority of cyclic AMP receptor proteins in hormone-independent tumors were found to be present free from the catalytic subunit of protein kinase (20), (29).

Based upon these data, we postulated that the cyclic AMP receptor protein which can penetrate into the nucleus must have two functional domains, one for cyclic AMP-binding and the other for an interaction with the catalytic subunit of protein kinase. The cyclic AMP receptor protein of the hormone-independent DMBA tumor is deficient in its ability to be phosphorylated and to interact with the catalytic subunit of protein kinase and, therefore, is incapable of migrating into the nucleus. The 39,000-dalton cyclic AMP receptor protein, the proteolytic fragment of the 56,000-dalton receptor (42), (118), which was found in a large amount in most of the tumors examined, is also incapable of penetrating into the nucleus (20), (21). This protein retains the intact cyclic AMP-binding but has reduced ability to be phosphorylated (self-phosphorylation) and to bind with the catalytic subunit of protein kinase (20), (42), (118). Another class of abnormal cyclic AMP receptor proteins, AuT-PK85, has been isolated from adrenocortical carcinoma by Sharma and co-workers (108); this receptor can bind cyclic AMP and be autophosphorylated but cannot interact with the catalytic subunit of protein kinase. Whether this receptor can penetrate the nucleus is not known.

The above data are consistent with the hypothesis (18), (20) that neoplastic growth, i.e., unrestrained growth, may be the consequence of an aberrant cyclic AMP-dependent protein kinase system in the cell which is primarily due to the decreased amount of holoprotein kinase. As presented schematically in Fig. 1, most of the cyclic AMP-dependent protein kinase in normal cells is present in the form of holoenzyme (RC) (72), thus the enzyme is stimulated by cyclic AMP _in vitro_ at least 5-fold (75). The amounts of subunits R and C and the proteolytic fragments of R, i.e., R' and R", are present in small fractions. In neoplastic cells, the cyclic AMP-dependent protein kinase holoenzyme (RC) is greatly decreased. In most experimental tumors examined, cyclic AMP-binding and cyclic AMP-dependent protein kinase activities have been found to be lower than in normal tissues, and in particular, the stimulatory effect of cyclic AMP on the enzyme was decreased (16). A decrease of cyclic

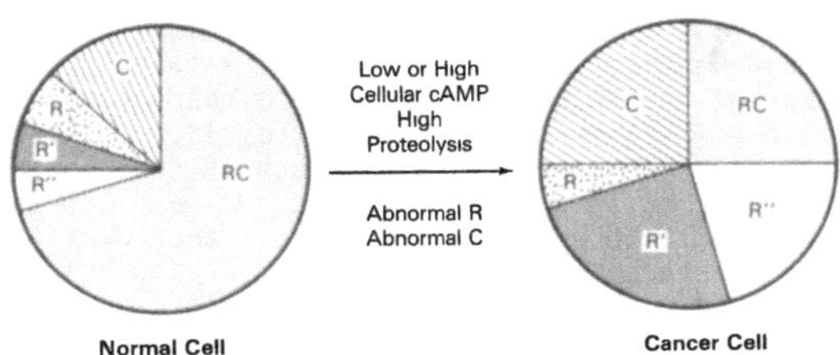

Fig. 1. Relative amount of holoenzyme to subunits of cyclic AMP-dependent protein kinase in normal and neoplastic cells. RC, holoenzyme; R, regulatory subunit (cyclic AMP receptor protein); R', R", proteolytic fragments of R; C, catalytic subunit.

AMP-dependent protein kinase, especially the type II enzyme, has also been reported in human primary mammary carcinomas (55). Compared with normal tissues, neoplastic tissues showed an impressively wide range of cyclic AMP levels from very low to very high (16). At low levels of cyclic AMP, the amount of total cyclic AMP-dependent protein kinase would be expected to be low, whereas at high levels of cyclic AMP, the amount of holoenzyme (RC) should decrease due to its separation to the subunits, R and C (72). Proteolysis potentiates the decrease of RC by an irreversible breakdown of the R subunit to the fragments R' and R" which cannot recombine with the C subunit (42). Indeed, R', the 39,000-dalton cyclic AMP receptor protein, is largely increased in tumors as compared with normal tissues (20), (29). The structural abnormality of R and C should also influence the interaction between the two subunits. Abnormal R has been shown to be correlated with resistance to dibutyryl cyclic AMP-induced cytolysis in S49 lymphosarcoma mutant cells (39), (40), (112), a clone of neuroblastoma cells (109), and hormone-independent dibutyryl cyclic AMP-unresponsive mammary tumors (20), (29). In hormone-independent mammary tumors, the alteration of R was indeed correlated with a decrease of the holoprotein kinase (RC).

Hormone-dependent mammary tumors, which possess intact but a decreased amount of cyclic AMP-dependent protein kinase, can undergo regression with the proper cyclic AMP stimulation and the holoprotein kinase in these regressing tumors increases, thereby mimicking normal cells (31). Thus, the biochemical reversion of neoplastic to normal-like cells appears to depend on the relative cellular concentration of cyclic AMP to cyclic AMP-dependent protein kinase holoenzyme.

Antagonism between cyclic AMP and estrogen

The regulation of hormone-dependent mammary tumor growth appears to depend on the antagonistic interaction between cyclic AMP and estrogen (7), (15), (17), (23). During growth, high estrogen-binding and low cyclic AMP-binding activities are found in DMBA-induced tumors. When DMBA tumors undergo growth arrest following either ovariectomy or dibutyryl cyclic AMP treatment of the host, cyclic AMP-binding markedly increases while estrogen-binding sharply decreases in the regressing tumors. These reciprocal changes in cyclic AMP- and estrogen-binding activities are detectable within 1 day after either ovariectomy or dibutyryl cyclic AMP treatment, when there is no appreciable change in tumor size, indicating that the changes are early events in the regression process rather than the result of tumor regression. The changes are reversed, however, when tumor growth is resumed following either the injection of 17β-estradiol or cessation of dibutyryl cyclic AMP treatment. The increased cyclic AMP-binding activity seems to be the result of new protein synthesis since the increase can be blocked by cycloheximide. The decrease of estrogen-binding activity is due to a decrease in total binding sites without any modification of either binding affinity or sedimentation characteristics.

Interestingly, we observed that the inverse relationship between cyclic AMP- and estrogen-binding activities was closely related to the hormone-dependency of tumor growth. In hormone-independent mammary tumors that continue to grow and fail to regress after hormonal deprivation, we found a wide range of estrogen and cyclic AMP-binding activities that do not change after ovariectomy or dibutyryl cyclic AMP treatment. It appears, therefore, that these binding proteins for cyclic AMP and estrogen may interact in the control of hormone-dependent mammary tumor growth. If so, a reliable assessment of the hormone-dependency of mammary carcinomas could be achieved by investigating both estrogen-binding and cyclic AMP-binding activities. Experiments carried out with rat mammary tumors showed that the hormone-dependency of the tumors was closely related to the relative concentrations of estrogen receptor (ER) and cyclic AMP receptor protein (CR) in the tumor cytosol (8). When ER and CR were expressed as the ER/CR ratio, 95% of hormone-dependent tumors (tumors regressing following ovariectomy) had ratios of 35 x 10^{-3} or greater, whereas 97% of autonomously growing tumors had ratios of less than 35 x 10^{-3}. When ER alone was measured, hormone-dependency was correctly predicted in only 60% of these tumors. The ratios of ER/CR were also elevated in normal estrogen target tissues as compared to non-target tissues. These data show that the relative concentrations of ER and CR reflect the hormone-dependency of mammary tumors and normal tissues more accurately than does the concentration of ER alone.

The apparent antagonism between ER and CR was also observed in their translocation from the cytosol to the nucleus (6). In a hormone-dependent MTW9 mammary tumor cell-free system, cytosol activated with either [^{3}H]17β-estradiol or [^{3}H]cyclic AMP was incubated with purified nuclei to determine the specific nuclear uptake of these receptor proteins. No competition was noted between estrogen and cyclic AMP for each other's specific binding protein in the cytosol. However, the presence of unlabeled cyclic AMP (5 x 10^{-7}M) inhibited the specific nuclear uptake of [^{3}H]17β-estradiol by 50% and the presence of unlabeled 17β-estradiol (10^{-8}M) inhibited the specific nuclear uptake of [^{3}H]cyclic AMP by 60%. Moreover, phosphorylation and dephosphorylation appeared to play a role during the nuclear translocation of these receptor proteins: phosphorylation enhanced nuclear uptake of cyclic AMP receptor but inhibited nuclear uptake of estrogen receptor.

From these data we proposed that the regulation of hormone-dependent mammary tumor growth is dependent upon the antagonistic action between cyclic AMP and estrogen, probably through their respective receptor proteins.

Nuclear protein phosphorylation

There is evidence that certain steroid and thyroid hormones mediate nuclear protein phosphorylation and regulation of DNA transcription primarily through stimulation of nuclear cyclic AMP-independent protein kinase. In the case of hormones and exogenous stimuli that act via cyclic AMP, however, nuclear protein phosphorylation and gene expression are stimulated by the cyclic AMP-mediated translocation of cytoplasmic cyclic AMP-dependent protein kinase to nuclear acceptor sites (11), (38), (43), (64). In both cases, hormone-mediated stimulation of nuclear cyclic AMP-dependent and -independent protein kinases could result in phosphorylative modification of certain nuclear proteins. Studies (36), (37) from our laboratory have shown a correlation between specific nuclear protein phosphorylation and growth arrest of hormone-dependent mammary tumors. In growing DMBA tumor nuclei, a low molecular weight basic protein species, GAP (growth-associated protein), was found to be the major endogenous substrate for nuclear protein kinase; whereas, in nuclei from tumors regressing after ovariectomy or dibutyryl cyclic AMP treatment, the phosphorylation of GAP decreases and a new non-histone basic protein species of higher molecular weight, RAP (regression-associated protein), becomes the predominant substrate of the endogenous kinase. These changes in phosphorylation take place within 1 day post ovariectomy or dibutyryl cyclic AMP treatment and are reversed by injection of 17ß-estradiol or cessation of dibutyryl cyclic AMP treatment. Phosphorylation of RAP was also induced in regressing DMBA tumors following tamoxifen or high dose estrogen injections (9) and _in vitro_ by incubation of growing DMBA tumor slices with cyclic AMP (32). Moreover, the exogenous substrate specificity and the effect of cyclic AMP-dependent protein kinase inhibitor protein on nuclear protein kinase activity indicated that phosphorylation of GAP and RAP is probably due to the presence of different kinases in the tumor nuclei; the former is due to cyclic AMP-independent protein kinase and the latter is due to cyclic AMP-dependent protein kinase. Since cyclic AMP-dependent protein kinase is undetectable in growing DMBA tumor nuclei but present in the tumor cytosol (31), the enzyme is probably transferred from the cytoplasm to the nucleus during regression.

Direct evidence that the cytoplasmic cyclic AMP-dependent protein kinase penetrates into the nucleus has been shown by experiments using tumor slices _in vitro_ and a cell-free system of DMBA tumors (21). When tumor slices were incubated with cyclic AMP, benzamidine and arginine, the 56,000-dalton cyclic AMP receptor protein initially increased markedly in the cytosol, mimicking _in vivo_ tumors regressing after ovariectomy or dibutyryl cyclic AMP treatment (7), and then penetrated into the nucleus, as shown by the photoaffinity cross-linking method using the photoaffinity label, 8-azido-[^{32}P]cyclic AMP (20). The nuclear binding of the 56,000-dalton cyclic AMP receptor protein was accompanied by stimulation of new phosphorylation of the 76,000-dalton nuclear protein, RAP (21). These events occurred maximally at a physiological level of cyclic AMP (10^{-8}M) and minimally at both sub- and supra-physiological levels of cyclic AMP (20), (21). In hormone-independent mammary tumors that fail to regress following ovariectomy or dibutyryl cyclic AMP treatment, neither nuclear translocation of cyclic AMP receptor protein nor phosphorylation of the 76,000-dalton nuclear protein occurred (7), (37). In an attempt to find an explanation for these results, a recombination experiment was carried out using activated cytosol and isolated nuclei from hormone-dependent and -independent DMBA tumors (20). It was found that the activated cytosol derived from a hormone-dependent DMBA tumor was able to induce phosphorylation of the 76,000-dalton protein in nuclei derived from both hormone-dependent and -independent tumors, whereas the activated cytosol derived from a hormone-independent DMBA tumor failed to induce phosphorylation of this protein in either hormone-dependent or -independent tumor nuclei. Moreover, the absence of phosphorylation of the 76,000-dalton protein correlated with diminished nuclear binding of the 56,000-dalton cyclic AMP receptor protein. We interpreted these data to indicate that both nuclear binding of cyclic AMP receptor and subsequent phosphorylation of the 76,000-daltons depend on the cyclic AMP receptor complex of cytosol but not on the nuclei. The hormone-independent tumor contains defective cytoplasmic cyclic AMP receptor protein (i.e., a charge alteration, decreased self-phosphorylation and decreased interacting ability with the catalytic subunit of protein kinase) which fails to penetrate into the nucleus and thus does not exhibit phosphorylation of the 76,000-dalton protein.

Evidence from the experiments described here supports the hypothesis that nuclear translocation of cyclic AMP receptor complex in the cytoplasm may be the triggering event leading to tumor regression _in vivo_.

CYCLIC NUCLEOTIDES IN TRANSFORMATION

If an alteration of cyclic nucleotide metabolism plays a role in the initiation of neoplastic transformation, then the change would be expected to occur very soon after exposure of a susceptible tissue to a carcinogenic stimulus.

The possibility that cyclic AMP serves as a negative signal for cell growth and cyclic GMP serves as a positive signal has received considerable attention (51), (57).

Since a single exposure to certain N-nitroso compounds by a susceptible host can induce neoplastic transformation (82), the early events following exposure of cells to the carcinogen must be critical to the expression of its oncogenic action. De Rubertis and Craven (47) reported that the cyclic GMP content of several human and rat tissues increased markedly within 5 min after exposure to N-methyl-N'-nitro-N-nitrosoguanidine (MNNG) _in vitro_. In contrast, the cyclic AMP content was not detectably altered in any of the tissues examined (47). The ability of MNNG to increase cyclic GMP is clearly shown _in vivo_ with rat colonic mucosa, where the carcinogenic action of MNNG is well established (111). Intrarectal administration of a single dose of this compound has been found to induce colonic cancer (87). Thus in colonic mucosa, a rise in cyclic GMP appears to be one of the earliest *in vivo* effects of this carcinogen and reflects activation of the synthetic enzyme, guanylate cyclase (47). The extent to which other chemical carcinogens activate guanylate cyclase, however, is not known and the role of cyclic GMP in cell proliferation remains to be elucidated.

Studies by Pastan and associates (91), (92) have disclosed considerable involvement of cyclic AMP in malignant transformation. In normal fibroblastic embryo cells, the level of cyclic AMP regulates cell shape, motility, adhesiveness to substratum, growth rate and the synthesis of many macromolecules. In transformation, the "transforming agent," whether it be a virus, carcinogen or ionizing radiation, lowers cyclic AMP levels. Consequently, all the properties under cyclic AMP control are altered. A fall in cyclic AMP level might be achieved by inactivation of the synthetic enzyme, adenylate cyclase, and/or activation of the degradative enzyme, cyclic AMP-phosphodiesterase. The first report of a change in adenylate cyclase in cultured cells following transformation was by Burk (10) who found decreased activity in a line of polyoma virus-transformed BHK cells. Following transformation of chick embryo fibroblast cells by Rous sarcoma virus, the cyclic AMP level and the adenylate cyclase activity also decreased (1), (90).

A convenient way to study the early events following transformation is to employ viral mutants that are temperature sensitive in transformation functions. When cells infected with the mutant are shifted from 41°C (nonpermissive) to 37°C (permissive), the morphology of some of the cells begins to change to that of transformed cells within 10-20 min. Just as rapidly the cyclic AMP levels fall (90) and the activity of adenylate cyclase decreases (1). Thus the changes in cyclic AMP metabolism parallel the change in phenotype. Studies with such mutants provide strong evidence that there is a close link between cellular transformation and cyclic AMP metabolism.

Another approach to study the role of cyclic AMP in transformation is to pretreat transformed cells *in vitro* with cyclic AMP or cyclic AMP derivatives, then implant the transformed cells into an appropriate host to examine their tumorigenicity. Smith and Handler (110) showed that the ability of human cancer cells (KB) to form a solid tumor in the hamster cheek pouch was lost when these cells were grown in 1 mM cyclic AMP prior to inoculation. This was attributed to the growth-inhibitory property of cyclic AMP and not to its toxicity, since if the same pretreated cells were allowed to grow in normal medium prior to animal inoculation, the cells reverted to the malignant state and tumor incidence increased.

It can be concluded from these studies that cyclic nucleotides seem to be important components involved in the expression of neoplastic transformation. Oncogenesis, however, is a complex process which probably involves multiple steps including the appearance of a new cell population.

It remains for future studies to provide the answers to how cyclic AMP is involved and what the sequence of steps is in the process of malignant transformation. It would be highly desirable to determine whether the transformation process could be prevented or reverted by manipulation of the cyclic AMP system. The possible role of cyclic AMP in reversion of malignancy is discussed below.

CYCLIC AMP IN REVERSION OF MALIGNANCY

Mouse neuroblastoma cells in culture have been used extensively as a model to study the problems of differentiation and malignancy. That the malignancy of nerve cells is the result of abnormal regulation of differentiation is evidenced by the expression in these cells to varying degrees (mostly at extremely low levels) of many differentiated functions. These properties include morphological differentiation (105), induction of neurotransmitter enzymes (4), (100), (117) and acquisition of excitable membranes (67).

Occasionally, neuroblastoma cells differentiate spontaneously and then regress completely. Prasad (96) suggested that cyclic AMP may be linked with the morphological differentiation of neuroblastoma cells since treatment of these cells with dibutyryl cyclic AMP, prostaglandin E_1 (PGE_1), and inhibitors of cyclic AMP-phosphodiesterase induces irreversible morphological differentiation. That this differentiation may be a reversion of malignancy is supported by the observation that no tumor is produced when these treated neuroblastoma cells are inoculated into animals (96). Agents that increase cellular cyclic AMP levels have therefore been used in the treatment of human neuroblastomas. Helson *et al.* (56) reported that patients with disseminated neuroblastomas that were unresponsive to any other known therapeutic agents underwent temporary regression of tumors after treatment with papaverine, an inhibitor of cyclic AMP-phosphodiesterase activity. In addition, they observed at autopsies of these patients that many neuroblastoma cells were transformed to ganglioneuroblastoma cells. Since papaverine induces an increased cyclic AMP level, cell death, differentiation and membrane changes in human neuroblastoma cells in culture (97), it was proposed (98) that the transformation of neuroblastoma cells to ganglioneuroblastoma cells may be mediated by cyclic AMP and cell death may be partly due to the differentiated cells acting as a strong antigen against the tumor cells.

Klein and Loizzi (70) reported on the effect of cyclic AMP on cell differentiation and growth in the hormone-responsive R3230AC rat mammary adenocarcinoma. Following daily subcutaneous injections of dibutyryl cyclic AMP beginning on day 1 after tumor implantation, the growth rate increased appreciably. R3230AC tumor is composed primarily of epithelial cells with a histologic organization resembling mammary gland alveoli (58). The ultrastructure of cells treated with dibutyryl cyclic AMP showed a rough endoplasmic reticulum in short dilated segments, proliferation of the Golgi complex with extensive membrane, dilated cisternae, and numerous vesicles of various sizes containing fine granular material indicative of cell differentiation. These data suggested that the increase in tumor size after dibutyryl cyclic AMP treatment is attributable to an increase in cell size rather than an increase in cell number.

In our recent study (25) with the human breast carcinoma cell line, MCF-7, we also observed cyclic AMP-induced growth arrest together with a change in cell morphology. The _in vitro_ growth of MCF-7 cells was inhibited by a daily supplement of L-arginine (1.0 mg/ml) which acted synergistically with dibutyryl cyclic AMP (10^{-6}M) to block cell replication completely within 2 days. The synergistic growth inhibitory effect of dibutyryl cyclic AMP and arginine was also observed when the arginine analogue, arginine methyl ester, was substituted at a concentration of 50 μg/ml; whereas other amino acids, such as lysine or tryptophan, combined with dibutyryl cyclic AMP exhibited no inhibitory effect. The growth inhibition by arginine was preceded by a sharp increase in cellular cyclic AMP which was attributed to the stimulation of NAD-dependent ADP-ribosylation and NAD-dependent activation of adenylate cyclase in the cell membrane. Moreover, the growth arrest by arginine was accompanied by a striking change in cell morphology. As shown in Fig. 2, the cytoplasm of arginine-treated cells was greatly enlarged without any appreciable change in the size of the nuclei. Upon cessation of arginine treatment, the cell number increased and the cell morphology returned to that of untreated cells. A similar growth inhibitory effect of arginine alone and the synergistic growth inhibitory action between arginine and dibutyryl cyclic AMP have also been shown in hormone-dependent mammary carcinomas DMBA and MTW9 _in vivo_ (26).

The evidence of malignant reversion summarized above is compatible with other _in vitro_ studies in which cyclic AMP-induced inhibition of cell proliferation is often associated with a change in morphology, synthesis of specialized cell products, and cell differentiation. These studies, therefore, suggest that cyclic AMP is capable of causing some transformed cells to revert to cells morphologically and biochemically similar to untransformed cells.

CONCLUSION

The objective of this chapter was to explore the role of cyclic AMP in controlling the growth of mammary tumors. The data presented support the hypothesis that the nuclear translocation of a complex consisting of cyclic AMP, its receptor binding protein and the catalytic unit of protein kinase is the indispensable event necessary to maintain normal or controlled growth. Thus the growth regulatory function of cyclic AMP depends upon both the structural integrity of the cyclic AMP receptor protein and an optimum cellular concentration (physiological level) of cyclic AMP.

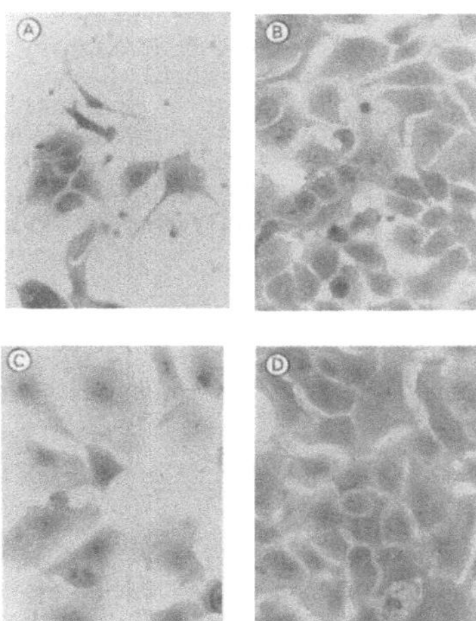

Fig. 2. L-arginine-induced growth arrest and morphological change in human breast carcinoma cells (MCF-7). A, MCF-7 cells grown in regular medium for 1 day; B, MCF-7 cells grown in regular medium for 5 days; C, MCF-7 cells grown for 5 days under the same conditions as B, except L-arginine·HCl (1 mg/ml) was added to the medium during growth; D, MCF-7 cells grown under the same conditions as C for 5 days, then grown in regular medium for 3 days. Cells were seeded as 1 x 10^6 cells/flask and the medium was changed every 48 hr. The photograph was taken after H & E staining (x 290).

Abnormal or neoplastic growth may be the phenotypic expression of a disrupted cyclic AMP-growth regulatory function, which may be the result of an alteration of the intracellular cyclic AMP level and/or the cyclic AMP receptor molecule. Under proper cyclic AMP stimulation, tumor regression does occur in hormone-dependent mammary carcinomas in which the integral cyclic AMP receptor protein is induced and then translocated into the nucleus. In hormone-independent mammary tumors, which contain a defective cyclic AMP receptor protein, nuclear translocation of the receptor does not occur and tumors continue to grow under the same cyclic AMP stimulation. Thus, cyclic AMP triggers regression of certain tumors in which cyclic AMP induces biochemical reversion of the neoplastic cells to normal-like cells. This finding could be of clinical significance in the treatment of hormone-dependent tumors.

The mechanism of cyclic AMP action at the nuclear level, as demonstrated by the nuclear translocation of the cyclic AMP receptor complex, is analogous to that of steroid hormone action at the nuclear level. Thus an interrelationship between the action of cyclic AMP and a steroid hormone in the expression of genetic information seems possible. During growth and regression of hormone-dependent mammary tumors, estrogen and cyclic AMP exert opposing actions, probably through their respective receptor proteins. The identification of the nuclear acceptor sites for cyclic AMP and estrogen receptors, together with the characterization of nuclear substrates for cyclic AMP-dependent and -independent protein kinases, should provide insight into the interaction of cyclic AMP and estrogen in the growth control of hormone-dependent mammary tumors.

ACKNOWLEDGEMENT

I am grateful to my collaborators for their help over the years.

REFERENCES

1. Anderson WB, Johnson GS, Pastan I. Transformation of chick-embryo fibroblasts by wild-type and temperature-sensitive Rous sarcoma virus alters adenylate cyclase activity. Proc Natl Acad Sci USA 70: 1055-1059, 1973.
2. Ashman DF, Lipton R, Melicow MM, Price TD. Isolation of adenosine 3',5'-monophosphate and guanosine 3',5'-monophosphate from rat urine. Biochem Biophys Res Commun 11: 330-334, 1963.
3. Beatson GT. On the treatment of inoperable cases of carcinoma of the mamma: Suggestions for a new method of treatment, with illustrative cases. Lancet 2: 104-107, 162-165, 1896.
4. Blume A, Gilbert F, Wilson S, Farber J, Rosenberg R, Nirenberg M. Regulation of acetylcholinesterase in neuroblastoma cells. Proc Natl Acad Sci USA 67: 786-792, 1970.
5. Bodwin JS, Cho-Chung YS. Interdependence of cyclic AMP binding protein and estrogen receptor in the growth control of hormone-dependent mammary carcinoma. Proc Am Assoc Cancer Res 20: 234, 1979.
6. Bodwin JS, Cho-Chung YS, Schneider WC. Nuclear translocation of estrogen receptor and cyclic AMP-binding protein in MTW9 mammary tumor. Proc Am Assoc Cancer Res 21: 36, 1980.
7. Bodwin JS, Clair T, Cho-Chung YS. Inverse relation between estrogen receptors and cyclic adenosine 3',5'-monophosphate-binding proteins in hormone-dependent mammary tumor regression due to dibutyryl cyclic adenosine 3',5'-monophosphate treatment or ovariectomy. Cancer Res 38: 3410-3413, 1978.
8. Bodwin JS, Clair T, Cho-Chung YS. Relationship of hormone-dependency to estrogen receptor and adenosine 3',5'-cyclic monophosphate-binding proteins in rat mammary tumors. J Natl Cancer Inst 64: 395-398, 1980.
9. Bodwin JS, Hirayama PH, Rego JA, Cho-Chung YS. Tamoxifen or pharmacological dose estrogen induced regression of hormone-dependent mammary tumors: Cyclic adenosine 3',5'-monophosphate mediated events. J Natl Cancer Inst 66: 321-326, 1981.

10. Burk R. Reduced adenyl cyclase activity in a polyoma virus transformed cell line. Nature 219: 1272-1275, 1968.
11. Byus CV, Russell DH. Possible regulations of ornithine decarboxylase activity in the adrenal medulla of the rat by a cAMP-dependent mechanism. Biochem Pharmac 25: 1595-1600, 1976.
12. Callentine MR. Nonsteroidal estrogen antagonists. Clin Obstet Gynecol 10: 74-87, 1967.
13. Chan PC, Cohen LA. Dietary fat and growth promotion of rat mammary tumors. Cancer Res 35: 3384-3386, 1975.
14. Cho-Chung YS. In vivo inhibition of tumor growth by cyclic adenosine 3',5'-monophosphate derivatives. Cancer Res 34: 3492-3496, 1974.
15. Cho-Chung YS. Interaction of cyclic AMP and estrogen in tumor growth control. pp 335-346 in Endocrine Control in Neoplasia, eds RK Sharma, WE Criss, Raven Press, New York, 1978.
16. Cho-Chung YS. Cyclic AMP and tumor growth in vivo. pp 55-93 in Influence of Hormones on Tumor Development, Vol I, eds JA Kellen, R Hilf, CRC Press, Boca Raton, 1979.
17. Cho-Chung YS. Minireview: On the interaction of cyclic AMP-binding protein and estrogen receptor in growth control. Life Sci 24: 1231-1240, 1979.
18. Cho-Chung YS. On the mechanism of cyclic AMP-mediated growth arrest of solid tumors. pp 111-121 in Advances in Cyclic Nucleotide Research, Vol 12, eds P Hamet, H Sands, Raven Press, New York, 1980.
19. Cho-Chung YS. Cyclic AMP and mammary tumor regression. Cell Mol Biol 26: 395-403, 1980.
20. Cho-Chung YS. Cyclic AMP and its receptor protein in tumor growth regulation in vivo. J Cyclic Nucleotide Res 6: 163-177, 1980.
21. Cho-Chung YS, Archibald D, Clair T. Cyclic AMP receptor triggers nuclear protein phosphorylation in a hormone-dependent mammary tumor cell-free system. Science 205: 1390-1392, 1979.
22. Cho-Chung YS, Bodwin JS, Clair T. Cyclic AMP-binding protein: Role in ovariectomy-induced regression of a hormone-dependent mammary tumor. J Natl Cancer Inst 60: 1175-1178, 1978.
23. Cho-Chung YS, Bodwin JS, Clair T. Cyclic AMP-binding protein: Inverse relationship with estrogen-receptors in hormone-dependent mammary tumor regression. Eur J Biochem 86: 51-60, 1978.
24. Cho-Chung YS, Clair T. Altered cyclic AMP-binding and db cyclic AMP-unresponsiveness in vivo. Nature 265: 452-454, 1977.
25. Cho-Chung YS, Clair T, Berghoffer B. L-arginine and dibutyryl cyclic AMP synergistically inhibit growth of murine mammary tumor in vivo and human breast cancer cells (MCF-7) in vivo. Proc Am Assoc Cancer Res 21: 39, 1980.
26. Cho-Chung YS, Clair T, Bodwin JS, Hill DM. Arrest of mammary tumor growth in vivo by L-arginine: Stimulation of NAD-dependent activation of adenylate cyclase. Biochem Biophys Res Commun 95: 1306-1313, 1980.
27. Cho-Chung YS, Clair T, Huffman P. Loss of nuclear cyclic AMP-binding in cyclic AMP-unresponsive Walker 256 mammary carcinoma. J Biol Chem 252: 6349-6355, 1977.

28. Cho-Chung YS, Clair T, Porper R. Cyclic AMP-binding proteins and protein kinase during regression of Walker 256 mammary carcinoma. J Biol Chem 252: 6342-6348, 1977.
29. Cho-Chung YS, Clair T, Schwimmer M, Steinberg L, Rego J, Grantham FH. Cyclic adenosine 3',5'-monophosphate receptor proteins in hormone-dependent and -independent rat mammary tumors. Cancer Res (in press).
30. Cho-Chung YS, Clair T, Yi PN, Parkison C. Comparative studies on cyclic AMP binding and protein kinase in cyclic AMP-responsive and -unresponsive Walker 256 mammary carcinomas. J Biol Chem 252: 6335-6341, 1977.
31. Cho-Chung YS, Clair T, Zubialde JP. Increase of cyclic AMP-dependent protein kinase type II as an early event in hormone-dependent mammary tumor regression. Biochem Biophys Res Commun 85: 1150-1155, 1978.
32. Cho-Chung YS, Doud FJ. Antagonistic action between cyclic AMP and estrogen in phosphorylation of mammary tumor nuclear proteins. Cancer Letters 5: 219-224, 1978.
33. Cho-Chung YS, Gullino PM. Mammary tumor regression. V. Role of acid ribonuclease and cathepsin. J Biol Chem 248: 4743-4749, 1973.
34. Cho-Chung YS, Gullino PM. Mammary tumor regression. VI. Synthesis and degradation of acid ribonuclease. J Biol Chem 248: 4750-4755, 1973.
35. Cho-Chung YS, Gullino PM. *In vivo* inhibition of growth of two hormone-dependent mammary tumors by dibutyryl cyclic AMP. Science 183: 87-88, 1974.
36. Cho-Chung YS, Redler BH. Dibutyryl cyclic AMP mimics ovariectomy: Nuclear protein phosphorylation in mammary tumor regression. Science 197: 272-275, 1977.
37. Cho-Chung YS, Redler BH, Lewallen RP. Nuclear protein phosphorylation and hormone-dependent mammary tumor regression following dibutyryl cyclic adenosine 3',5'-monophosphate treatment or ovariectomy. Cancer Res 38: 3405-3409, 1978.
38. Chuang DM, Hollenbeck RA, Costa E. Protein phosphorylation in nuclei of adrenal medulla incubated with cyclic adenosine 3',5'-monophosphate-dependent protein kinase. J Biol Chem 252: 8365-8373, 1977.
39. Coffino P, Bourne HR, Friedrich U, Hochman J, Insel PA, Lamaire I, Melmon KL, Tomkins GM. Molecular mechanisms of cyclic AMP action: A genetic approach. pp 669-684 in *Recent Progress in Hormone Research*, Vol 32, ed RO Greep, Academic Press, New York, 1976.
40. Coffino P, Yamamoto KR. Somatic genetic studies of steroid and cyclic AMP receptors. pp 57-66 in *Control Mechanisms in Cancer*, eds WE Criss, T Ono, JR Sabine, Raven Press, New York, 1976.
41. Cohen LA, Chan PC. Intracellular cAMP levels in normal rat mammary gland and adenocarcinoma. *In vivo* vs *in vitro*. Life Sci 16: 107-115, 1975.
42. Corbin JD, Sugden PH, West L, Flockhart DA, Lincoln TM, McCarthy D. Studies on the properties and mode of action of the purified regulatory subunit of bovine heart adenosine 3',5'-monophosphate-dependent protein kinase. J Biol Chem 253: 3997-4003, 1978.

43. Costa E, Kurosawa A, Guidotti A. Activation and nuclear translocation of protein kinase during transsynaptic induction of tyrosine 3-monooxygenase. Proc Natl Acad Sci USA 73: 1058-1062, 1976.
44. Daniel V, Litwack G, Tomkins GM. Induction of cytolysis of cultured lymphoma cells by adenosine 3',5'-cyclic monophosphate and the isolation of resistant variants. Proc Natl Acad Sci USA 70: 76-79, 1973.
45. Dao TL. Nature of hormonal influence in carcinogenesis studies in vivo and in vitro. pp 503-514 in Chemical Carcinogenesis, Part B, eds POP Ts'O, JA DiPaolo, Marcel Dekker, Inc., New York, 1974.
46. Dao TL, Sinha D. Oestrogen and prolactin in mammary carcinogenesis in vivo and in vitro studies. pp 189-194 in Prolactin and Carcinogenesis, eds AR Boyns, K Griffiths, Alpha Omega Alpha, Cardiff, Wales, 1972.
47. De Rubertis FR, Craven PA. Cyclic nucleotides in carcinogenesis: Activation of the guanylate cyclase-cyclic AMP system by chemical carcinogen. pp 97-109 in Advances in Cyclic Nucleotide Research, Vol 12, eds P Hamet, H Sands, Raven Press, New York, 1980.
48. Erlichman J, Rosenfeld R, Rosen OM. Phosphorylation of a cyclic adenosine 3',5'-monophosphate-dependent protein kinase from bovine cardiac muscle. J Biol Chem 249: 5000-5003, 1974.
49. Gericke D, Chandra P. Inhibition of tumor growth by nucleoside cyclic 3',5'-monophosphates. Hoppe Seyler's Z Physiol Chem 350: 1469-1471, 1969.
50. Goldberg ND, Dietz SB, O'Toole AG. Cyclic guanosine 3',5'-monophosphate in mammalian tissues and urine. J Biol Chem 244: 4458-4466, 1969.
51. Goldberg ND, Haddox MK. Cyclic AMP metabolism and involvement in biological regulation. Ann Rev Biochem 46: 823-896, 1977.
52. Guerinot F, Delarue JC, Contesso G, Bohuon C. Adenosine 3',5'-cyclic monophosphate and guanosine 3',5'-cyclic monophosphate levels in human breast cancer tissue. Oncology 34: 261-263, 1977.
53. Gullino PM, Pettigrew HM, Grantham FH. N-Nitrosomethylurea as mammary gland carcinogen in rats. J Natl Cancer Inst 54: 401-404, 1975.
54. Haddow A, Watkinson JM, Paterson E, Koller PC. Influence of synthetic oestrogens upon advanced malignant disease. Br Med J 2: 393-398, 1944.
55. Handschin JC, Eppenberger U. Altered cellular ratio of type I and type II cyclic AMP-dependent protein kinase in human mammary tumors. FEBS Lett 106: 301-304, 1979.
56. Helson L, Helson C, Peterson RF. A rationale for the treatment of metastatic neuroblastoma. J Natl Cancer Inst 57: 727-729, 1976.
57. Hickie RA. Regulation of cyclic AMP and cyclic GMP in Morris hepatomas and liver. Adv Exp Med Biol 92: 451-488, 1977.
58. Hilf R, Inge M, Carlton B. Biochemical and morphologic properties of a new lactating mammary tumor line in the rat. Cancer Res 25: 286-297, 1965.
59. Huggins C, Bergenstal DM. Inhibition of human mammary and prostatic cancers by adrenalectomy. Cancer Res 12: 134-141, 1952.

60. Huggins C, Grand LC, Brillantes FP. Mammary cancer induced by a single feeding of polynuclear hydrocarbons, and its suppression. Nature 189: 204-207, 1961.
61. Hoffmann F, Beavo JA, Bechtel PJ, Krebs EG. Comparison of adenosine 3',5'-monophosphate-dependent protein kinase from rabbit skeletal and bovine heart muscle. J Biol Chem 250: 7795-7801, 1975.
62. Ishikawa E, Ishikawa S, Davis JW, Sutherland EW. Determination of guanosine 3',5'-monophosphate in tissues and guanyl cyclase in rat intestine. J Biol Chem 244: 6371-6376, 1969.
63. Jensen EV, DeSombre ER. Mechanism of action of the female sex hormones. Annu Rev Biochem 789: 203-230, 1972.
64. Jungmann RA, Lee SG, DeAngelo AB. Translocation of cytoplasmic protein kinase and cyclic adenosine monophosphate-binding protein to intracellular acceptor sites. pp 281-306 in Advances in Cyclic Nucleotide Research, Vol 5, eds GI Drummond, P Greengard, GA Robison, Raven Press, New York, 1975.
65. Keller R. Suppression of normal and enhanced tumor growth in rats by agents interfering with intracellular cyclic nucleotides. Life Sci 11 (part 2): 485-491, 1972.
66. Kim U, Furth J. Relation of mammotropes to mammary tumors. IV. Development of highly hormone dependent mammary tumors. Proc Soc Exp Biol Med 105: 490-492, 1960.
67. Kimhi Y, Palfrey C, Spector I, Barak Y, Littauer UZ. Maturation of neuroblastoma cells in the presence of dimethylsulfoxide. Proc Natl Acad Sci USA 73: 462-466, 1976.
68. King RJB, Mainwaring WIP. V. Glucocorticoid. VI. Mineralicorticoids. III. Estrogens. VIII. Progesterone. pp 102-287 in Steroid Cell Interactions, eds RJB King, University Park Press, Baltimore, 1974.
69. King RJB, Smith JA, Steggles AW. Oestrogen-binding and the hormone responsiveness of tumors. Steroidologia 1: 73-88, 1970.
70. Klein DM, Loizzi RF. Enhancement of R3230AC rat mammary tumor growth and cellular differentiation by dibutyryl cyclic adenosine monophosphate. J Natl Cancer Inst 58: 813-818, 1977.
71. Konijn TM. Cyclic AMP as a first messenger. pp 17-31 in Advances Cyclic Nucleotide Res, Vol 1, eds P Greengard, GA Robison, R Paoletti, Raven Press, New York, 1972.
72. Krebs EG. Protein kinase. Curr Top Cell Regul 5: 99-133, 1972.
73. Kuehl FA Jr, Ham EA, Zanetti ME, Sanford CH, Nicol SE, Goldberg ND. Estrogen-related increases in uterine guanosine 3',5'-cyclic monophosphate levels. Proc Natl Acad Sci USA 71: 1866-1870, 1974.
74. Kung W, Bechtel E, Geyer E, Salokangas A, Preisz J, Huber P, Torhorst J, Jungmann RA, Talmadge K, Eppenberger U. Altered levels of cyclic nucleotides, cAMP-phosphodiesterase and adenylyl cyclase activities in normal, dysplastic and neoplastic human mammary tissue. FEBS Lett 82: 102-106, 1977.
75. Kuo JF, Greengard P. Cyclic nucleotide-dependent protein kinase. IV. Wide-spread occurrence of adenosine 3',5'-monophosphate-dependent protein kinase in various tissues and phyla of the animal kingdom. Proc Natl Acad Sci USA 64: 1349-1355, 1969.

76. Kyser KA. The tissue, subcellular and molecular binding of estradiol to dimethylbenzanthracene-induced rat mammary tumors. Ph.D. Dissertation, The University of Chicago, 1970.

77. Lerner LJ, Holthaus FJ Jr, Thompsen CR. A non-steroidal estrogen antagonist 1-(p-2-diethylaminoethoxyphenyl)-1-phenyl-2-p-methoxyphenyl ethanol. Endocrinology 63: 295-318, 1958.

78. Leung BS, Sasaki GH, Leung JS. Estrogen-prolactin dependency in 7, 12-dimethylbenz(α)anthracene-induced tumors. Cancer Res 35: 621-627, 1975.

79. Liao W. Cellular receptors and mechanism of action of steroid hormones. pp 87-172 in International Review of Cytology, Vol 41, eds GH Bourne, JF Danielli, KW Jeon, Academic Press, New York, 1975.

80. Liu AYC, Greengard P. Regulation by steroid hormones of phosphorylation of specific protein common to several target organs. Proc Natl Acad Sci USA 73: 568-572, 1976.

81. Maeno H, Reyes PL, Ueda T, Rudolph SA, Greengard P. Autophosphorylation of adenosine 3',5'-monophosphate-dependent protein kinase from bovine brain. Arch Biochem Biophys 164: 551-559, 1974.

82. Magee PN. In vivo reactions of nitroso compounds. Ann NY Acad Sci 163: 717-730, 1969.

83. Matusik RJ, Hilf R. Relationship of adenosine 3',5'-cyclic monophosphate and guanosine 3',5'-cyclic monophosphate to growth of dimethylbenz[α]anthracene-induced mammary tumors in rats. J Natl Cancer Inst 56: 659-661, 1976.

84. McGuire WL. Current status of estrogen receptors in human breast cancer. Cancer 36: 638-644, 1975.

85. McGuire WL, Julian J. Comparison of macromolecular binding of estradiol in hormone-dependent and hormone-independent rat mammary carcinoma. Cancer Res 31: 1440-1445, 1971.

86. Minton JP, Wisenbaugh TW, Matthews RH. Elevated adenosine 3',5'-monophosphate levels in human breast cancer tissue. J Natl Cancer Inst 53: 283-284, 1974.

87. Narisawa T, Magadia NE, Weisburger JH, Wynder EL. Promoting effect of bile acids on colon carcinogenesis after intrarectal instillation of N-methyl-N'-nitro-N-nitrosoguanidine in rats. J Natl Cancer Inst 53: 1093-1097, 1974.

88. Oertel GW, Benes P, Hoffman G, Shuy E. Interaction between dehydroepiandrosterone, glucose-6-phosphate dehydrogenase, and cyclic adenosine 3',5'-monophosphate in neoplastic and normal human mammary tissue. Experientia 31: 1124-1125, 1975.

89. O'Malley BW, Means AR. Female steroid hormones and target cell nuclei. The effects of steroid hormones on target cell nuclei are of major importance in the interaction of new cell functions. Science 183: 610-620, 1974.

90. Otten J, Bader J, Johnson GS, Pastan I. A mutation in a Rous sarcoma virus gene that controls adenosine 3',5'-monophosphate levels and transformation. J Biol Chem 247: 1632-1633, 1972.

91. Pastan I, Johnson GS. Cyclic AMP and the transformation of fibroblasts. Adv Cancer Res 19: 303-329, 1974.

92. Pastan I, Johnson GS, Anderson WB. Role of cyclic nucleotides in growth control. Annu Rev Biochem 44: 491-522, 1975.

93. Pastan I, Perlman RL. Regulation of gene transcription in E. coli by cyclic AMP. pp 11-16 in Advances in Cyclic Nucleotide Research, Vol 1, eds P Greengard, GA Robison, R Paoletti, Raven Press, New York, 1972.
94. Perry JW, Oka T. Cyclic AMP as a negative regulator of hormonally induced lactogenesis in mouse mammary gland organ culture. Proc Natl Acad Sci USA 77: 2093-2097, 1980.
95. Pomerantz AH, Rudolph SA, Haley BE, Greengard P. Photoaffinity labeling of a protein kinase from bovine brain with 8-azidoadenosine 3',5'-monophosphate. Biochemistry 14: 3858-3862, 1975.
96. Prasad KN. Cyclic AMP-induced differentiated mouse neuroblastoma cells lose tumourigenic characteristics. Cytobios 6: 163-166, 1972.
97. Prasad KN, Kumar S. Role of cyclic AMP in differentiation of human neuroblastoma cells in culture. Cancer 36: 1338-1343, 1975.
98. Prasad KN, Sahu SK, Sinha PK. Cyclic nucleotides in the regulation of expression of differentiated functions in neuroblastoma cells. J Natl Cancer Inst 57: 619-631, 1976.
99. Rangel-Aldao R, Kupiec JW, Rosen OM. Resolution of the phosphorylated and dephosphorylated cAMP-binding proteins of bovine cardiac muscle by affinity labeling and two-dimensional electrophoresis. J Biol Chem 254: 2499-2508, 1979.
100. Richelson E. Stimulation of tyrosine hydroxylase activity in an adrenergic clone of mouse neuroblastoma by dibutyryl cyclic AMP. Nature New Biol 242: 175-177, 1973.
101. Rubin CS, Rosen OM. Protein phosphorylation. Annu Rev Biochem 44: 831-887, 1975.
102. Sapag-Hagar M, Greenbaum AL. The role of cyclic nucleotides in the development and function of rat mammary tissue. FEBS Lett 46: 180-183, 1974.
103. Sapag-Hagar M, Greenbaum AL, Lewis DJ, Hallowes RC. The effect of DI-butyryl cAMP on enzymatic and metabolic changes in explants of rat mammary tissue. Biochem Biophys Res Commun 59: 261-268, 1974.
104. Schinzinger A. Ueber Carcinoma mammae. Verh Deutsch Ges Chir 18: 28-29, 1889.
105. Schubert D, Humphreys S, Baroni C, Cohn S. In vitro differentiation of a mouse neuroblastoma. Proc Natl Acad Sci USA 64: 316-323, 1969.
106. Segaloff A. Hormones and breast cancer. Recent Prog Horm Res 22: 351-379, 1966.
107. Shafie SM, Cho-Chung YS, Gullino PM. Cyclic adenosine 3',5'-monophosphate and protein kinase activity in insulin-dependent and and -independent mammary tumors. Cancer Res 39: 2501-2504, 1979.
108. Shanker G, Ahrens H, Sharma RK. Novel protein kinase, AUT-PK85, isolated from adrenocortical carcinoma: Purification and characterization. Proc Natl Acad Sci USA 76: 66-70, 1979.
109. Simantov R, Sachs L. Temperature sensitivity of cyclic adenosine 3',5'-monophosphate-binding proteins and the regulation of growth and differentiation in neuroblastoma cells. J Biol Chem 250: 3236-3242, 1975.
110. Smith EE, Handler AH. Apparent suppression of the tumorigenicity of human cancer cells by cyclic AMP. Res Commun Chem Pathol Pharmacol 5: 863-866, 1973.

111. So BT, Magadia NE, Wynder EL. Induction of carcinomas of the colon and rectum in rats by N-methyl-N-nitro-N-nitrosoguanidine. J Natl Cancer Inst 50: 927-932, 1973.
112. Steinberg RA, O'Farrell PH, Friedrich U, Coffino P. Mutations causing charge alterations in regulatory subunits of the cyclic AMP-dependent protein kinase of cultured S49 lymphoma cells. Cell 10: 381-391, 1977.
113. Sutherland EW. Studies on the mechanism of hormone action. Science 177: 401-408, 1972.
114. Tisdale MJ, Phillips BJ. Cyclic nucleotide metabolism in Walker carcinoma cells resistant to alkylating agents. Biochem Pharm 27: 947-952, 1978.
115. Turkington RW. Hormone-dependent differentiation of mammary gland in vitro. pp 199-218 in Current Topics in Developmental Biology, Vol 3, eds AA Moscona, A Monroy, Academic Press, New York, 1968.
116. Walter U, Uno I, Liu AY-C, Greengard P. Study of autophosphorylation of isozymes of cyclic AMP-dependent protein kinases. J Biol Chem 252: 6588-6590, 1977.
117. Waymire JC, Weiner N, Prasad KN. Regulation of tyrosine hydroxylase activity in cultured mouse neuroblastoma cells. Elevation induced by analogs of adenosine 3',5'-cyclic monophosphate. Proc Natl Acad Sci USA 69: 2241-2245, 1972.
118. Weber W, Hilz H. Adenosine 3',5'-monophosphate-binding proteins from bovine kidney. Isolation by affinity chromatography and limited proteolysis of the regulatory subunit of protein kinase II. Eur J Biochem 83: 215-225, 1978.
119. Wittliff JL. Steroid binding proteins in normal and neoplastic mammary cells. Methods Cancer Res 11: 293-354, 1975.
120. Wu C. Hormonal regulation of glutamine synthetase and ornithine aminotransferase in normal and neoplastic rat tissues. pp 125-138 in Control Mechanisms in Cancer, eds WE Criss, T Ono, JR Sabine, Raven Press, New York, 1976.

Chapter 9

PROSTAGLANDINS, FATTY ACIDS AND PHOSPHOLIPIDS IN NORMAL AND NEOPLASTIC BREAST TISSUES

Grace Y Sun, Benjamin S Leung

INTRODUCTION

Regulation of mammary functions by hormonal factors is a complex phenomenon. Consequently, many of the biochemical mechanisms underlying various functional changes are not yet well understood. It is realized, however, that a disturbance of the regulatory mechanisms may result in abnormal functioning of the gland. Fatty acids and phospholipids are important not only as structural components of the mammary cell membranes, but also in regulating the membrane functions (72). Metabolism of the membrane lipids is generally governed by membrane-bound enzymes, some of which are hormonally regulated. The mammary gland lipids are altered during physiological changes such as from non-pregnant to pregnant states, pregnancy to lactation or neoplastic transformation of the gland. In this chapter, the compositional and metabolic changes of fatty acids and phospholipids of the mammary gland under different physiological conditions will be described and a comparison of the changes of neoplastic tissues with normal tissue will be made. Neoplastic cell transformation and tumor growth are also correlated to effects exerted by dietary lipids. A discussion of the mammary gland prostaglandins is included because these molecules are derived from polyunsaturated fatty acids, and they may play an important role in regulating the glandular functions, as well as tumorigenesis.

CONTENT OF FATTY ACIDS AND PHOSPHOLIPIDS

Normal mammary tissues.

The types of phospholipids found in the mammary tissue of non-ruminants are generally not different from those present in other organs of the body. The mammary tissue, however, contains a notable amount of ethanolamine and choline plasmalogens, and lyso-phospholipids. Metabolism of phospholipids in normal mammary tissue can be divided into four physiologically distinct periods: pregnancy, early lactation, lactation and post weaning. Changes in phospholipids and fatty acids are known to be associated with these various stages (73). For example, the proportion of phosphatidylcholine (PC) in the rat mammary gland increases during early lactation and again after weaning (Table 1). On the other hand, the proportion of phosphatidylethanolamines (PE) increases during lactation, especially towards the late lactating period. During lactation, a slight decrease in the proportion of ethanolamine plasmalogens and an increase in lysolecithin are also noted. Following weaning, there is a decrease in the levels of the acidic phospholipids such as phosphatidylserines (PS) and phosphatidylinositols (PI). These compositional changes are possibly related to altered activities of hormone-regulated enzymes which are involved in the metabolism of these lipids.

Table 1. Phospholipid Composition of Rat Mammary Tissue During Pregnant, Lactating and Post-Weaning Periods.

Phospholipids	Pregnant	Early Lactation 1-3 days	Lactation 7-19 days	Post-Weaning 2-5 days
		% mole distribution		
Sph	13.5 ± 2.3	13.6 ± 1.07	9.9 ± 1.84	20.1 ± 2.31
PI	9.9 ± 1.2	7.9 ± 1.19	10.6 ± 1.34	8.2 ± 2.20
PS	9.2 ± 1.7	6.7 ± 0.47	6.1 ± 0.66	--
PCp	2.9 ± 0.5	3.5 ± 0.25	3.1 ± 0.40	--
PC	31.6 ± 0.5	40.2 ± 1.15	33.6 ± 3.42	49.8 ± 2.83
PEp	13.4 ± 0.7	5.6 ± 0.75	6.7 ± 1.21	5.6 ± 3.42
PE	13.9 ± 0.9	15.0 ± 2.2	22.0 ± 1.59	6.5 ± 0.41
PA	1.1 ± 0.8	0.9 ± 0.40	1.3 ± 0.64	--
LPC	4.3 ± 2.7	6.4 ± 0.31	7.0 ± 1.37	8.4 ± 1.24
	(n=5)	(n=3)	(n=4)	(n=4)

Values are obtained from Table 1 of Sun and Leung (73), after grouping and recalculation. Lipids extracted from each sample were separated by a reactional two-dimensional thin-layer chromatographic procedure according to Horrocks and Sun (25). Abbreviations: Sph, sphingomyelin; PI, phosphatidylinositols; PS, phosphatidylserine; PCpl, phosphatidylcholine plasmalogens; PC, phosphatidylcholines; PEpl, phosphatidylethanolamine plasmalogens; PA, phosphatidate; LPC, lyso-phosphatidylcholines.

Marked acyl group changes are also observed in the phospholipids and triacylglycerols (TG) of the mammary gland in conjunction with the changes in physiological stages (73). During pregnancy, acyl groups of PC and PE in the rat mammary gland contain relatively low proportion of 18:2 and high proportion of 20:4. This relationship is reversed shortly after parturition (Table 2). The fatty acids of TG in pregnant rat mammary gland are comprised mainly of 16:0, 18:1 and 18:2, with only trace amounts of 20:4 and 18:0. During lactation, the proportion of 18:2 in TG increases and is accompanied by a gradual increase of medium chain fatty acids (Table 3). Thus, the increase of 18:2 in the lactating gland can be found in both TG and phospholipids, whereas medium chain fatty acids are esterified mainly to TG. The acyl group levels in TG and phospholipids returns rapidly to levels of the pre-pregnant state shortly after weaning (Sun and Leung, unpublished results).

Table 2. Acyl Group Composition (percent weight) of Phosphatidylcholine and Phosphatidylethanolamines in Mammary Gland During Pregnant, Lactating and Post-Weaning Periods.

Acyl groups	Preg 21 d	Lact 1 d	Lact 10 d	Lact 18 d	Lact 21 d	Post 1 d
			Phosphatidylcholines			
12:0	-	0.4	-	0.6	-	-
14:0	-	0.3	0.4	0.4	1.1	-
16:0	34.2	42.1	29.0	23.1	21.0	-
18:0	15.3	21.6	29.4	24.0	23.5	-
18:1	24.3	21.2	14.9	14.2	12.4	-
18:2	10.6	9.5	19.1	22.5	26.0	-
20:3	-	-	-	0.8	1.5	-
20:4	15.6	5.0	7.1	12.2	11.9	-
U[a]	-	-	-	2.3	2.6	-
			Phosphatidylethanolamines			
16:0	7.0	5.1	4.2	4.8	4.6	10.9
18:0	23.7	39.9	26.2	29.0	26.9	28.1
18:1	25.0	28.3	23.3	20.6	18.3	16.6
18:2	8.2	5.3	21.8	18.8	21.2	15.7
20:3	-	-	-	0.3	0.9	-
20:4	36.1	21.4	24.6	23.7	23.6	28.7
U	-	-	-	2.9	4.6	-

[a]Unidentified fatty acids with retention times longer than that for 20:4. Procedures for analysis was same as described in Sun and Leung (73) that the data were obtained from analysis of a different group of rats. Abbreviations: Preg, pregnant; lact, lactation; post, post-weaning; d, days.

Table 3. Acyl Group Composition of Triacylglycerols from Rat Mammary Gland During Pregnant, Lactating and Post-Weaning Periods.

Acyl groups	Preg 10 d	Preg 18 d	Lact 1 d	Lact 5 d	Lact 10 d	Lact 18 d	Lact 21 d	Post 1 d
				%, wt.				
12:0	-	1.1	1.5	1.9	2.3	4.4	3.5	1.3
14:0	1.3	2.0	2.7	2.5	4.9	6.4	7.7	1.9
14:1	-	0.9	0.8	0.3	0.8	1.1	1.1	0.7
16:0	28.5	25.7	25.6	24.2	22.7	21.7	25.1	23.9
16:1	7.5	6.9	6.8	4.2	4.9	4.0	4.4	4.9
18:0	4.6	5.4	5.1	5.8	5.5	6.9	6.4	5.6
18:1	42.8	40.8	39.9	41.8	38.3	34.3	30.7	39.8
18:2	14.1	12.5	12.6	15.8	17.0	17.2	17.9	17.9
18:3	1.2	1.2	1.1	1.4	2.3	3.2	3.0	2.0
20:4	-	2.5	2.4	1.3	1.2	0.8	0.3	2.0

Procedures for sample analyses are same as described in Table 2.

Apart from the gross acyl group changes in TG and phospholipids described above, some small but significant changes in the 20:4 of PC and TG are observed in the mammary gland around the time of parturition. The change in 20:4 level (Fig 1) during parturition is different from that of 18:2 (Fig 2). Immediately before delivery, there is a rapid decline of 20:4 level of PC which is followed by a marked increase during the first two days of lactation (Fig 1). Although the 20:4 level of TG in the normal gland is generally very low (sometimes undetectable), a sharp rise in this fatty acid is shown at the time of parturition (Fig 1). The increase in 20:4 of TG is short-lived and can only be detected during parturition. Rillema and Mulder (60) also observed a small but significant increase in 20:4 from the neutral lipid fraction of the gland around the mid-pregnant period. The transient increase in 20:4 level during parturition may imply a metabolic correlation between fatty acids and prostaglandin biosynthesis, although the mechanism underlying these changes is not known.

In contrast, changes of 18:2 in TG in the mammary glands before and after parturition are distinctly different (Fig 2). Increase of 18:2 continues until mid-lactation and this maximal level is sustained to the end of lactation.

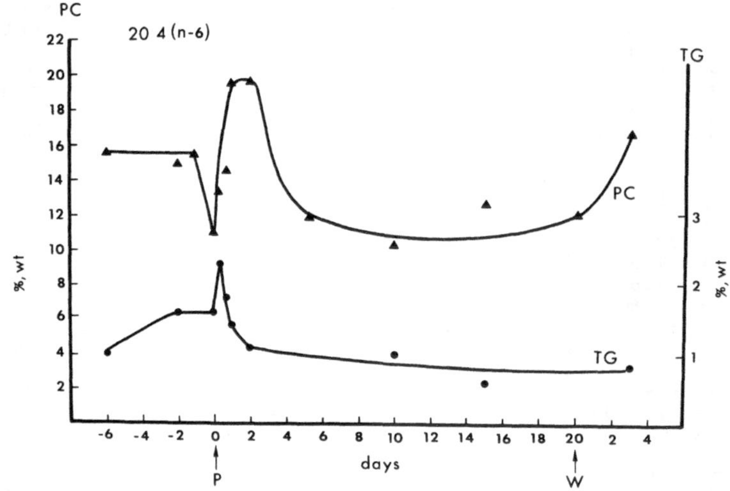

Fig 1. Percent distribution of 20:4 in phosphatidylcholines (PC) and triacylglycerols (TG) of rat mammary gland as a function of time before and after parturition (P).

Mammary tumors.

Unlike normal tissue, the lipids in mammary tumors lack the neutral glycerides, especially TG (76). On the contrary, most tumors show elevated levels of free fatty acids (FFA) (77) and lyso-phospholipids (46). Accumulation of FFA and lyso-phospholipids is a frequent indication of phospholipid degradation due to the pathophysiological insult. This explains why women with metastatic breast carcinoma have higher serum levels of FFA than controls (18). Changes in phospholipid and acyl group profiles occur in mammary tumors induced in Sprague Dawley rats by intragastric feeding of DMBA (46). In general, the mammary tumors show a greater variability in their lipid composition as compared to control tissues, probably relating to different degrees of neoplastic transformation. As compared to apparently "normal" tissues taken from the contralateral gland, the tumor phospholipids are characterized by a lower proportion of PC and a higher proportion of PE, and the decrease in PC/PE ratio is more apparent in malignant tumors than in benign tumors (Table 4). The former tissue seems to have a higher level of lyso-phospholipids than the latter or "normal" tissues. However, we would like to confirm this finding by better quantitative method for lyso-phospholipid assay now available in our laboratory.

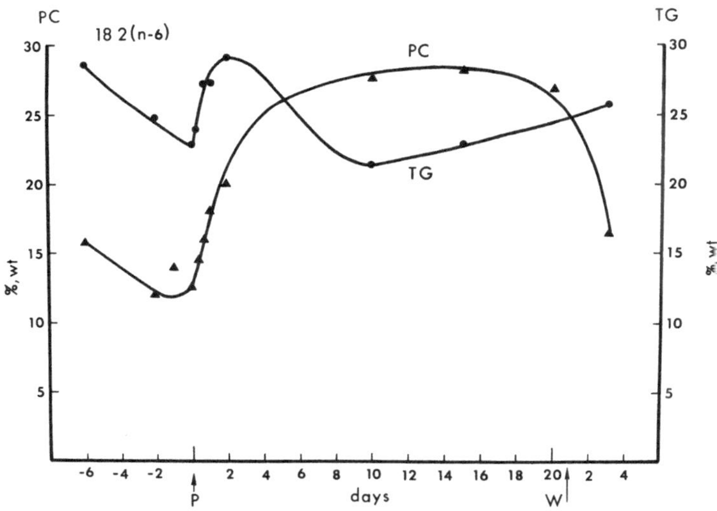

Fig 2. Percent distribution of 18:2 in phosphatidylcholines (PC) and triacylglycerols (TG) of rat mammary gland as a function of time before and after parturition (P).

The acyl group composition of phospholipids in DMBA-tumors is different from "normal" mammary tissues taken from the same tumor-bearing rats. The tumor phospholipids exhibit a decrease in the proportion of 18:2 and an increase in 18:1. The proportions of other longer chain polyunsaturated fatty acids, however, do not show appreciable changes (46). Other changes such as a decrease in 18:2 and a concurrent increase of 20:4 in the total tissue fatty acids from the tumors has been reported (76), and the increase in 20:4 appears to be related to the degree of metastatic transformation (56). The 20:4 levels are several fold higher in DMBA-induced tumors and in mid-pregnant rats in comparison with the mammary lipids from virgin rats (60). This increase is attributed to the change in diacylglycerols which increase from an undetectable level in normal mammary tissues to about 19% of total fatty acids in the tumors (60). In some of our studies, we also observe an increase in 20:4 level in the tumors, but the increase is mainly shown in TG which rise from a trace level to a noticeable 3% (Sun and Leung, unpublished data). The increase in 20:4 in the neutral glycerides of tumors should be further substantiated, because this change may have important physiological implications in providing the substrates for prostaglandin biosynthesis.

Table 4. A Comparison of the Phospholipid Composition of Mammary Tissue and Tumors.

Phospholipids	17u N	17u B	17z N	17z B	18A N	18A M	18B N	18B M
			% mole distribution					
Sph	20.3	18.9	18.3	11.9	20.3	12.7	12.0	14.9
PI	5.0	6.1	4.7	6.3	5.8	9.7	6.3	7.8
PS	8.2	11.7	9.3	8.4	11.2	9.5	8.8	8.1
PCpl	5.3	-	4.1	-	4.6	2.3	4.5	3.9
PC	46.9	42.1	41.6	42.2	40.7	30.4	42.5	31.5
PEpl	5.5	8.2	10.6	15.7	8.3	15.9	15.8	16.9
PE	6.3	8.7	8.2	12.8	7.6	14.3	10.1	13.2
PA	3.0	4.3	2.9	2.7	1.5	1.2	-	-
LPC	1.1	-	1.1	-	-	3.9	-	3.7

Lipids were extracted from the tissue by chloroform-methanol 2:1 (v/v) and were separated by the reactional two-dimensional thin layer chromatographic procedure according to Horrocks and Sun (27). Abbreviations for phospholipids are same as in Table 1. In each analysis of the tumor (B, benign and M, malignant), apparently normal tissue (N) was obtained from the contralateral gland for comparison.

METABOLISM OF PHOSPHOLIPIDS

Normal mammary gland

Since phosphatidate is the precursor for biosynthesis of all glycerol-containing lipids, it is important to understand the biochemical mechanisms for regulating the acylation of α-glycerophosphates in the mammary gland (Fig 3). Kinsella and Gross (39) found that palmitoyl-CoA is a highly preferred substrate for the acylation of α-glycerophosphates as well as 1-palmitoyl-glycerophosphates, and suggested that these acyltransferases are the key enzymes in controlling bovine milk fat production. Tanioka et al. (78) also showed that palmitate is a better preferred substrate for this transfer reaction. The fact that a maximal rate of acylation may occur at or below the critical micellar concentration (CMC) of the acyl-CoA suggests that only the monomeric molecules are accepted by the enzyme. When mammary gland microsomes are incubated with fatty acids in the presence of CoASH, ATP and Mg^{++} (BSA and NaF), the phosphatidate formed contains oleate and palmitate at the first and second positions, respectively (14). This type of acyl group specificity is different from that exhibited by the liver microsomes.

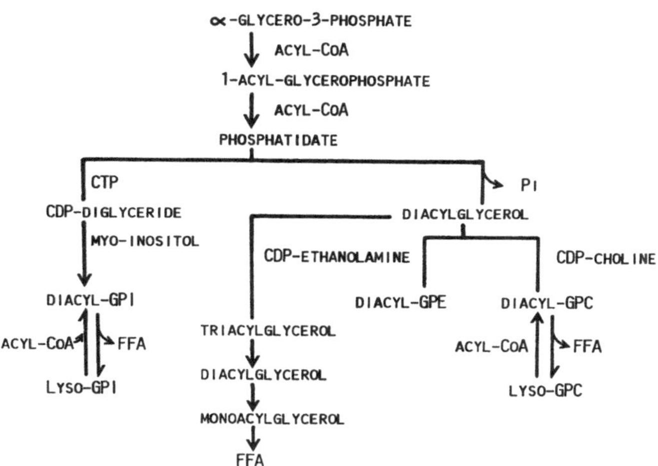

Fig 3. A scheme depicting the metabolism of phospholipids and triacylglycerols in the mammary gland.

The acyltransferase responsible for acylation of lyso-phosphatidic acid (LPAT) has been studied in substantial detail by Kinsella (38). This enzyme is present in the microsomal fraction of the lactating bovine mammary gland and is shown to prefer palmitoyl-CoA as the acyl-donor. However, in the lactating mammary gland, the enzyme can also accept medium chain fatty acids ranging from C_8 to C_{18}, but not those below C_8 (51). Caffrey et al. (6) observed a biphasic substrate curve upon assay of the LPAT activity in mammary gland microsomes during late pregnant and early lactation states. However, during early pregnancy, the enzyme is only active with substrates in the monomeric form. Since the two isoenzymes exhibit disparate thermal stabilities and sensitivities towards different types of detergents (8), physiological surfactants are thought to play a role in regulating their activities (7).

Although activities of the enzymes involved in fatty acid activation and esterification in mammary homogenates are low before parturition, activity increases during lactation (66). The incorporation of fatty acids directly into membrane phospholipids is mediated by fatty acid:CoASH ligase and lyso-phospholipid acyltransferase (74). Unlike lysophosphatidate acyltransferase, acyl-CoA: 1-acyl-glycero-3-phosphocholine acyltransferase in the mammary gland prefers oleate and linoleate as the acyl acceptor donor. Biosynthesis of PC in the mammary gland is normally 3-6 fold more active than that for PE. Therefore, most labeled precursors, whether they be ^{32}P-phosphate, glycerol or fatty acids, are more rapidly directed towards the synthesis of PC (36).

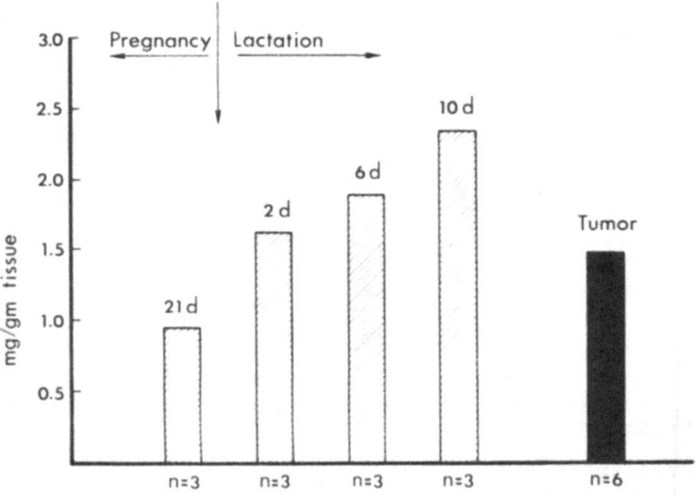

Fig. 4. Amount of microsomes yielded per gm tissue in pregnant and lactating mammary gland, and in mammary adenocarcinomas.

The synthesis and metabolism of mammary gland phospholipids occur mainly in the microsomal fraction. As shown in Fig 4, the amount of microsomes yielded from the mammary tissue (based on per gm of tissue) increases shortly after parturition, reaching a maximum at 10 days of lactation. The amount of microsomal proteins obtained from the tumors is higher than the non-lactating tissue but lower than the lactating tissue. The activities of oleoyl-CoA transfer to 1-acyl-glycerophosphocholines (GPC) and 1-acyl-glycerophosphate by the mammary gland microsomes were determined during these different physiological states. As shown in Fig 5 and 6, both types of acyltransferases increase dramatically shortly after parturition and reach a maximum around mid-lactation. Both events also return to pre-parturition state shortly after weaning. Apparently, a rapid turnover of the acyl groups of membrane phospholipids is occurring in the tissue during lactation. Not only the increase in enzymic activities is needed for synthesis of milk fat, but an active acyl group turnover is probably important for the secretory event as well.

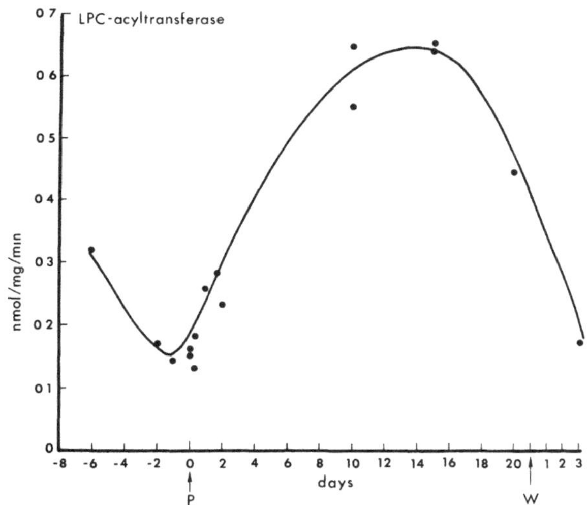

Fig 5. Activity of the oleoyl-CoA:1-palmitoyl-GPC acyltransferase in microsomes of rat mammary gland as a function of time before and after parturition (P). Assay procedure for this enzyme is same as in Sun et al. (75).

During lactation, TG in blood is taken up preferentially by the mammary gland, and then hydrolyzed within the gland by lipase before reassembling as milk fat. Triacylglycerol synthesis by the mammary gland microsomes can be influenced by glycerol-3-phosphate which is the initial precursor for the acylation reactions (55). In the absence of glycerol-3-phosphates, microsomal acyl-CoA is directed to form phospholipids, whereas in its presence, acyl-CoA is directed to the synthesis of TG instead.

The TG in lactating mammary gland is characterized by the presence of medium chain fatty acids, which seem to appear in late pregnancy and increase rapidly during early lactation, but disappear within 3 days after weaning (Sun, unpublished observation), (13). The TG with medium chain fatty acids is thought to be synthesized by acylation of medium chain acyl-

CoA to diacylglycerols containing the long chain fatty acids. Lin et al. (50) showed that TG in milk has more long chain saturated fatty acids in the 2-position of the glycerol moiety than the 1 and 3 position. However, when the specificity of diacylglycerol acyltransferase towards acyl-CoA was examined using 1,2-dipalmitoylglycerol as substrate (52), enzyme in the lactating mammary gland seems to lack specificity for transferring medium chain acyl-CoA.

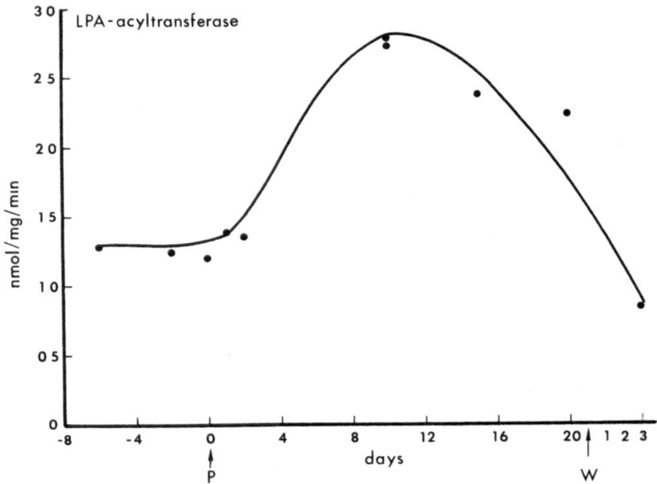

Fig 6. Activity of the oleoyl-CoA:1-palmitoyl-GP acyltransferase in microsomes of rat mammary gland as a function of time before and after parturition (P). Assay procedure for this enzyme is the same as in Sun et al. (75).

Mammary tumors

Many factors may have contributed to the changes in phospholipid composition in the tumors. First, the decrease in PC and increase in PE in tumors may be due to an inhibition of some enzymes (e.g., methyltransferases) which are responsible for the conversion of PE to PC. High activity of methyltransferase is exhibited in normal mammary tissues and this methylation process may be related to the increase in binding of growth hormone to its receptor (3).

Table 5. Oleoyl-CoA:1-acyl-GPC Acyltransferase and Oleoyl-CoA Hydrolase Activities in Tumors and Normal Mammary Tissues.

Tissue type	Description	acyl-transferase	Acyl-CoA hydrolase
		nmole/mg/min	
Normal	21 day pregnant	0.5	1.6
"	2 day lactation	1.6	4.5
"	6 day lactation	2.9-4.2	3.0-7.7
"	10 day lactation	9.7-13.2	8.2-11.6
Tumor 15	Rapid growing	0.32	0.47
" 21	"	1.35	0.69
" 23	"	0.38	0.98
" 18	Slow growing	2.96	1.97
" 20	"	5.13	1.48
" 24	"	9.08	1.95

Mammary tissue and tumors were homogenized in 0.32M sucrose with 50mM Tris (pH 7.4) and microsomes were isolated by differential centrifugation. The microsomal proteins were adjusted to 1mg/ml and 0.1ml was taken to assay for acyltransferase and hydrolase activities using labeled acyl-CoA as substrate (75). Tumor growth was determined by daily measurements of the two maximal diameters of the tumor.

Secondly, the increase in FFA and lyso-phospholipids in tumors may be due to either an increase in phospholipase A activity or an inhibition of lyso-phospholipid acyltransferase which is responsible for reacylating lyso-phospholipids (Fig 3). The DMBA induced mammary tumors are low in lyso-phospholipid acyltransferase activity as compared to "normal" mammary tissues of virgin rats (Table 5). Within the group of tumors being analyzed, up to several fold higher enzymic activities (especially acyltransferase) is found in the slow growing tumors as compared to the fast growing tumors (Table 5). The deacylation-reacylation process is considered an important cellular event for the maintenance of the normal turnover of membrane phospholipids (43). Apparently the normal rate of turnover is curtailed in the fast growing tumors. The result is in good agreement with previous observations that lysolecithin is accumulating more readily in the malignant tumors (Table 4). Lyso-phospholipid accumulation may, in turn, give rise to alterations of a number of membrane functions because of their potent membrane perturbing properties (81).

EFFECTS OF DIETARY LIPIDS

Mammary tumorigenesis and growth.

A number of studies have indicated that mammary milk secretion (5) and mammary tumor induction in experimental animals can be affected by the dietary fat intake. Kidwell et al. (32) showed that unsaturated fatty acids are required for the maintenance and growth of mammary tumor cells. Linoleic acid is needed to maintain tumor cell growth *in vitro* in a medium supplemented with delipidized serum. The levels of dietary fats, regardless of the type of fatty acids in them, can affect tumorigenesis (11), presumably through an increase in transport of the lipophilic carcinogens, such as DMBA, to the target sites. However, high dietary fat intake also promotes a higher incidence of tumors induced by water-soluble carcinogens, such as N-nitrosomethylurea (12). Gammal et al. (19) showed that DMBA-induced mammary tumors develop more readily in rats fed a diet containing a high level of corn oil (20%) than diets containing either a high level of coconut oil (20%) or a low level of corn oil (0.5%). The more recent study of Carroll and Hopkins (10) also showed that polyunsaturated fatty acids (PUFA) are more effective than saturated fat in promoting tumor development in the mammary gland. A diet containing 3% cottonseed or sunflower seed oil stimulates twice as many DMBA-tumors as a diet containing 20% corn oil. Similar observations have been reported for the growth of transplantable mammary carcinoma in host tissues (56), (24), (25), (26).

The tumor promoting property of a high fat diet appears to be related to the susceptibility of the cell membranes to peroxidative changes. Thus, the amount of antioxidant in the fat can influence tumor formation (33); and more antioxidant is required when animals are fed with unsaturated fat. For example, when the antioxidant butylated hydroxytoluene (BHT) is included in high fat diet, the incidence of tumor induction and growth reduce markedly (33).

Effects on tumor lipids.

The effect of dietary fats on the fatty acid composition of a number of mouse and rat mammary adenocarcinomas has been examined by Hillyard et al. (25). Dietary polyunsaturated fatty acids enhance the growth of these transplantable rat and mouse mammary adenocarcinomas (24). The dietary polyunsaturated fatty acids do not alter the composition of tumor lipids, but do induce changes in the fatty acid composition of the tumors (25). Thus, tumors derived from rats fed a fat free diet show a decrease in 18:2 and an increase in 18:1 and 16:1 as compared to those derived from a high corn oil diet. The arachidonate level seems to vary more than any other fatty acid in response to dietary intervention. A small dietary supplement (0.5%) of this fatty acid can double its concentration in tumors, and a dietary addition of 5,8,11,14-eicosatetranoic acid (TYA), an inhibitor for the desaturase, can cause an expected increase of 18:2 and a decrease of 20:4 levels.

EFFECTS OF DIETARY CARBOHYDRATES

Feeding rats with a diet high in carbohydrate and low in fat can cause an increase in lipogenesis in the liver and adipose tissues (83). Similarly, a 2-fold and 7-fold increase of TG in the R3230AC mammary adenocarcinoma and in the liver are noted, respectively, when fed high carbohydrate diet. These increases may be attributed to the rise in levels of hormones regulating lipogenesis. Estrogen is known to induce an increase in FFA and TG in the mammary tumors (22), (23). Interestingly, the FFA levels in tumor and in liver increase to a similar extent regardless of whether animals are fed with high or low levels of carbohydrates. There are also changes of the acyl group profiles of FFA and TG in tumors, mainly from an increase in medium chain fatty acids, such as C10, 11 and 12, due to the high carbohydrate diet. A similar increase of medium chain fatty acids is observed during lactation, a physiological state noted for high levels of lipogenic hormones.

LIPID INDUCERS OF CELL TRANSFORMATION

Essential fatty acids (EFA) are required for proper development of the mammary gland (40). Long-term EFA deficiency tends to cause atrophy of the mammary alveolar structure, a condition which may be more susceptible to carcinogenic transformation. Specific inducers are produced by mammary cells in culture to regulate cellular differentiation (17). Some of the inducers are lipophilic compounds such as medium chain saturated fatty acids (C_4 to C_{14}), myristoyl and palmitoyl lysolecithins, myristic acid methyl esters. Kano-Sueoka et al. (31) recently identified phosphoethanolamine as the pituitary-derived growth-promoting material which, at less than 1 nmole/ml in the medium, could induce growth of a pituitary-dependent, rat mammary carcinoma cell line 64-24. Since the original tumor responds partially to growth stimulation by prolactin *in vivo*, the *in vitro* result implies that phosphoethanolamine may have similar hormone-like effect in promoting tumor growth in the animal.

FATTY ACID SYNTHESIS

The biochemical basis for the induction of specific fatty acid synthesis during lactation is a challenging problem which has not been resolved. During lactation, cytoplasmic materials, which include enzymes for lipid and carbohydrate biosynthesis, are present in milk secretion (34), (54).

The lipid composition of milk fat is quite different from that of the gland. The milk fat is comprised of about 84-91% TG with 2-4% FFA and <1% PL (35), and the lactating mammary cell is comprised of 77% TG and 15% phospholipids. The milk phospholipids normally contain 3% LPC, 38% PC, and 32% PE, whereas the phospholipid composition of the lactating cells is 45% PC, 24% PE, 8.5% PI, 6.0% PS, 11% Sph, 2.8% CL and 2.6% LPC.

Lactating mammary cells are capable of incorporating acetate to form short and medium-chain fatty acids and TG *in vitro* (37) and *in vivo* (9). Some of the properties of fatty acid synthetase system in lactating rat mammary gland has been described by Smith and Abraham (67), (68). This enzyme complex in guinea pig mammary gland is present in the soluble fraction of the gland and is labile upon cold storage (69), (70). Following purification to homogeneity, the enzyme has a molecular weight of 4.0×10^5, and is capable of synthesizing fatty acids ranging from C_4 to C_{18}, with a large proportion of C_{16}. Termination of fatty acid synthesis is aided by thioesterase which effectively cleaves the acyl-CoA from the synthetase. The levels of different acetyl-CoAs available to the gland are thought to be an important factor in influencing the type of fatty acids synthesized during lactation (41). For example, the synthesis of short chain fatty acids in the mammary glands of the cow increases when the concentration of malonyl-CoA in the system decreases.

Lin and Smith (49) observed that there are two thioesterase domains in the fatty acid synthetase. Thioesterase I activity can be selectively removed from the multi-enzyme complex by limited proteolysis using serine esterase inhibitor, thus enabling the investigation of thioesterase II, which may be required for the biosynthesis of medium chain fatty acids (47). Acyl-enzyme thioesters formed by the modified fatty acid synthetases are effective substrates for thioesterase II. During the loading process, thioesterase II can terminate the elongation process at chain lengths as short as 6 carbons. Activity profiles of fatty acid synthetase and thioesterase II can be distinguished during pregnancy and lactation; fatty acid synthetase activity is low throughout pregnancy but increases shortly after parturition, whereas activity of thioesterase II begins to rise during the second and third week of pregnancy, reaching a maximum at parturition and remains high throughout lactation. Consequently, the maximal activity of thioesterase II is better correlated with the usual increase in medium chain fatty acids of TG during the mid-pregnancy. However, the contention that thioesterase II is responsible for synthesis of medium chain fatty acids has not been settled because phenylmethane sulphoryl fluoride, an inhibitor of the terminating thioester hydrolase of the fatty acid synthetase complex, does not inhibit the synthesis of short chain products (i.e., C_4-C_6) (21). The synthesis of these short chain products, according to Hansen and Knudsen (21), involves the reverse of the "loading" reaction.

Fatty acid synthetase activity in mammary adenocarcinoma is, in general, very low (50); the normal mammary gland has 30 times the level present in tumors. Other than this difference, properties of the fatty acid synthetase in tumors are similar to that in normal tissue. Thioesterase II activity is apparently not present in mammary adenocarcinomas of rodents (48), although it was previously thought that medium chain fatty acids in adenocarcinomas might be derived from the same mechanism.

PHOSPHOLIPASES AND PROSTAGLANDINS

Relatively little is known about the phospholipases (A, C and D) in mammary gland. Phospholipase A activity is detected in virgin and mid-pregnant mammary gland and in mammary tumors, in both the membrane pellet and supernatant fractions (62). Its activity in the supernatant fraction increases during mid-pregnancy. A regulatory role of the enzyme in secretory functions of the gland is implicated, since prolactin enhances the phosholipase A activity of the mammary tissue (61). Phospholipase A activity is an order of magnitude higher in tumors than in normal gland; this increase corresponds to the higher levels of FFA and lyso-phospholipids in tumors we described earlier, and activity may also explain for the general increase in prostaglandin levels in tumors (76).

There is little doubt that prostaglandins can play an important role in mediating many known physiological functions of mammary glands and tumors. However, the exact mode of action(s) has not been clearly defined. Hwang et al. (28) reported a 50-fold increase in the thromboxane B_2 level in serum of lactating cow as compared to bulls or ovariectomized cows. Prostaglandin production is higher in human breast tumors than in normal mammary tissues, especially those tumors exhibiting a high cell density (64). In fact, the amount of increase in prostaglandin level in tumors has been suggested as an index for predicting the metastatic potential of breast cancers.

Prostaglandin synthesis in human breast tumors is localized mainly in the microsomes which produces mainly PGE_2. This prostaglandin is then converted to PGF_{2a} by 9-keto-reductase in the cytosol fraction (63). Both types of prostaglandin synthesizing enzymes are detected in human mammary tumors. PGF_{2a} is known for its luteolytic action. Induction of lactogenesis in pregnant rabbits by PGF_{2a} is abolished by the administration of progesterone. The inhibitory effect of PGF_{2a} on the growth of a hormone-dependent rat mammary adenocarcinoma is also associated with a marked reduction of serum progesterone concentration (30).

The increase in prostaglandins in mammary tumors has prompted Leaper et al. (44) to test the effects of non-steroidal inhibitors of prostaglandins as a possible approach to palliate breast cancer. A daily administration of 2.5 mg/kg of Flurbiprofen reduces tumor growth and lengthens the survival time of the animal. This drug also retards the growth of a metastasizing mammary cancer transplanted into mice (1,2).

Arachidonic acid and some other polyunsaturated fatty acids have been shown to exert a biphasic effect on guanylate cyclase activity in homogenates of mammary gland obtained from mid-pregnant mice (57). Low concentrations of 20:4 stimulate a 2-fold increase in activity, but high concentrations inhibit it. This stimulatory effect is abolished by indomethacin and aspirin, suggesting a conversion of 20:4 to prostaglandins. Direct addition of prostaglandins to the tissue, however, fails to elicit a stimulatory action on guanylate cyclase activity.

Mammary gland lipids in response to hormonal regulation

A comprehensive review of the hormonal factors in lipogenesis of mammary gland and tumors has recently been presented by Mayer (53). In this section, we will describe briefly the hormonal regulation on mammary gland lipids and also present some recent findings from our laboratories.

Although it is generally known that the process of lactation is directed by hormones, the exact mechanism underlying this secretory event is not yet fully understood. Strong et al. (70) demonstrate that prolactin stimulates the synthesis of milk fatty acids in mammary explants. Mammary gland explants of pregnant or virgin mice also exhibit marked differentiation in culture in the presence of insulin, cortisol and prolactin. These hormones also stimulate the incorporation of [^{14}C]acetate into the fatty acids in mammary gland explants of pregnant mice (79). Without prolactin, fatty acids formed in explants resemble those found in adipose tissue, whereas in the presence of these three hormones, fatty acids of explants resemble those of milk fat. Following a 24-hr incubation in medium 199 without hormone, the rate of fatty acid synthesis in mammary explants is reduced; the reduction can be reversed by insulin (20). Other hormones, such as corticosterone, prolactin and growth hormone, can also elicit a response on the rate of mammary fatty acid synthesis.

Hormones play a pivotal role in metabolic and functional events of the mammary gland. In most cases, a concerted action of several hormones are required. This fact has been well demonstrated in other chapters of this monograph. The initiation of lactogenesis, for example, requires prolactin and is signaled by the sharp decline of ovarian progesterone at the end of pregnancy (16), (42). PGF_2 induces lactogenesis and also advances parturition when it is injected into pregnant rats (82).

Dhami et al. (15) believe that steroid hormones which are important in mediating the physiological events in mammary tissue can also affect the lipid metabolism of other organs. Thus, the phospholipid content in liver is altered in conjunction with the physiological status of the mammary gland; i.e., it decreases during pregnancy but returns to normal values after delivery.

The mechanism of prolactin action on its target tissues has been investigated by Rillema (58) who presents evidence showing that prolactin is internalized into the target cells and elicits a number of intracellular actions which include: (1) increasing the intracellular concentration of potassium and decreasing the level of sodium, (2) changing the cellular level of cyclic nucleotides, and (3) enhancing the prostaglandin biosynthesis through stimulation of phospholipase A_2 activity. Extracellular Ca^{++} is required for the action of prolactin on the cell surface receptors. Phospholipase A added to the mammary gland explants can stimulate uridine incorporation into RNA in a manner similar to that of prolactin (59). Serum prolactin levels may also be correlated with the incidence of DMBA tumor induction. Boyns et al. (4) indicated that the mouse strain showing the highest incidence of circulating prolactin levels also gives a higher incidence of tumor induction. Suppression of prolactin secretion has been correlated with an inhibition of mammary tumorigenesis in the rats (80).

It is generally known that certain breast cancers from human and experimental animals are stimulated by exogenous steroid hormones. In this situation, deletion of hormones by surgical ablation may lead to a prompt regression of these tumors. The regression of human mammary carcinoma after ovariectomy has been linked to the presence of estrogen receptor (29). The relationship of estrogen receptor to tumorigenesis is complex and possibly relates to many other cellular events (65). The growth of CAMA-1 cell line, which was obtained from a human mammary adenocarcinoma, depends on estradiol for growth (45). Addition of estradiol at low levels (10 pM to 10 nM) to a culture stimulates an increase in the incorporation of labeled precursors into proteins, DNA and RNA while high levels (10 uM) decrease uptake. Cell growth is also inhibited by high levels of estradiol.

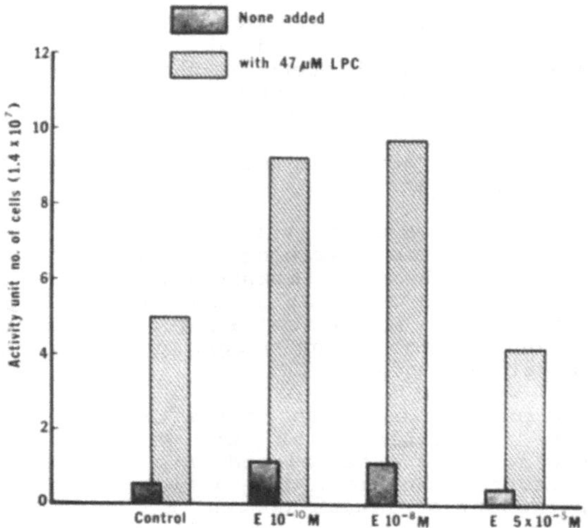

Fig 7. The effect of estradiol on the incorporation of oleoyl-CoA into phosphatidylcholine of mammary cancer cells (CAMA-1) in the presence or absence of 1-palmitoyl-GPC (LPC). In this experiment, CAMA-1 cells were plated in a medium supplemented with bovine fetal calf serum stripped of endogenous steroids by dextran-coated charcoal. Estradiol (0, 10^{-10}, 10^{-8} and 5 x 10^{-5}) were then added to cells during plating. After 4 days, cells were harvested by EDTA-trypsinization and cells were homogenized in 0.32 M sucrose in 50 mM Tris-HCl (pH 7.4). The homogenates were centrifuged at 12,000 g for 30 min after which the supernates were used for metabolic study.

An increased turnover of membrane phospholipids in response to estrogen is also noted. As shown in Fig 7, the post-mitochondrial supernatant membranes are active in transferring labeled oleoyl-CoA to 1-acyl-GPC, and the acyltransferase activity in this fraction is stimulated by low levels of estradiol, but is inhibited by high levels of the steroid. The endogenous acylating activity is low in the absence of added lyso-substrate, and is affected proportionally by estradiol as in the case of added lyso-phospholipids. These results indicate that CAMA-1 cells are capable of turning over membrane phospholipids through the deacylation-reacylation mechanism (Fig 3), and activity of this enzymatic process is affected by estradiol.

Since phospholipase A_2-mediated deacylation of phospholipids is normally a Ca^{++} mediated event, the effect of this divalent cation on production of endogenous lyso-phospholipids was examined. Results in Fig 8 showed that addition of 1mM Ca^{++} to the incubation medium elicits an increase of phospholipid acylating activity, probably due to an increase in endogenous lyso-phospholipids. The stimulatory effect of Ca^{++} seems to be more pronounced in the acylation of phosphatidylinositols; and cells which are supplemented with low levels of estradiol potentiates this response. These results show that a suitable amount of estradiol is needed to promote growth of the CAMA-1 cells, and for the increase in cellular metabolism, including membrane phospholipid turnover.

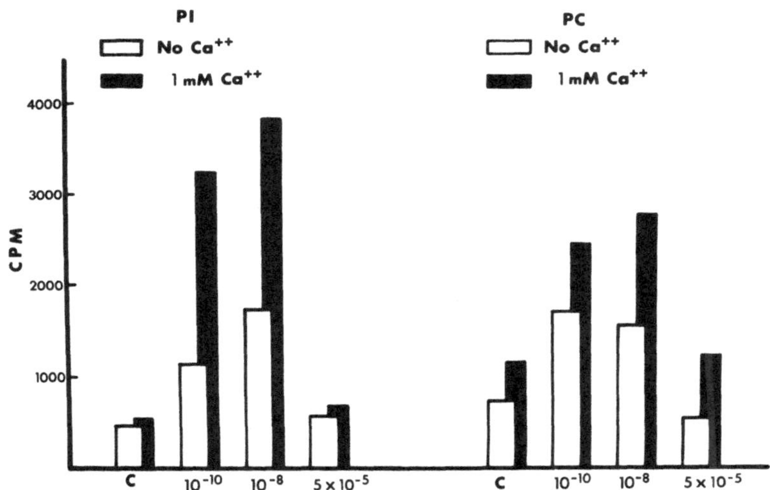

Fig 8. The effect of estradiol on the incorporation of oleoyl-CoA into phosphatidylinositols (PI) phosphatidylcholines (PC) of CAMA-1 cells. Assays were carried out without addition of exogenous lyso-phospholipid substrates but in the presence or absence of Ca^{++} in the incubation mixture.

ACKNOWLEDGEMENT

The studies reported in this chapter were supported in part by National Cancer Institute 1R01 CA25998 and the National Science Foundation NSF BNS76 24338.

REFERENCES

1. Bennett A, Berstock DA, Raja B, Stamford IF. Survival time after surgery is inversely related to the amounts of prostaglandins extracted from human breast cancers. Br J Pharmacol 66: 451P, 1979.

2. Bennett A, Houghton J, Leaper DJ, Stamford IF. Cancer growth, response to treatment and survival time in mice: Beneficial effect of the prostaglandin synthesis inhibitor flurbiprofen. Prostaglandins 17: 179-191, 1979.

3. Bhattacharya A, Vonderhaar BK. Phospholipid methylation stimulates lactogenic binding in mouse mammary gland membranes. Proc Natl Acad Sci USA 76: 4489-4492, 1979.

4. Boyns AR, Buchan R, Cole EN, Forrest APM, Griffiths, K. Basal prolactin blood levels in three strains of rat with differing incidence of 7,12-dimethylbenz(a)anthracene induced mammary tumors. Eur J Cancer 9: 169-171, 1973.

5. Brandorff NP. The effect of dietary fat on the fatty acid composition of lipids secreted in rats' milk. Lipids 15: 276-278, 1980.

6. Caffrey M, Infante JP, Kinsella JE. Isoenzymes of an acyltransferase from rabbit mammary gland: evidence from biphasic substrate saturation kinetics. FEBS Lett 52: 116-120, 1975.

7. Caffrey M, Kinsella JE. Isoenzymes of an acyltransferase from rabbit mammary gland: solubilization of the micelle-specific species with Triton X-100. Biochem Biophys Res Commun 71: 484-491, 1976.

8. Caffrey M, Kinsella JE. Properties of palmitoyl-CoA:Monopalmitoyl-_sn_-glycerol 3-phosphate palmitoyl-transferase from rabbit mammary gland. Int J Biochem 9: 239-248, 1978.

9. Carey EM, Dils R. The pattern of fatty acid synthesis in lactating rabbit mammary gland studied _in vivo_. Biochem J 126: 1005-1007, 1972.

10. Carroll KK, Hopkins GJ. Dietary polyunsaturated fat in relation to mammary carcinogenesis. Lipids 14: 155-158, 1979.

11. Carroll KK, Khor HT. Effects of level and type of dietary fat on incidence of mammary tumors induced in female Sprague-Dawley rats by 7,12-dimethylbenz(a)anthracene. Lipids 6: 415-420, 1971.

12. Chan PC, Head JF, Cohen LA, Wynder EL. Influence of dietary fat on the induction of mammary tumors by N-nitrosomethylurea: associated hormone changes and differences between Sprague-Dawley and F344 rats. J Natl Cancer Inst 59: 1279-1283, 1977.

13. Cooper SM, Grigor MR. Stereospecific biosynthesis of triacylglycerols in mammary glands from lactating rats. Biochem J 174: 659-662, 1978.

14. Cooper SM, Grigor MR. Fatty acid specificities of microsomal acyltransferases esterifying positions-1 and -2 of acylglycerols in mammary glands from lactating rats. Biochem J 187: 289-295, 1980.

15. Dhami MSI, Feuer CF, Feuer G. Fatty acid changes in the hepatic endoplasmic reticulum during pregnancy in the rat. Res Commun Chem Pathol Pharmacol 23: 383-394, 1979.

16. Dies RP. Oxytocin test to demonstrate the initiation and end of lactation in rats. J Endocrin 40: 133-134, 1968.

17. Dulbecco R, Bologna M, Unger M. Control of differentiation of a mammary cell line by lipids. Proc Natl Acad Sci USA 77: 1551-1555, 1980.

18. Feldman EB, Carter AC. Circulating lipids and lipoproteins in women with metastatic breast carcinoma. J Clin Endocrinol Metab 33: 8-13, 1971.

19. Gammal EB, Carroll KK, Plunkett ER. Effects of dietary fat on mammary carcinogenesis by 7,12-dimochylbenz(a)-anthracene in rats. Cancer Res 27: 1737-1742, 1967.

20. Hallowes RC, Wang DY, Lewis DJ, Strong CR, Dils R. The stimulation by prolactin and growth hormone of fatty acid synthesis in explants from rat mammary glands. J Endocrinol 57: 265-276, 1973.

21. Hansen JK, Knudsen J. Transacylation as a chain-termination mechanism in fatty acid synthesis by mammalian fatty acid synthetase. Synthesis of butyrate and hexanoate by lactating cow mammary gland fatty acid synthetase. Biochem J 15: 287-294, 1980.

22. Hilf R, Michel I, Bell C. Dose responses of R3230AC mammary tumor and mammary tissue to estrogen: Enzymes, nucleic acids, and lipids. Cancer Res 26: 865-870, 1966.

23. Hilf R, Michel I, Gibbs CC, Bell C. NADP-linked enzymes and lipids in normal and neoplastic tissue: Effects of estrogen and dietary glucose. Biochim Biophys Acta 116: 589-592, 1966.

24. Hillyard LA, Abraham S. Effect of dietary polyunsaturated fatty acids on growth of mammary adenocarcinomas in mice and rats. Cancer Res 39: 4430-4437, 1979.

25. Hillyard LA, Rao GA, Abraham S. Effect of dietary fat on fatty acid composition of mouse and rat mammary adenocarcinomas (40781). Proc Soc Exp Biol Med 163: 376-383, 1980.

26. Hopkins GJ, West CE. Effect of dietary polyunsaturated fat on the growth of a transplantable adenocarcinoma in $C3HA_fB$ mice. J Natl Cancer Inst 58: 753-756, 1977.

27. Horrocks LA, Sun GY. Ethanolamine plasmalogens. pp 223-231 in Research Methods in Neurochemistry, Vol. 1, eds N Marks, R Rodnight. Plenum Publishing Co, New York, 1972.

28. Hwang DW, Godke RA, Rings RW. Species variation in serum levels of prostaglandins and their precursor acids. Lipids 15: 597-600, 1980.

29. Jensen EV, Desombre ER. Mechanism of action of the female sex hormones. Annu Rev Biochem 41: 203-230, 1972.

30. Jubiz W, Frailey J, Smith JB. Inhibitory effect of prostaglandin F_2 alpha on the growth of a hormone-dependent rat mammary tumor. Cancer Res 39: 998-1000, 1979.

31. Kano-Sueoka T, Cohen DM, Yamaizumi Z, Nishimura S, Mori M, Fujiki H. Phosphoethanolamine as a growth factor of a mammary carcinoma cell line of rat. Proc Natl Acad Sci USA 11: 5741-5744, 1979.

32. Kidwell WR, Monaco ME, Wicha MS, Smith GS. Unsaturated fatty acid requirements for growth and survival of a rat mammary tumor cell line. Cancer Res 38: 4091-4100, 1978.

33. King MM, Bailey DM, Gibson DD, Pitha JV, McCay PB. Incidence and growth of mammary tumors induced by 7,12-dimethylbenz[a]anthracene as related to the dietary content of fat and antioxidant. J Natl Cancer Inst 63: 657-663, 1979.

34. Kinsella JE. Glycerolipid synthesis in milk: Evidence of glycerol kinase and other biosynthetic enzymes. Int J Biochem 3: 89-92, 1972.

35. Kinsella JE. Lipid composition and fatty acid metabolism by mammary cells of rat. Int J Biochem 4: 549-556, 1973.

36. Kinsella JE. Preferential labeling of phosphatidylcholine during phospholipid synthesis by bovine mammary tissue. Lipids 8: 393-400, 1973.

37. Kinsella JE. Biosynthesis of fatty acids in rat mammary cells. Int J Biochem 5: 417-421, 1974.

38. Kinsella JE. Monoacyl-sn-glycerol 3-phosphate acyltransferase specificity in bovine mammary microsomes. Lipids 11: 680-684, 1976.

39. Kinsella JE, Gross, M. Palmitic acid and initiation of mammary glyceride synthesis *via* phosphatidic acid. Biochim Biophys Acta 316: 109-113, 1973.

40. Knazek RA, Liu SC, Bodwin JS, Vonderhaar BK. Requirement of essential fatty acids in the diet for development of the mouse mammary gland. J Natl Cancer Inst 64: 377-382, 1980.

41. Knudsen J. Fatty acid synthetase from cow mammary gland tissue cells. Biochim Biophys Acta 280: 408-414, 1972.

42. Kuhn J. Progesterone withdrawal as the lactogenic trigger in the rat. J Endocrinol 44: 39-54, 1969.

43. Lands WEM, Crawford CG. Enzymes of membrane phospholipid metabolism in animals. pp 3-85 in *The Enzymes of Biological Membranes*, Vol. 2, ed A Martonosi. Plenum Press, New York, 1976.

44. Leaper DJ, French BT, Bennett A. Breast Cancer and prostaglandins: A new approach to treatment. Br J Surg 66: 683-686, 1979.

45. Leung BS. Hormonal dependency of experimental breast cancer. pp 219-261 in *Hormones, Receptors, and Breast Cancer*, ed WL McGuire. Raven Press, New York, 1978.

46. Leung BS, Sun GY. Acyl group composition of membrane phospholipids in mammary tissues and carcinoma induced by dimethylbenz(a)anthracene (39465). Proc Soc Exp Biol Med 152: 671-676, 1976.

47. Libertini LJ, Smith S. Purification and properties of a thioesterase from lactating rat mammary gland which modifies the product specificity of fatty acid synthetase. J Biol Chem 253: 1393-1401, 1978.

48. Libertini LJ, Lin CY, Abraham S, Hilf R, Smith S. Medium chain fatty acid synthesis in rodent mammary adenocarcinomas *in vitro*. Biochim Biophys Acta 618: 185-191, 1980.

49. Lin CY, Smith S. Properties of the thioesterase component obtained by limited trypsinization of the fatty acid synthetase multienzyme complex. J Biol Chem 253: 1954-1962, 1978.

50. Lin CY, Smith S, Abraham S. Fatty acid synthetase from a mouse mammary adenocarcinoma. Cancer Res 35: 3094-3099, 1975.

51. Marshall MO, Knudsen J. The specificity of 1-acyl-sn-glycerol 3-phosphate acyltransferase in microsomal fractions from lactating cow mammary gland towards short, medium and long chain acyl-CoA esters. Biochim Biophys Acta 489: 236-241, 1977.

52. Marshall MO, Knudsen J. Specificity of diacylglycerol acyltransferase from bovine mammary gland, liver and adipose tissue towards acyl-CoA esters. Eur J Biochem 94: 93-98, 1979.

53. Mayer RJ. Hormonal factors in lipogenesis in mammary gland. Vit Hormones 36: 101-163, 1978.

54. McCarthy RD, Patton S. Biosynthesis of glycerides in freshly secreted milk. Nature (London) 202: 347-349, 1964.

55. Rao GA, Abraham S. Fatty acid desaturation by mammary gland microsomes from lactating mice. Lipids 9: 269-271, 1974.

56. Rao GA, Abraham S. Brief Communication: Enhanced growth rate of transplanted mammary adenocarcinoma induced in C3H mice by dietary linoleate. J Natl Cancer Inst 56: 431-432, 1976.

57. Rillema JA. Activation of guanylate cyclase by activation in mammary gland homogenates from mice. Prostaglandins 15: 857-865, 1978.

58. Rillema JA. Mechanism of prolactin action. Fed Proc 39: 2593-2598, 1980.

59. Rillema JA, Anderson LD. Phospholipases and the effect of prolactin on uridine incorporation into RNA in mammary gland explants of mice. Biochim Biophys Acta 428: 819-824, 1976.

60. Rillema JA, Mulder JA. Arachidonic acid distribution in lipids of mammary glands and DMBA-induced tumors of rats. Prostaglan Med 1: 31-38, 1978.

61. Rillema JA, Wild EA. Prolactin activation of phospholipase A activity in membrane preparations from mammary glands. Endocrinology 100: 1219-1222, 1977.

62. Rillema JA, Osmialowski EC, Linebaugh BE. Phospholipase A_2 activity in 9,10-dimethyl-1,2-Benzanthracene-induced

mammary tumors of rats. Biochim Biochem Acta 617: 150-155, 1980.

63. Rolland PH, Martin PM, Rolland AM, Toga M. Prostaglandins in human breast cancer. Identification of a cytosolic prostaglandin-9-keto-reductase activity. Biomedicine 31: 178-182, 1979.

64. Rolland PH, Martin PM, Jacquemier J, Rolland AM, Toga M. Prostaglandin in human breast cancer: Evidence suggesting that an elevated prostaglandin production is a marker of high metastatic potential for neoplastic cells. J Natl Cancer Inst 64: 1061-1070, 1980.

65. Shafie SM. Estrogen and the growth of breast cancer: New evidence suggests indirect action. Science 209: 701-702, 1980.

66. Short VJ, Brindley DN, Dils R. Co-ordinate changes in enzymes of fatty acid synthesis, activation and esterification in rabbit mammary gland during pregnancy and lactation. Biochem J 162: 445-450, 1977.

67. Smith S, Abraham S. Fatty acid synthetase from lactating rat mammary gland. Studies on the termination sequence. J Biol Chem 246: 2537-2542, 1971.

68. Smith S, Abraham S. Fatty acid synthetase from lactating rat mammary gland. III. Dissociation and reassociation. J Biol Chem 246: 6428-6435, 1971.

69. Strong CR, Dils R. Fatty acids synthesized by mammary gland slices from lactating guinea pig and rabbit. Comp Biochem Physiol 43B: 643-652, 1972.

70. Strong CR, Dils R. The fatty acid synthetase complex of lactating guinea-pig mammary gland. Int J Biochem 3: 369-377, 1972.

71. Strong CR, Forsyth I, Dils R. The effects of hormones on milk fat synthesis in mammary gland explants from pseudopregnant rabbits. Biochem J 128: 509-519, 1972.

72. Sun AY, Sun GY. Functional roles of phospholipids of synaptosomal membrane. pp 169-197 in _Function and Metabolism of Phospholipids in CNS and PNS_, eds G Porcellati, L Amaducci, C Galli. Plenum Press, New York, 1976.

73. Sun GY, Leung BS. Changes in phospholipids and acyl group composition of rat mammary gland during pregnant, lactating, and post-weaning periods. Lipids 11: 322-327, 1976.

74. Sun GY, Su KL, Der OM, Tang W. Enzymic regulation of arachidonate metabolism in brain membrane phosphoglycerides. Lipids 14: 229-235, 1979.

75. Sun GY, Smith RE, Chan K, MacQuarrie R. Inhibition of acyl-CoA hydrolase activity in liver microsomes by lysophospholipids. Biochem Biophys Res Commun 94: 1278-1284, 1980.

76. Tan WC, Chapman C, Takatori T, Privett OS. Studies of lipid class and fatty acid profiles of rat mammary tumors induced by 7,12-dimethylbenz(a)anthracene. Lipids 10: 70-74, 1974.

77. Tan WC, Privett OS, Goldyne ME. Studies of prostaglandins in rat mammary tumors induced by 7,12-dimethylbenz(a)-anthracene. Cancer Res 34: 3229-3231, 1974.

78. Tanioka H, Lin CY, Smith S, Abraham S. Acyl specificity in glyceride synthesis by lactating rat mammary gland. Lipids 9: 229-234, 1974.

79. Wang DY, Hallowes RC, Bealing J, Strong CR, Dils R. The effect of prolactin and growth hormone on fatty acid synthesis by pregnant mouse mammary gland in organ culture. J Endocr 53: 311-321, 1972.

80. Welsch CW, Brown CK, Goodrich-Smith M, Van J, Denenberg B, Anderson TM, Brooks CL. Inhibition of mammary tumorigenesis in carcinogen-treated Lewis rats by suppression of prolactin secretion. J Natl Cancer Inst 63: 1211-1214, 1979.

81. Weltzien HU. Cytolytic and membrane-perturbing properties of lysophosphatidylcholine. Biochim Biophys Acta 559: 259-287, 1979.

82. Vermouth NT, Dies RP. Inhibitory effect of progesterone on the lactogenic and abortive action of prostaglandin F_{2a}. J Endocrinol 66: 21-29, 1975.

83. Zalenski D, Hilf R. Effect of dietary carbohydrate on fatty acids in the R3230AC mammary adenocarcinoma (37193). Proc Soc Exp Biol Med 142: 1137-1140, 1973.

Chapter 10

POLYAMINES IN NORMAL AND NEOPLASTIC GROWTH OF MAMMARY GLAND

Takami Oka, John W. Perry, Toshiyuki Takemoto, Tadashi Sakai, Nobuyuki Terada, Hideo Inoue

INTRODUCTION

The diamine putrescine and the polyamines spermidine and spermine are small aliphatic nitrogenous bases which are present in all mammalian cells. The structures of these polycations are presented below:

$$\overset{+}{N}H_3CH_2CH_2CH_2CH_2\overset{+}{N}H_3$$

PUTRESCINE

$$\overset{+}{N}H_3CH_2CH_2CH_2\overset{+}{N}H_2CH_2CH_2CH_2CH_2\overset{+}{N}H_3$$

SPERMIDINE

$$\overset{+}{N}H_3CH_2CH_2CH_2\overset{+}{N}H_2CH_2CH_2CH_2CH_2\overset{+}{N}H_2CH_2CH_2CH_2\overset{+}{N}H_3$$

SPERMINE.

Because the amino groups of these compounds are fully charged at physiological pH, the polyamines can interact with negatively charged cellular constituents such as nucleic acids, proteins, and phospholipids. This electrostatic binding is believed to be the basis of some of the known effects that polyamines have in various cell-free systems. Although the discovery of the polyamines dates back to several decades, their biological and physiological importance have only recently been recognized. Increased polyamine biosynthesis and accumulation occur in the early phase of all growth processes. A high concentration of polyamines is also found in tissues with a high rate of protein synthesis such as prostate gland, pancreas, and the lactating mammary gland. A number of hormones including estrogens, progesterone, glucocorticoid, growth hormone, insulin, and prolactin stimulate polyamine biosynthesis in various target tissues. In addition, it has been shown that carcinogens such as methylcholanthrene and tumor promoting agents increase the level of polyamines through stimulation of ornithine decarboxylase. Furthermore clinical studies suggest that alterations in polyamines in some body fluids may serve the diagnosis or prognostic evaluation of certain diseases. These studies, together with the numerous observed effects of polyamines on the synthesis of macromolecules, on the activities of various enzymes and on the function of biological membranes in cell-free systems, suggest an essential role for polyamines in the regulation of cell growth and function. In this chapter we will review primarily our studies on the biosynthesis and function of polyamines in growth and differentiation of the mouse mammary gland.

The mammary gland provides an excellent model system for the study of cell growth and differentiation. The growth and development of mammary gland are virtually arrested in the adult, non-pregnant state. During pregnancy mammary epithelial cells undergo extensive proliferation to form a net work of lobulo-alveolar cells that synthesize the characteristic milk components during lactation period. Earlier studies (41) have shown that such morphological and biochemical changes that occur during pregnacy and lactation can be induced in culture by cultivating mammary tissue explants in a chemically-defined synthetic medium containing appropriate combination of hormones. This organ culture system has proved to be useful model system for the study of the fundamental mechanisms involved in the hormone-dependent growth and development of the mammary gland because it provides a well-controlled cellular enviroment and eliminates certain problems that are inherent in experiments performed in vivo.

DEVELOPMENTAL CHANGES IN THE SYNTHESIS AND ACCUMULATION OF POLYAMINES IN MAMMARY GLAND

As shown in Fig. 1, the concentrations of the polyamines spermidine and putrescine in mouse (25) and rat (33) mammary gland remained low in the virgin state, when mammary cells are developmentally dormant. The concentrations of spermidine and putrescine in mammary cells begin to rise during pregnancy when cell proliferation occurs, and it reaches maximal level during the lactation period when milk proteins are formed. The increase in spermidine concentartion is two- to three-fold during pregnancy and six-to eight-fold during lactation, while the concentration of putrescine increases five-fold and two-fold, respectively during the same periods. In contrast, little change in spermine levels is found throughout the development of mammary tissue. The increases in the concentration of putrescine and spermidine are accompanied by a rise in the activities of a group of polyamine biosynthetic enzymes, arginase, ornithine decarbxylase (ODC), S-adenosyl-L-methionine decarboxylase (S-ado-met DC) and spermidine synthase (25) (see Fig. 2 for the biosynthetic pathway of polyamines).

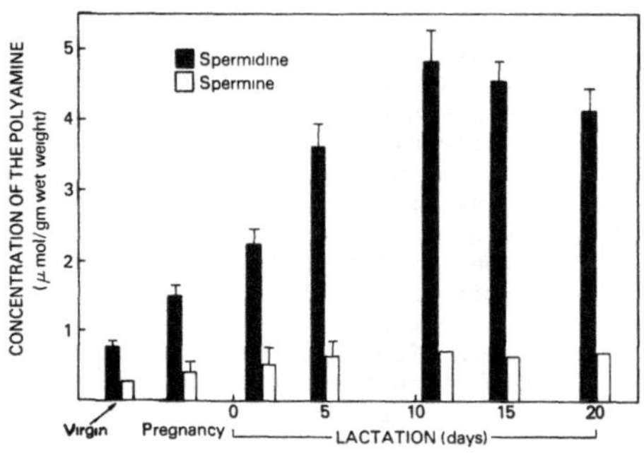

Fig. 1 Concentration of polyamines in mouse mammary gland during pregnancy and lactation.

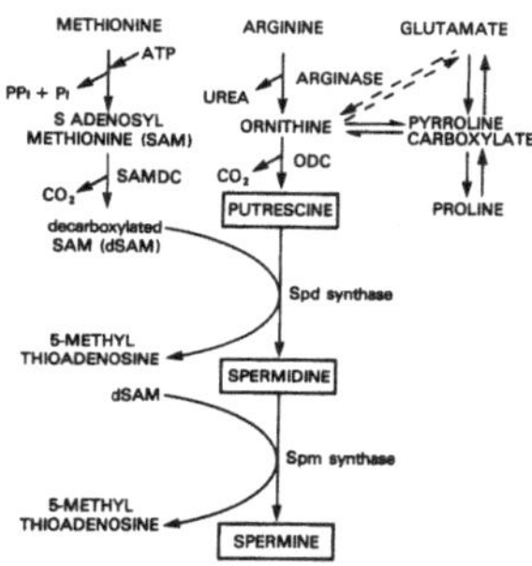

Fig. 2 Biosynthetic pathway of polyamines in mammalian cells.

The Control of Polyamine Biosynthesis During Cell Proliferation of Mammary Gland in vitro. The non-proliferating mammary cells in virgin mice can be induced to undergo DNA synthesis and cell division in vitro in the presence of insulin (39). Time course studies on polyamine biosynthesis and DNA synthesis showed (34) that insulin elicits sequential stimulation of the activity of ODC, S-ado-met DC and spermidine synthase, and increases in the concentrations of putrescine and spermidine prior to the augmentation of DNA synthesis(Fig. 3). In explants cultured with insulin, the activity of ODC began to increase as early as three hours, with a peak at about ten hours. Explants cultured without insulin showed also a substantial increase in ODC activity during 54 hours of culture. The activity of S-ado-met DC in explants treated with insulin began to increase at 10 to 12 hours, reached a peak at 20 hours, and thereafter remained at an elevated level. In the absence of insulin small increases in the S-ado-met-DC activity were observed. Spermidine synthase activity in explants cultured with insulin began to increase within 24 hours and thereafter continued to rise for the next 40 hours, whereas in the absence of insulin, the increase occurred more slowly and to a lesser extent. As predicted from the changes in the activities of the above enzymes, insulin caused a rapid increase in the concentration of putrescine between 6 and 20 hours, and subsequent accumulation of spermidine. After 68 hours of culture, the concentration of spermidine doubled to the level, approximately 150 pmol/mg tissue, that was found in the mammary gland of midpregnant mice. In explants cultured without insulin, putrescine concentration was increased about 3-fold at 6 hours and spermidine concentration at 68 hours was 12-15% higher than that of the uncultured control. Throughout the culture period, there was

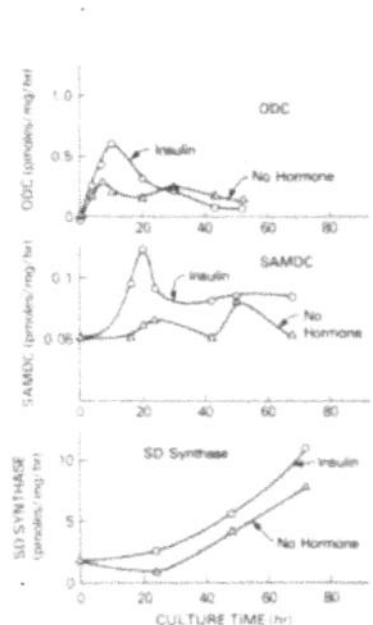

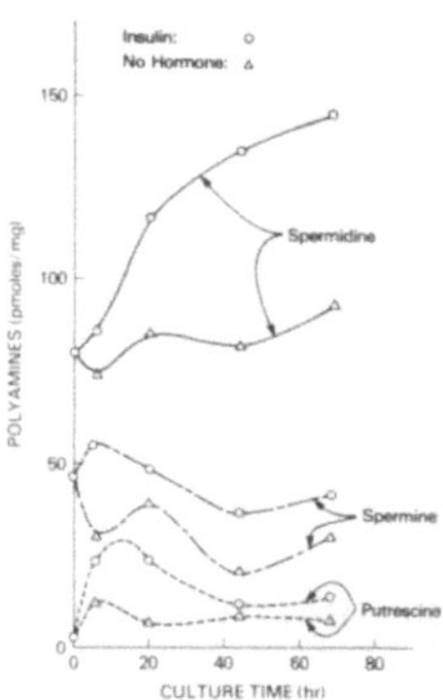

Fig. 3 Time course of activities of polyamine biosynthetic enzymes and the concentrations of polyamines in virgin C3H/HeN mouse mammary explants cultured with or without insulin.

a gradual decline in the concentration of spermine, although the explants cultured with insulin contained higher amounts of spermine than those without insulin. As will be described later, an organ culture of mammary gland of virgin mice appears to be ideal for studying the function of the polyamines in the proliferation of mammary epithelium.

<u>The Control of Polyamine Biosynthesis During Differentiation in vitro</u>. When mammary tissue from mid-pregnant mouse was cultured with insuin, cortisol, and prolactin, mammary cells synthesize the milk proteins casein and alpha-lactalbumin (41). As shown in Fig. 4, the concentration of spermidine increased significantly prior to the accelerated production of milk-proteins, amounting to about a 3-fold increase at 48 hours, when the milk-protein synthesis was maximal (20). The concentration of spermine increased only slightly during a 48 hour culture. In order to study the mechanism whereby the interplay of insulin, cortisol and prolactin increases the accumulation of spermidine in mammary cells during lactogenesis <u>in</u>

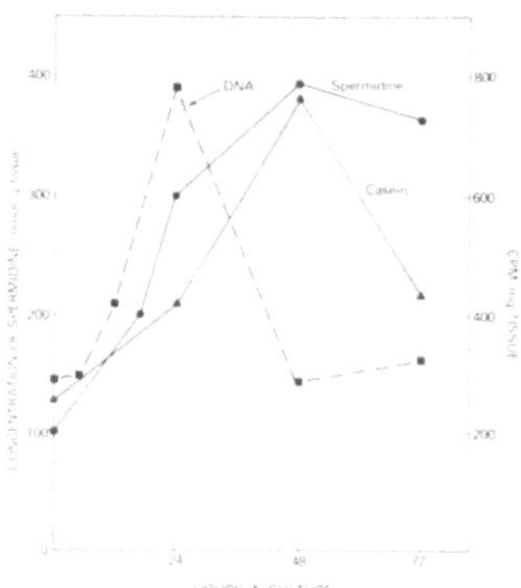

Fig. 4 Time course of DNA synthesis, spermidine accumulation and casein synthesis in mid-pregnant mouse mammary explants cultured with insulin, cortisol and prolactin.

vitro, the effect of hormones on the activities of polyamine biosynthetic enzymes was examined. Mammary epithelium of rat (43) and mouse (25) contains two forms of arginase, one being associated with mitochondrial fraction and the other with cytosol fraction. Of the two forms of mammary arginase, only the activity of the soluble enzyme was increased several-fold by the action of insulin and prolactin, while the particulate enzyme was essentially unresponsive (25). Time course studies which compared the increase in soluble arginase activity with the formation of spermidine from arginine shows a close temporal relationship, indicating the involvement of the soluble arginase in polyamine biosynthesis (25).

The activity of ODC increases biphasically during the hormone-dependent development of mouse mammary epithelium in vitro (25). As shown in Fig. 5, the first peak of activity occurred at 3-4 hours and the increase was mainly elicited by incubating mammary explants in a serum-free culture medium without any added hormones. Addition of insulin or prolactin or both caused a greater increase in the first peak of the activity and also induced the second peak of activity at about 12 hours. Studies with actinomycin D and cycloheximide suggest that the first increase in ODC is effected at a post-transcriptional level, whereas a second increase is

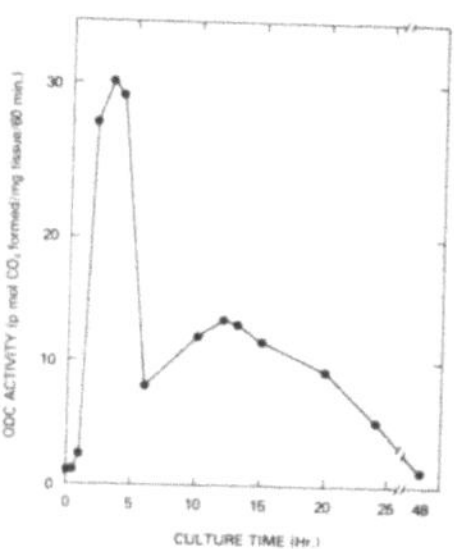

Fig. 5 Time course of ODC activity in mid-pregnant mouse mammary explant cultured with insulin, cortisol and prolactin.

at both transcriptional and translational levels.

In order to better understand the control mechanism of ODC in cultured mammary cells, we have examined the regulatory factor(s) responsible for the hormone-independent increase in enzyme activity. The results shown in Fig. 6 indicate that a change in the osmolarity of the cellular enviroment is the major contributing factor for the emergence of the hormone-independent ODC activity in mammary explants (29). Thus, incubation of mammary explants for 3 hours in a medeum diluted 53% with distilled water results in approximately 1000-fold stimulation of enzyme activity over the initial level, whereas a similar dilution with 0.18M NaCl or 0.3M sucrose blocks the increase.

Fig. 6 Increase of ODC activity in mouse mammary explants as a function of the dilution of culture medium.

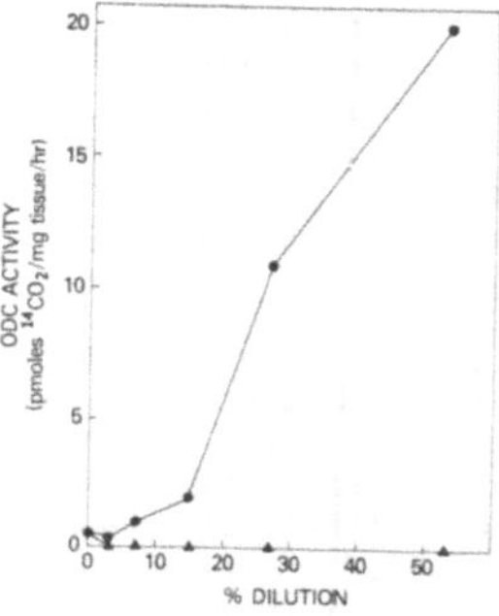

The increase in enzyme activity is similarly induced by a reduction in the concentration of NaCl in the culture medium. The hypoosmotic stimulation of ODC activity appears to be affected at a post-transcriptional level, and is enhanced further by the addition of insulin and prolactin. The hypoosmotic enhancement of ODC activity produces a large increase in the intracellular concentration of putrescine in mammary explants. However, neither the concentration of spermidine and spermine nor the activity of S-ado-met DC is affected. The immunological studies, using anti-S-ado-met DC raised against pure enzyme preparation from mouse mammary tissue (36) showed that the amount of S-ado-met DC in cultured tissue remained at the basal level of uncultured tissue. The additional studies (36) revealed an apparent inverse relationship between the intracellular concentration of putrescine and the activity of S-ado-met DC, suggesting that putrescine can exert a negative regulatory influence.

The hypoosomotic enhancement of ODC activity produces a large increase in the intracellular concentration of putrescine in mammary explants. This observation suggested a possibility that the cellular demand for putrescine may be increased when mammary cells are exposed to hypoosomotic enviroment. Since mammary cells have been previously shown to possess a transport system for putrescine and other polyamines (13), such a possibility was examined by studying uptake and accumulation of exogenously added putrescine in cultured explants. These studies (29) showed that hypotonicity causes an increase in the rate of influx and a decrease in efflux of putrescine with enhancement of intracellular putrescine accumulation. On the other hand, the uptake of spermidine, spermine, amino acids, and sugars is unaffected. The results suggest that osmotic alteration in cellular enviroment causes an increased need for putrescine in mammary cells, resulting in stimulation of ODC activity.

The activity of S-ado-met DC in cultured mammary cells is stimulated two-to-three fold by the synergistic action of insulin and cortisol (20). The increase in enzyme activity parallels the rise in the concentration of spermidine in the cells(Fig. 7). The enzyme has been purified to apparent homogeneity from mouse mammary gland and liver (35). The purified enzyme from the two tissues was identical with respect to specific activity, physicochemical and immunological properties. The apparent molecular weight of native enzyme was approximately 68000-74000 daltons, whereas the molecular weight determined under denaturing conditions was 32000 daltons, indicating that the native protein is a dimer. Some of these characteristics of mouse S-ado-met DC are similar to those reported earlier for enzyme from other sources (3)(4)(6)(29). The activity of purified enzyme from mammary tissue is stimulated by physiological concentration of putrescine (Ka=0.5 uM), which decreases the apparent Km for the substrate and also prevents inactivation of the enzyme (35). In contrast, spermine, but not spermidine, inhibits the enzyme activity by reducing the Vmax of the enzyme reaction at physiological concentrations (Ki=0.5 mM). These data suggest that the precursor putrescine and the end product spermine in polyamine biosynthetic path may act as positive and negative regulatory factors, respectively, in cellular control of polyamine biosynthesis via their action on S-ado-met DC. Additional

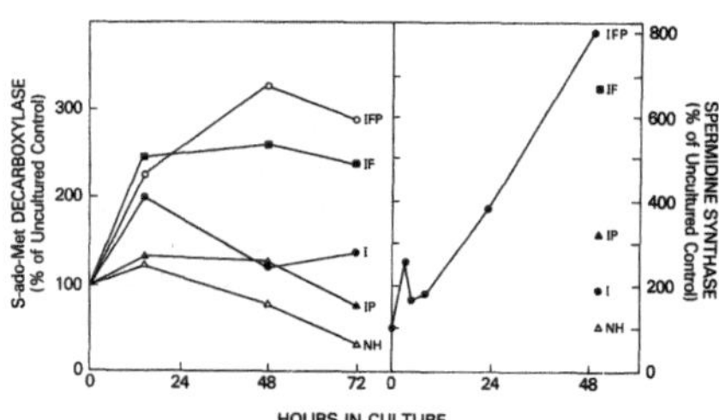

Fig. 7. Changes in the activities of S-ado-met DC and spermidine synthase in midpregant mouse mammary explants cultured with various combination of insulin (I), cortisol (F) and prolactin (P).

studies using a monospecific mouse antibody to the enzyme indicated that the enhanced activity of S-ado-met DC during the development of mouse mammary gland is primarily due to alteration in synthesis and degradation of enzyme molecule rather than modulation of the activity of the enzyme (36).

Since mammary gland contains two major cell types, fat cells and epithelial cells, it is important to ascertain that any biochemical changes observed with the tissue reflects the response of epithelial cells. When changes in spermidine synthase activity in cultured mammary tissue were examined, the enzyme activity in whole explants remained essentially constant during 72 hours of culture with insulin, cortisol and prolactin (34). In contrast, the same hormone treatment stimulated the enzyme activity in epithelial cell fraction, which comprises only a small percentage of the activity in whole tissue. The increase in enzyme activity occurred rapidly within 3 hours of culture and continued upto 72 hours (Fig. 7), amounting to about a three-to five-fold increase over the initial level. The epithelial enzyme activity remained unchanged in the absence of the hormones during culture. These results indicate that spermidine synthase activity of epithelial cells and fat cells of mammary explants respond differently to the actions of hormones. The stimulatory effect of hormones on the epithelial cell enzyme would not have been detected if whole explants alone were assayed, because of the high basal enzyme activity in fat cells and their unresponsiveness to the hormones. Addition of actionmycin D or cycloheximide at the onset of culture inhibited completely the hormonal stimulation of spermidine synthase activity, suggesting that the increase in enzyme activity may require both new RNA and protein synthesis (23).

The delayed addition of cycloheximide at any time during culture prevented a further increase in enzyme activity, but caused no significant decline of enzyme activity for 12 hours. This suggests a half-life for the mammary synthase of at least 12 hours, as observed earlier with rat liver enzyme (5). Additional studies to determine the role of insulin, cortisol and prolactin in stimulation of spermidine synthase activity showed that insulin and cortisol are largely responsible for the increase in enzyme activity (23).

The data presented above show that the interplay of insulin, glucocorticoid and prolactin causes the stimulation of a group of enzymes involved in the biosynthesis of the polyamines. The increase of the various enzyme activities is not synchronous and differs in extent and stimulatory agents involved. It is note-worthy that the activities of the last two enzymes in spermidine biosynthesis, S-ado-met decarboxylase and spermidine synthase are regulated by the action of both insulin and glucocorticoid. Further, the pattern of regulation of polyamine biosynthesis during the mammary differentiation _in vitro_ is also different from that observed during the insulin-dependent proliferation of cultured mammary cells.

THE FUNCTIONS OF POLYAMINES DURING MAMMARY CELL PROLIFERATION

Spermidine. As described above, the concentrations of putrescine and spermidine increase during the proliferation of mammary epithelial cells. To examine the causal relationship between spermidine accumulation and mammary cell proliferation, the effect of methyl glyoxal bis (guanylhydrazone) (MGBG), a potent inhibitor of spermidine biosynthesis (42), on DNA synthesis was studied. (Fig. 8) Addition of MGBG with insulin to the medium at the onset of culture completely prevented increases in both the concentration of spermidine and DNA synthesis. When MGBG was added at 24 and 48 hr, the inhibitory effect of the drug on DNA synthesis was substantially reduced. The resumption of DNA synthesis by the addition of spermidine to the culture containing insulin and MGBG is preceded by the rapid accumulation of spermidine in mammary cells, as occurs in the case of stimulation of DNA synthesis by insulin in the absence of MGBG (34). Following the addition of spermidine, mammary cells take up the polyamine rapidly and restore the intracellular level of spermidine to the control level within 4 hr, and DNA synthesis resumes in about 10 hr. The inhibitory effect of MGBG is specific for DNA synthesis since the drug produced only slight ($<$20%) inhibition of RNA and protein synthesis in cultured explants (34). In contrast, when mammary explants from mid-pregnant mice, which are in an active proliferative phase with a higher endogenous level of spermidine, were cultured with insulin and MGBG, little inhibition of DNA synthesis was observed, in spite of complete inhibition of spermidine biosynthesis by MGBG (34).

If the inhibitory effect of MGBG on DNA synthesis was the result of an intracellular deficiency of spermidine, the effect should be abolished by an exogenous supply of spermidine to the cells. Concomitant addition

Fig. 8 Effect of MGBG and spermidine on insulin-induced DNA synthesis. Mammary explants from virgin mice were cultured in the presence of insulin (○) or insulin(I) plus MGBG added at 0 (▲), 24 (△), and 48 (△) hours after explantation. Spermidine (100 μM, Sd) was added at 24 or 48 hours after the culture with insulin and MGBG. DNA synthesis was determined by labeling the explants with [^{3}H]thymidine (2 μCi/ml) for 24 hours.

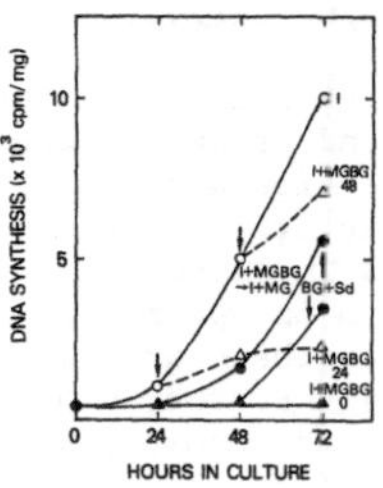

TABLE 1. Effect of HAVA on DNA synthesis in mammary explants from virgin mice cultured in various hypotonic media

Mammary explants were cultured for 48 h under the indicated conditions. DNA synthesis was determined by labeling the explants for 2 days with [^{3}H]thymidine (1 uCi/ml).

Culture system	DNA synthesis with isotonicity of			
	1	0.75	0.67	0.5
	cpm/mg tissue			
No hormone	817	1,083	609	358
Insulin	3,414	3,192	3,146	1,508
Insulin + HAVA (1 mM)	3,239	2,542	1,941	561

of spermidine (10^{-5}M) with MGBG at 0 hr completely eliminated the inhibition of DNA synthesis. The addition of spermidine at 24 hr or even 48 hr of culture with both insulin and MGBG allowed resumption of DNA synthesis. Spermidine was effective at concentrations between 10^{-6} and 10^{-3} M. Addition of spermidine (10^{-7} – 10^{-5} M) to the insulin-containing medium resulted in approximately a 20% increase in DNA synthesis, but spermidine, in the absence of insulin, did not stimulate DNA synthesis at all (34). Additional studies (34) showed that inhibition of DNA synthesis by MGBG can also be reversed by exogenous addition of other polyamines such as putrescine (10^{-4} – 10^{-3} M), and spermine (10^{-6} – 10^{-4} M). However, analysis of the intracellular concentration of each polyamine involved in the reversal process indicated that spermidine was the only polyamine that was effective at the physiological concentration, i.e., 100-150 pmol/mg tissue, found in the explants cultured with insulin for 72 hr.

Putrescine. During the induction of DNA synthesis by insulin in cultured mammary cells, the concentration of putrescine has also been found to increase substantially prior to the increase in DNA synthesis. While putrescine plays an indispensable role in the biosynthesis of spermidine as a precursor of the polyamine, it is also conceivable that putrescine may have an additional function in DNA synthesis. This is suggested by its ability to negate the inhibitory effect of MGBG on mammary DNA synthesis. Our previous observation (34) that an "osmolarity-sensitive" increase in ornithine decarboxylase activity with a subsequent rise in putrescine level invariably precedes induction of mammary cell proliferation by insulin *in vitro* led us to investigated the possible involvement of putrescine in the hormonal stimulation of DNA synthesis in cultured mammary explants. We have employed various culture conditions in which the intracellular level of putrescine was varied by alterations in the osmolarity of culture medium (22), use of DL-α-hydrazino-δ-aminovarleric acid, (HAVA), as an inhibitor of ornithine decarboxylase (11), and use of mammary explants derived from virgin and midpregnant mice, which contained initially a low and a high level of putrescine, respectively (34).

In cultured mammary explants from both virgin and midpregnant mice which contained a low and a high initial level of putrescine, respectively, HAVA at the onset of culture prevented an early, "osmolarity-sensitive" rise in the putrescine level that occurred prior to induction of DNA synthesis by insulin. In the presence of the drug, hormonal stimulation of DNA synthesis occurred normally in virgin mouse mammary explants cultured in isotonic medium and in midpregnant mouse mammary explants cultured in both isotonic and hypotonic media. However, in virgin mouse mammary explants cultured in hypotonic medium, the drug caused varying degrees of inhibition of DNA synthesis which were inversely related to the osmolarity of the medium (Table 1). The inhibitory effect of the drug on DNA synthesis was also dependent at the time of its addition, being most effective within the first 2 h of culture, but virtually ineffective at 12 h. Inhibition of DNA synthesis by the drug was reversible by addition of putrescine (0.5 to 1 μM), which was most effective within 1 h of culture and thereafter became less effective. (Fig. 9). The polyamines, spermidine, spermine, and cadaverine were ineffective in this respect. Similar results were obtained with another ornithine decarboxylase inhibitor, α-methylornithine. In contrast to the effect on DNA synthesis, HAVA inhibited neither protein synthesis nor the uptake of amino acids or glucose and caused a much smaller degree of inhibition of RNA synthesis. These results suggest that an osmolarity-sensitive increase in putrescine concentration is important for hormonal induction of DNA synthesis in mammary cells containing a low, initial level of putrescine which are cultured in hypotonic medium. Accordingly, both the initial cellular level of putrescine and the developmental state of cells appear to be important factors for the efficacy of HAVA in inhibition of DNA synthesis. The requirement for putrescine may not be apparent in those instances when the cellular levels of putrescine are initially high enough for subsequent DNA synthesis even though the drug inhibited an increase in putrescine. A similar view was presented in earlier studies on the role of spermidine in cell proliferation (8), (14), (34). Such consideration may be important in cases where inhibitors of polyamine biosynthesis are found to be effective in preventing DNA synthesis (7), (16),(38).

Fig. 9 Time course of DNA synthesis in virgin mouse mammary explants in hypotonic culture medium. Mammary explants were cultured for 5 days in 0.67 isotonic medium containing [^{3}H]thymidine (1 μCi/ml) and the following additions; insulin (□), or insulin + HAVA 1 mM (○), or insulin + HAVA + putrescine 1 μM (▲) or no addition (●). At the indicated time points, incorporation of [^{3}H]thymidine into DNA in cultured explants was determined.

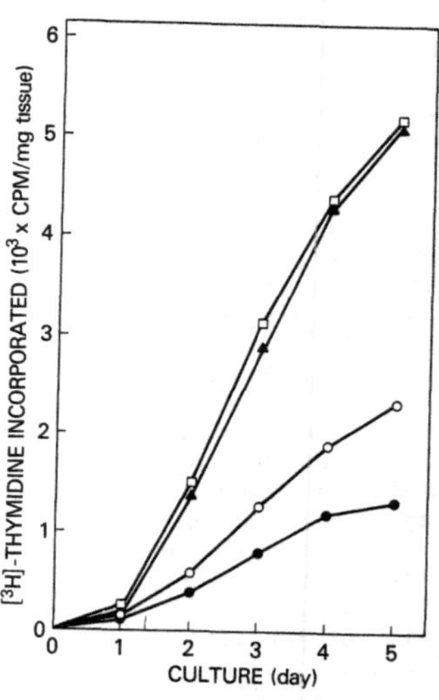

The precise mode of involvement of putrescine in mammary DNA synthesis in hypotonic culture remains to be elucidated. Since putrescine itself was ineffective in stimulating DNA synthesis in mammary explants, direct involvement of putrescine as a mitogenic factor is unlikely. Time course studies suggest that the diamine may be required for events occurring within a few hours of culture. A rapid osmolarity-sentitive increase in ODC and in the accumulation of putrescine may represent an adaptive response of mammary cells in culture. It is possible that alteration on the osmolarity of medium causes pertubation of the normal balance of intracellular ionic enviroment. The above results suggest that putrescine has an essential function in early phase of cell cycle prior to the initiation of DNA synthesis.

THE ROLE OF POLYAMINES IN THE DIFFERENTIATION OF MAMMARY GLAND

Milk protein synthesis. The hormone-dependent, terminal development of mammary gland culminates in the production of the milk proteins casein and α-lactalbumin during lactation. Casein is a group of acidic phosphoproteins which comprises over 50% of milk protein, whereas α-lactalbumin is a whey protein capable of modifying the substrate specificity of galactosyl transferase to include glucose, thus enhancing the biosynthesis of milk sugar, or lactose (41). These two proteins have often been used as specific markers for the differentiated function of mammary epithelium.

As mentioned above, the concentration of spermidine in mammary tissue increased markedly during lactogenesis in vivo as well as in vitro. In order to assess the role of spermidine in hormonal induction of milk-protein synthesis, MGBG was used (Table 2). When the drug was added to

TABLE 2. Effect of methylglyoxal bis(guanylhydrazone),MGBG, on milk protein formation and spermidine accumulation in mammary explants from mid-pregnant mice during 2-day culture.

Culture conditions	Spermidine (mol/g wet wt)	α-Lactalbumin[a] activity	Casein[b]
Uncultured control	150	50	230
Insulin + cortisol + prolactin	400	235	1100
Insulin + cortisol + prolactin + 10 μM MGBG	70	15	160
Insulin + cortisol + prolactin + 10 μM MGBG + spermidine[c]	Not Done	210	950

[a] pmol lactose formed/mg wet wt tissue/30 min.
[b] cpm/mg wet wt tissue/3 hours.
[c] 0.4 mM used

midpregnant mouse mammary gland cultured with the three hormones, the hormonal stimulation of both the concentration of spermidine and the accumulation of casein and α-lactalbumin was blocked (20). However, the inhibitory effect of the drug on milk protein synthesis was completely reversed by the addition of spermidine, but not of spermine or putrescine. Similar results were obtained by other investigators (2)(32). When mammary explants were cultured in medium in which the concentration of arginine was reduced by 20-fold to 0.2 mM, the concentration of spermidine and the formation of milk-proteins did not rise (21). However, addition of ornithine, putrescine or spermidine restored the increase in milk-protein synthesis, whereas the addition of spermine, proline and lysine was ineffective. These results suggest that spermidine may be necessary for milk protein synthesis.

Spermidine and glucocorticoid action. Direct evidence for the involvemnt of spermidine in milk-protein synthesis was obtained by cultivation of mammary tissue on media containing several combinations of spermidine, insulin, cortisol and prolactin (17)(20). The addition of spermidine, in place of cortisol, to a medium containing insulin and prolactin, markedly enhanced milk-protein synthesis. The increase in α-lactalbumin was similar to that produced by the combination of insulin, cortisol and prolactin, whereas the increase in casein synthesis was about half of that in the three-hormone system. Spermidine alone, or in combination with any one of the three hormones or with both insulin and cortisol, was ineffective. The effective spermidine concentration was as low as 0.4 mM, which is in the range found in the cells that are actively synthesizing milk proteins under the influence of insulin, cortisol and prolactin. Spermine, putrescine and divalent cations such as Mg^{++} had no stimulatory effect on the synthesis of milk proteins.

The effect of spermidine on cellular components. The effect of spermidine appears to be specific for glucocorticoid since this polyamine does not replace the requirement for insulin or prolactin. Earlier studies (18) of the role of glucocorticoid in this system have shown that the steroid, in the presence of insulin, facilitates sustained accumulation of rough endoplasmic reticulum (RER), an organelle which is vital for the formation of secretory milk-proteins. In the absence of the steroid hormone, accumulation of RER is only transient and disappears by the fourth day of culture. Additional studies (19) have shown that other cellular components are also subject to a similar stabilizing effect of glucocorticoid. For instance, glucose-6-phosphate dehydrogenase is a soluble enzyme that accumulates markedly during the lactation period and plays an important role in the lactogenesis. In mammary cells cultured with insulin, the activity of this enzyme increased by 50-100% during the first two days of culture, and then declined to the control level during day 3 and 4. Addition of glucocorticoid prevented the decline and maintained the elevated new steady-state level (Fig. 10). This effect of glucocorticoid can also be mimicked by exogenous addition of spermidine with insulin. Spermine or putrescine was not effective in this respect.

Fig. 10 Glucose 6-phosphate dehydrogenase in mammary gland in culture. Mammary explants from mid-pregnant mice were cultured in media containing insulin (I, ○), insulin and cortisol (IF, □), insulin and prolactin (IP, △), insulin, cortisol, and prolactin (IFP, ●), and insulin, cortisol, and 4 mM spermidine (ISP, ■). At indicated times, the enzyme activity in mammary epithelial cell fraction was determined.

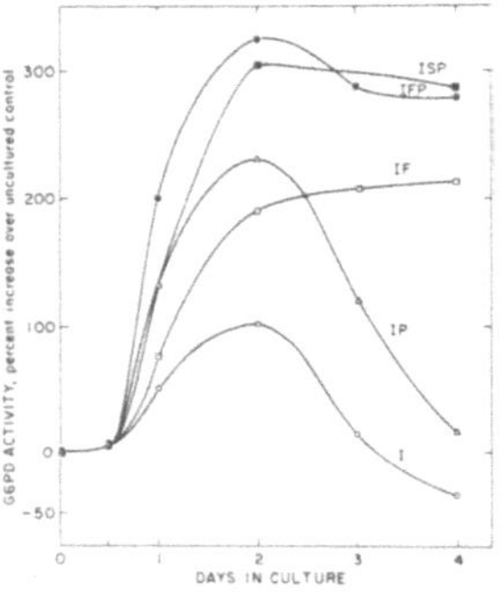

Studies on the glucocorticoid-dependent accumulation of RER in mammary cells have shown that such action of the steroid hormone involves augmentation of the biosynthesis of phosphatidylcholine, a major phospholipid component of RER of mammary cells (23). The increased formation of phosphatidylcholine has been shown to be mediated by the stimulation of the activity of choline kinase, the first enzyme involved in the biosynthesis of phosphatidylcholine (23) (31). In cultured mammary tissue, the increase in enzyme activity is dependent on the synergistic actions of insulin and cortisol and is blocked by the addition of MGBG (23) (Table 3). Inhibition by the drug, however, was overcome by the exogenous addition of 0.04 mM spermidine. Furthermore, spermidine, when added in place of cortisol, mimicked the stimulatory action of the steroid hormone on choline kinase by acting synergistically with insulin. The above results suggest that spermidine mediates several important actions of glucocorticoid on the differentiation of mammary cells. Since spermidine can stimulate the choline kinase in the enzyme assay system, it is tempting to speculate that cortisol increases the activity of choline kinase through the formation of spermidine, which

TABLE 3. Effect of insulin, cortisol, prolactin, spermidine and methylglyoxyal bis(guanylhydrazone), MGBG, on choline kinase activity in mouse mammary gland.

Mammary explants from mid-pregnant mice were cultured for 2 days under the indicated conditions.

Culture conditions	Activity (pmole/min/mg of explants)
Uncultured control	3.0
Insulin + cortisol + prolactin	16.8
Insulin + cortisol + prolactin + MGBG	7.5
Insulin + cortisol + prolactin + MGBG + spermidine(4 mM)	17.0
Insulin + spermidine(4 mM)	14.9

in turn, stimulates the enzyme activity leading to the accumulation of rough endoplasmic reticulum.

Differential actions of glucocorticoid and spermidine. As shown earlier (17)(20), exogenous spermidine can largely mimic the effect of cortisol on the accumulation of α-lactalbumin, whereas spermidine does not completely simulate the action of cortisol on casein synthesis. To gain some insight into these differential actions of spermidine, we have further investigated the role of cortisol in induction of milk-protein synthesis with use of a new immunochemical procedure to determine casein synthesis and a modified quantitative assay method to measure the amount of α-lactalbumin (15)(26)(27). As shown in Fig. 11, these studies revealed a striking difference between the optimal concentrations of cortisol required for maximal induction of the two milk proteins in culture: 3 x 10^{-8} molar for α-lactalbumin and 3 x 10^{-6}molar for casein. Moreover, $10^{-7}$to 10^{-5} molar cortisol caused progressive inhibition of α-lactalbumin accumulation. It was further shown that the differential effects of cortisol can be modulated by the concentration of prolactin (28). Thus, when a suboptimal concentration of prolactin was used, the stimulatory effect of cortisol on α-lactalbumin accumulation became manifested greatly and the inhibitory effect of cortisol at higher concentrations became smaller, as compared to the corresponding effect observed in the presence of an optimal concentration of prolactin (26)(27). The observed differential effect of cortisol indicate that the action of cortisol is mediated by different mechanisms with respect to the accumulation of casein and α-lactalbumin. Furthermore these results can provide an explanation for the differential ability of spermidine to mimic the action of cortisol on the accumulation of the two milk proteins in cultured mammary tissue (17).

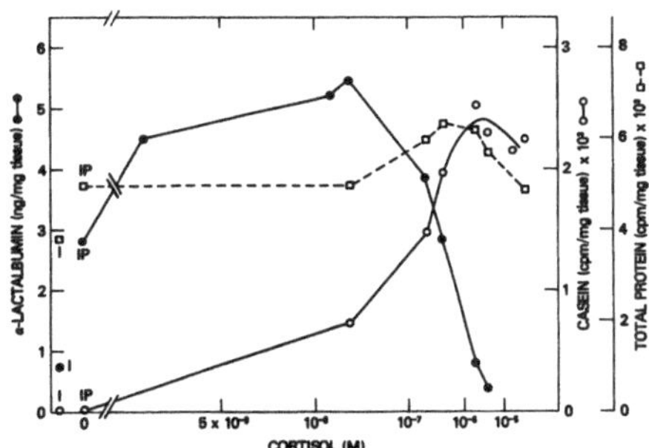

Fig. 11 Effect of cortisol concentration on casein synthesis, α-lactalbumin content, and total protein synthesis in mammary explants in culture. Mammary explants from mature virgin mice were cultured in medium containing combination of insulin(I), prolactin(P), and various concentration of cortisol. Casein synthesis was determined on the 3 rd day of culture by the method of Ono and Oka (27). α-Lactalbumin was determined by the assay of its activity in the lactose synthetase system (15). Total protein synthesis was determined by the incorporation of [^{3}H]-labeled amino acid mixture into trichloroacetic acid-insoluble materials.

<u>Spermidine and cell-free translation of mammary mRNAs</u>. Studies with the organ culture system have indicated that spermidine is necessary for the hormonal stimulation of milk protein synthesis. However, the molecular mechanisms involved in the action of spermidine on milk protein synthesis remained undefined. Numerous studies have demonstrated that spermidine stimulates polypeptide synthesis in various cell-free systems (1)(9)(10) (38). Spermidine plays a fundamental role in protein synthesis at the translational level by facilitating the synthesis of full size polypeptide chains (1) (9). To gain better understanding of the mechanisms whereby spermidine stimulates milk protein synthesis in mammary cells, we have studied its effect on the translation of the mammary mRNAs inclding casein mRNA in a cell-free system derived from wheat germ.

In the wheat germ cell-free system, spermidine at 0.4 mM in the presence of 1.5 mM Mg^{++} and 74 mM KCl elicited maximal <u>in vitro</u> translation of poly $(A)^+$-mRNA from lactating mouse mammary glands(Fig. 12). The <u>in vitro</u> synthesis of casein polypeptides as directed by total poly $(A)^+$-mRNA was also stimulated by increasing concentrations of spermidine, amounting to nearly 50% of total polypeptides at 0.3-0.6 mM spermidine. The level of incorporation of isotopic leucine into total and casein polypeptides in the presence of 0.4 mM spermidine was about two times higher than that found in the presence of an optimal concentration of Mg^{++} alone. The stimulatory effect of spermidine was dependent on the concentration of KCl in the translation system where 62-74 mM KCl allowed maximal <u>in vitro</u> translation, whereas higher concentrations of KCl markedly reduced the

Fig. 12 Effect of spermidine and Mg^{++} on the translation of poly(A)$^+$ RNA from lactating mouse mammary glands in the wheat germ system. Each 100 µl reaction contained 0.15 A_{260} unit/ml of poly(A)$^+$ RNA, 2.5 µCi of tritium-labeled leucine and other essential components for *in vitro* polypeptide synthesis. Incubation was performed at 25°C for 90 min. The insert figure shows the percent change in casein polypeptide synthesis as a function of the concentration of spermidine.

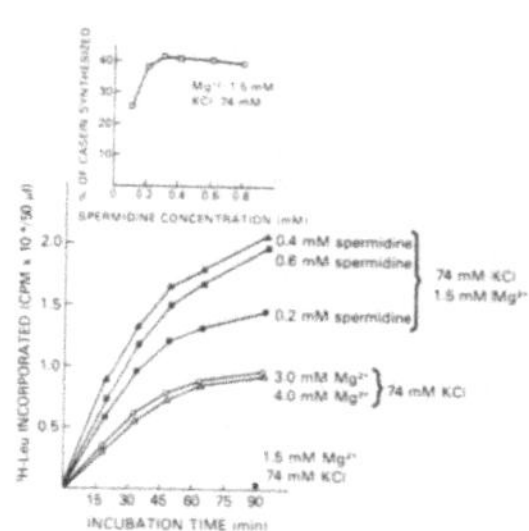

polypeptide synthesis. Conversely, spermidine was found to affect the sensitivity of the translation system to KCl. Further analysis revealed that spermidine enhances the rate of peptide chain elongation in the presence of the optimal concentrations of KCl whereas the polyamine can augment the inhibitory effect of high KCl on peptide chain initiation. These results indicate that the *in vitro* translation of mammary mRNAs is modulated by the interaction of spermidine and KCl.

Comparison of the effect of spermidine on the *in vitro* translation of partially purified casein and the other non-casein mRNAs showed a significant difference in the rate of chain elongation of polypeptides directed by the two mRNAs. In the presence of 0.4 mM spermidine, elongation of casein polypeptides was much faster than that of non-casein peptides. On the other hand, when the concentration of spermidine was reduced to 0.2 mM, the chain elongation became a rate-limiting step in casein polypeptide synthesis while the synthesis of non-casein polypeptides was less affected. This difference was more evident when high concentrations of KCl were used. Thus, maximal translation of casein mRNA *in vitro* appears to require adequate amount of spermidine which allows efficient elongation of casein peptide chain. At present, however, the reasons for the observed difference between the two mRNAs remain unknown. The population of non-casein mRNAs, like casein mRNA, was isolated on the basis of the presence of poly (A) tail at 5-terminus. These mRNAs were found to initiate multiple rounds of peptide synthesis and direct the formation of hitherto unidentified polypeptide of apparent molecular weight of 16000 to 20000 daltons. In preliminary experiments specific mRNA activity of this mRNA was found to be 20-30% lower than that of casein mRNA. It would be of interest to identify the translational product(s) of the non-casein mRNA(s) and further examine whether the observed difference in the characteristics of the translation of the two mRNAs can also occur at the cellular level.

The concentration of spermidine has been shown to increase markedly during the period of lactation. The above results indicating that spermidine, at concentrations comparable to those in lactating mammary cells (25), stimulates synthesis of casein polypeptides in a wheat germ ststem suggest possible involvement of the polyamine in milk protein synthesis at the translational level. Development of a homologous cell-free protein synthesizing system for milk protein would be most desirable to elucidate the mode of action of spermidine in milk protein synthesis.

POLYAMINE TRANSPORT

The observation that exogenous spermidine can replace the action of glucocorticoid has led us to examine the uptake and metabolism of polyamines in mammary explants. Studies on the uptake of spermidine showed that the mammary tissue possesses a transport system for spermidine and other polyamines which is a time-dependent, energy-requiring process, and is stimulated by insulin and prolactin (13). The stimulatory effect of insulin involves both enhancement of Vmax for spermidine influx and prevention of efflux of the polyamine, whereas prolactin elicits a greater increase in Vmax than insulin. Thus mammary cells can attain a level of spermidine sufficient for the formation of milk-protein by transporting it from the external medium under the influence of insulin and prolactin. It is of interest that the transport of spermidine is not stimulated by glucocorticoid, whose action can be replaced by exogenous spermidine.

As shown above, the intracellular level of the polyamines increases markedly during cell growth and development. Because such increases are often accompanied by enhanced activities of polyamine biosynthetic enzymes, it has been customory to ascribe an increase in the polyamine largely to its enhanced biosynthesis. However, the observations that the polyamines are taken up and released through transport systems in mammary cells may suggest another means of modulating the cellular polyamine level. It has been shown (25) that the concentration of polyamines increases significantly in maternal blood of pregnant rat. During lactation blood spermidine levels increase further to reach their highest level and then declined to the concentration of virgin animals toward the end of lactation. The cellular elements of blood from virgin, pregnant and lactating rats contain over 89% of the total blood polyamine. On a cell to cell basis, leukocytes contain over 160 times as much spermidine as erythrocytes. However, erythrocytes contain over 76% of the total blood spermidine. Although a definitive origin, fate and role for increased polyamines in blood during pregnancy and lactation remain to be clarified, it is possible that the blood polyamine may play a role in the growth and differentiation of mammary gland. Possible interaction between circulating polyamines and mammary transport system needs to be examined.

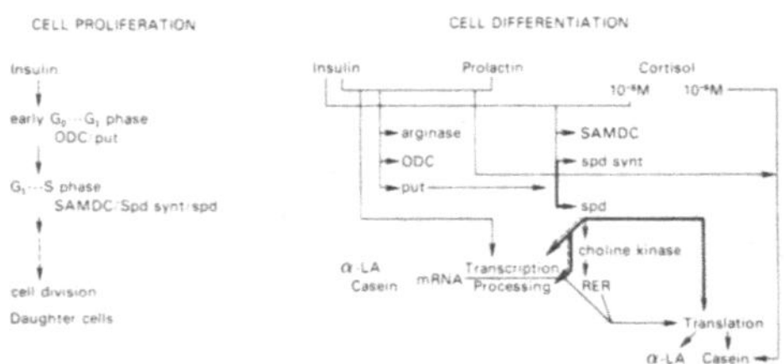

Fig. 13 The mode of involvement of polyamines in the development of mouse mammary gland. Put;putrescine, spd;spermidine, α-LA;α-lactalbumin Dotted lines refer to possible site of action.

CONCLUDING REMARK

Mammary gland organ culture system provides a useful model for studying the regulatory mechanisms of the biosynthesis of polyamines and their roles in the hormonal induction of cell growth and differentiation. Our studies indicate that polyamines are important for the regulation of both cell proliferation and differentiation in the mammary tissue. In cell proliferation, putrescine and spermidine are necessary component of the insulin-responsive DNA synthesis system. The polyamines, however, can not substitute for insulin as a mitogen (Fig. 13). The requirement of polyamines for DNA synthesis is apparent only in the case of mammary cells of virgin mice which are non-proliferative and contain low levels of the polyamines. The mammary cells of the mid-pregnant animal, however, are already in a proliferative phase with a sufficient amount of the polyamine for DNA synthesis, but do require more spermidine to synthesize milk-proteins. In this case, spermidine can substitute for some action of glucocorticoid, a hormone necessary for lactogenesis. It appears that the specific requirement for the polyamines in the biochemical processes of mammary cells may vary depending on the different phases of development and to some extent on the different species(2). Although the precise molecular mechanisms involved in the actions of polyamines remain unknown, it should be possible to extend these studies at molecular levels.

The use of the inhibitors of polyamine biosynthesis proved to be very useful to assess the role of polyamines in cell growth and metabolism. Because of the close association of polyamine accumulation with cell proliferation, chemical intervention of polyamine metabolism offers a possible clinical application, especially in the treatment of proliferative disorders including cancer. In fact, MGBG was used in cancer chemotherapy. Several inhibitors of ODC including DL-alpha-difluoromethylornithine have undergone some preclinical trial as an anti-tumor agent. Recently the ODC inhibitor has been shown to arrest the growth of EMT 6, a murine mammary tumor. At present other types of the inhibitor of polyamine biosynthesis have been in development.

Although a great deal of attention has been given to polyamines in relation to the diagnosis and prognosis of various cancer, there appears to be no specific pattern ascribable to cancer. For example,elevated urinary excretion of polyamines is observed in patients with advanced tumors including mammary gland, stomach and pancreas. Elevated levels of polyamines have been also found in various extracelluair fluids of tumor-bearing subjects. The rise in polyamine appears to result from tumor-cell death rather than from enhanced production and excretion of polyamines by growing tumors. At present, the clinical usefulness of polyamine analysis of body fluids in various pathological states remains equivocal.

During the past decade research on polyamines have increased strikingly, and much valuable information has been obtained. However, many important questions remain unanswered and it is hoped that future work will soon provide information necessary for the progress in polyamine research.

REFERENCES

1. Atkins JF, Lewis JB, Anderson CW, Gesteland RF. Enhanced differential synthesis of proteins in a mammalian cell-free system by addition of polyamines. J Biol Chem 250: 5688-5695, 1975.

2. Bolander FF, Topper YJ. Relationships between spermidine, glucocorticoid and milk proteins in different mammalian species. Biochem Biophs Res Commun 90: 1131-1135, 1979.

3. Cohn MS, Tabor CW, Tabor H. Identification of pyruvyl residue in S-adenosylmethionine decarboxylase from Saccharamyces cervisiae. J Biol Chem 252: 8212-8216, 1977.

4. Demetriou AA, Cohn MS, Tabor CW, Tabor H. Identification of pyruvate in S-adenosylmethionine decarboxylase from rat liver. J Biol Chem 253: 1684-1686, 1978.

5. Hannonen P, Raina A, Janne J. Polyamine synthesis in the regenerating liver: stimulation of S-adenosylmethionine decarboxylase and spermidine and spermine synthases after partial hepatectomy. Biochim Biophys Acta 273: 84-90, 1972.

6. Hannonen P. Enzymic decarboxylation of S-adenosyl-L-methionine in rat liver: possible interaction of putrescine with prosthetic group. Acta Chemica Scandinavica B 29: 295-299, 1975.

7. Harik SI, Hollenberg MD, Snyder SH. α-Hydrazino-ornithine blocks net synthesis of putrescine but not of RNA and DNA. Nature 249: 250-251, 1974.

8. Holtta E, Pohjanpelto P, Janne J. Dissociation of the early antiproliferative action of methylglyoxal bis(guanylhydrazone) from polyamine depletion. FEBS Letter 97: 9-13, 1979.

9. Hunter AR, Farrell PJ, Jackson RJ, Hunt T. The role of polyamine in cell-free protein synthesis in the wheat germ system. Eur J Biochem 75: 149-157, 1977.

10. Igarashi K, Yabuki M, Yoshioka Y, Eguchi K, Hirose S. Mechanism of stimulation of polyphenylalanine synthesis by spermidine. Biochem Biophys Res Commun 75: 163-171, 1977.

11. Inoue H, Kato Y, Takigawa M, Adachi K, Takeda Y. Effect of DL-α-hydrazino-aminovaleric acid, an inhibitor of ornithine decarboxylase, on polyamine metabolism in isoproterenol-stimulated mouse parotid glands. J Biochem (Tokyo) 77: 879-893, 1975.

12. Inoue H, Oka T. The effect of inhibitors of ornithine decarboxylase on DNA synthesis in mouse mammary gland in culture. J Biol Chem 255: 3308-3312, 1980.

13. Kano K, Oka T. Polyamine transport in mouse mammary gland. General properties and hormonal regulation. J Biol Chem 251: 2795-2800 1976.

14. Mamont PS, Bohlen J, Milann P, Bey P, Schuber F, Tardiff C. α-Methyl ornithine, a potent competitive inhibitor of ornithine decarboxylase, blocks proliferation of rat hepatoma cells in culture. Proc Natl Acad Sci USA 73: 1626-1630, 1976.

15. Nagamatsu Y, Oka T. Mouse α-lactalbumin; purification, characterization and the antibody formation. Biochem J 185: 227-237, 1980.

16. Newton NE, Abdel-Monen MM. Inhibitors of polyamine biosynthesis. Effect of α-methyl-ornithine and methylglyoxal Bis(guanylhydrazone) on growth and polyamine content of L1210 leukemic cells of mice. J Med Chem 20: 249-253, 1977.

17. Oka T. The role of spermidine in hormone-dependent differentiation of mammary gland *in vitro*. Science 184: 78-80, 1974.

18. Oka T, Topper YJ. Hormone-dependent accumulation of rough endoplasmic reticulum in mouse mammary epithelial cells *in vitro*. J Biol Chem 246: 7701-7707, 1971.

19. Oka T, Perry JW. Studies on the function of glucocorticoid in mouse mammary cell differentiation *in vitro*: stimulation of glucose-6-phosphate dehydrogenase. J Biol Chem 249: 3586-3591, 1974.

20. Oka T, Perry JW. Spermidine as a possible mediator of glucocorticoid effect on milk protein synthesis in mouse mammary epithelium *in vitro*. J Biol Chem 249: 7647-7652, 1974.

21. Oka T, Perry JW. Arginase affects lactogenesis through its influence on the biosynthesis of spermidine. Nature 250: 660-661, 1974.

22. Oka T, Perry JW. Studies on regulatory factors of ornithine decarboxylase activity during development of mouse mammary epithelium in vitro. J Biol Chem 251: 1738-1744, 1976

23. Oka T, Perry JW. Glucocorticoid stimulation of choline kinase activity during the development of mouse mammary gland. Devel Biol 68: 311-318, 1979

24. Oka T, Perry JW, Kano K. Hormonal regulation of spermidine synthase during the development of mouse mammary epithelium in vitro. Biochem Biophys Res Commun 79: 979-986, 1977.

25. Oka T, Sakai T, Lundren DW, Perry JW. Polyamines in growth and development of mammary gland. pp 301-323 in Hormones, Receptors and Breast Cancer, ed WL McGuire. Raven Press, New York 1978.

26. Ono M, Oka T. α-Lactalbumin-casein induction in virgin mouse mammary explants: dose-dependent differential action of cortisol. Science 207: 1367-1369, 1980.

27. Ono M, Oka T. The differential actions of cortisol on the accumulation of α-lactalbumin and casein in midpregnant mouse mammary gland in culture. Cell 19: 473-480, 1980.

28. Ono M, Perry JW, Oka T. The concentration-dependent differential effects of cortisol on the synthesis of α-lactalbumin and casein in cultured mouse mammary gland explants: The importance of prolactin concentration. In Vitro 17: 121-128, 1981.

29. Perry JW, Oka T. Regulation of ornithine decarboxylase in cultured mouse mammary gland by the osmolarity in the cellular enviroment. Biochim Biophys Acta 629: 24-35, 1980.

30. Pegg AE. Purification of rat liver S-adenosyl-L-methionine decarboxylase. Biochem J 141: 581-583, 1974.

31. Poso H, Sinervirta R, Janne J. S-adenosyl-L-methionine from baker's yeast. Biochem J 151: 67-73, 1975.

32. Rillema JA, Linebaugh BE, Mulder JA. Regulation of casein synthesis by polyamines in mammary gland explants of mice. Endocrinology 100: 529-536, 1977.

33. Russell DH, McVicker T. Polyamine biogenesis in the rat mammary gland during pregancy and lactation. Biochem J 130: 71-76, 1972.

34. Sakai T, Ludgren DW, Oka T. Polyamine biosynthesis and DNA synthesis in cultured mammary gland explants from virgin mice. J Cell Physiol 95: 259-268, 1978.

35. Sakai T, Hori C, Kano K, Oka T. Purification and characterization of S-adenosyl-L-methionine decarboxylase from mouse mammary gland and liver. Biochemistry 18: 5541-5548, 1979.

36. Sakai T, Perry JW, Hori C, Oka T. Putrescine and the regulation of S-adenosyl-L-methionine decarboxylase in cultured mouse mammary gland. Biochim Biophys Acta 614: 577-582, 1980.

37. Salden M, Bloemendal H. Polyamine can replace the dialyzable component from crude reticulocyte intiation factors. Biochem Biophys Res Commun 68: 157-161, 1976.

38. Seidenfeld J, Marton LJ. Depletion of intracellular putrescine and spermidine by α-difluoromethylornithine does not inhibit proliferation of 9L rat brain tumor cells. Biochem Biophys Res Commun 86: 1192-1198, 1979.

39. Stockdale FE, Topper YJ. The role of DNA synthesis and mitosis in hormone-dependent differentiation. Proc Natl Acad Sci USA 56: 1283-1289, 1966.

40. Takemoto T, Nagamatsu Y, Oka, T. Casein and α-lactalbumin mRNAs during the development of mouse mammary gland: isolation, partial purification and translation in a cell-free system. Develop Biol 78: 247-257, 1980.

41. Topper YJ, Oka T. Some aspects of mammary gland development in the mature mouse. pp 327-348 in Lactation I, eds GL Larson, VR Smith, Academic Press, New York, 1974.

42. Williams-Ashman HG, Schenone A. Methylglyoxal Bis(guanylhydrazone) as a potent inhibitor of mammalian and yeast S-adenosylmethionine decarboxylases. Biochem Biophys Res Commun 46: 288-295, 1972.

43. Yip MCM, Knox WE. Function of arginase in lactating mammary gland. Biochem J 127: 893-899, 1972.

HORMONAL REGULATION OF CASEIN GENE EXPRESSION IN NORMAL AND NEOPLASTIC CELLS IN MURINE MAMMARY GLANDS

M R Banerjee, Ranjan Ganguly, Nozer M Mehta, Nivedita Ganguly

I. INTRODUCTION

Contemporary advances of knowledge and technology in the areas of cellular and molecular biology have revealed that selective gene expression plays a definitive role in the regulation of cellular differentiation. In conventional terms, selective gene expression denotes a regulated transcription of different structural genes producing the respective mRNAs. During recent years it has also become evident that the physical structure of eukaryotic genes are composed of expressed (exons) and unexpressed (introns) segments along the DNA strand and this requires splicing and processing of the initial transcripts into the final mRNA (20), (50), (119). Moreover, post-translational processing of the polypeptides may also modify the final product and hence influence gene expression (108). Thus, selective gene expression during a developmental process may be subject to modulation at any of these complex series of events. Based on the observation that the insect steroid hormone, ecdysone, is capable of inducing specific puffs in polytene chromosomes of *Drosophila* larvae, Karlson (55) proposed that hormonal modulation of specific gene expression may influence developmental processes in the target tissue. Demonstration of ecdysone-induced synthesis of the enzyme, dopa decarboxylase in the larvae (101), correlation between transcription and puff formation in the polytene chromosomes (31), and cell-free translation of ecdysone-induced mRNA for dopa decarboxylase (56) now appear to corroborate Karlson's original thesis.

Hormonal induction of specific gene activation in vertebrates has been observed in different endocrine target organs eliciting specialized proteins. Notable examples are estrogen regulation of the egg white proteins, ovalbumin and conalbumin, in the chick oviduct (76), (80), (99). It is now clear that synthesis of the egg white proteins is the result of steroid hormone-induced specific gene expression in the tubular gland cells, although the mechanism(s) of the specific interaction(s) of the steroid hormone, or the estrogen-receptor complex with the gene itself yet remain to be elucidated (15), (108), (136). Vitellogenin is another estrogen-dependent specific protein. The complex regulatory processes at the transcriptional, post-transcriptional and post-translational level of control of the estrogen-dependent vitellogenin gene is also being unfolded in studies using frog liver as a model system (112), (113).

The mammary gland in female mammals represents a major endocrine target organ. A complex mixture of steroid and polypeptide hormones are involved in the regulation of morphogenesis and functional differentiation of the mammary parenchyma and the specific hormones needed at various stages of development have been described (7), (23), (27), (62), (69), (72), (127). The hormone regulated functional differentiation of the mammary epithelium is marked by lactogenesis which involves production of several specific proteins, including casein. Casein, a complex group of phospho-proteins constitutes the major component (60-80%) of the milk proteins (24), (51), (65). The adrenal steroid hormone, cortisol (or corticosterone), and the pituitary polypeptide hormone, prolactin, are the two principal hormones required for mammary cell specific production of casein (7), (27), (35). Thus, the multi-hormonal regulation of the casein synthesis in the mammary gland presents a model for understanding the mechanism(s) of the synergistic action between steroid and polypeptide hormones modulating specific gene expression in a mammalian cell population. In this chapter we will review primarily our recent studies concerning the role of prolactin and glucocorticoid in the regulation of casein gene expression during normal and neoplastic development of the murine (BALB/c mice) mammary gland.

II. GENERAL MACROMOLECULAR ACTIVITY

Hormonal infleunces on mammary gland macromolecules have been extensively discussed in several recent reviews (7), (28), (90), (124), (129). The brief account presented in this section is to provide the background information for the reader. Studies measuring labeled precursor incorporation determined mostly in acid insoluble material, have shown that RNA, protein and DNA synthesis as well as DNA-polymerase activity remain relatively high in the mammary gland of pregnant animals. The ovarian steroids can significantly influence these macromolecular activities in the gland. Analysis of the RNA in the gland during alveolar morphogenesis further revealed that synthesis of both heterogenous nuclear RNA (HnRNA) and ribosomal RNA (rRNA) are influenced by the ovarian hormones (5), (6). Pregnancy-like, alveolar morphogenesis of the mammary parenchyma in the whole mammary gland *in vitro*, is also accompanied by increased macromolecular activity (70). Presence of the ovarian and/or the adrenal steroids in the medium with prolactin stimulates RNA (including HnRNA), protein and DNA synthesis, including DNA polymerase activity in the gland *in vitro*.

Lactogenesis is associated with a pronounced increase of RNA in the post-partum mammary gland (28). The increase of RNA content also corresponds to a high level of RNA synthesis in the early lactating glands (4), (10). Precursor (^{3}H-uridine) uptake into RNA is ten-fold higher in 5 day lactating glands than in mammary tissue of virgin mice. This pronounced increase of RNA synthesis with the onset of lactogenesis includes a preferential increase of rRNA (4), (7). The processing of the ribosomal precursor RNA and the cytoplasmic migration of the 28S and 18S rRNAs is similar to other eukaryotic cells (35). The increased level of RNA in the lactating mammary gland is sensitive to adrenal ablation and cortisol treatment of the animal (4), (7). Studies *in vivo* have further shown that prolactin also plays a regulatory role on mammary RNA synthesis in lactating animals and glucocorticoid and/or prolactin stimulation of mammary RNA is concomitant with increased secretory activity in the post-partum gland (2), (28). The transition of the animal from pregnancy to parturition is also marked by an increase in the amount of larger polysomes in the mammary cells and the maintenance of the polysomes in the post-partum mammary gland is influenced both by cortisol and prolactin treatment of the animals (7), (28). Recent studies have also shown that cortisol treatment can influence the synthesis of poly(A) RNA in the mammary gland of non-hypophysectomizec lactating mice (11), (12). Since the hormone stimulated secretory material observed in most of these earlier studies was not analyzed for the milk proteins, a relationship between the hormone-induced RNA and production of the milk proteins remained unclear. Moreover, systemic complexities of the hormone environment made it difficult to make a reliable assessment of the results obtained after endocrine ablation and exogenous hormone therapy of the animal. Nevertheless, the studies *in vivo* did establish that mammary cell macromolecular activities associated with the developmental process of the gland, are responsive to these hormones. It is particularly relevant to point out that the increase in the amount of mammary cell RNA associated with the expression of functional differentiation of the parenchyma, is influenced by adrenal glucocorticoid and prolactin, the two hormones needed for lactogenesis.

In a short-term organ culture model derived from pieces of mammary tissue from pregnant mice or rats the explants are capable of eliciting milk-like secretory material in the presence of prolactin and cortisol with insulin in a synthetic culture medium (15), (34), (41), (89). Subsequently, it was established that under similar culture conditions the mammary explants from pregnant mice produce the milk proteins, casein plus α-lactalbumin (53), (121), (128). The demonstration that mammary tissue elicits a hormone-inducible, specific protein in a serum-free synthetic medium, markedly advanced the feasibility of studying the mecahnisms of the multiple hormone regulation of mammary cell specific gene expression.

During the initial years, studies in several laboratories have attempted to establish a temporal relationship between the hormonal stimulation of increase in RNA synthesis and the production of the milk proteins in mammary explants *in vitro* (37), (122), (129). It was observed that both prolactin and cortisol were required for (i) the maximum stimulation of RNA synthesis, including HnRNA, and (ii) the maintenance of high level of RNA content. Incubation of the explants initially with cortisol does not stimulate RNA synthesis to a significant level, but subsequent addition of prolactin to the medium stimulates both RNA and casein synthesis. Inhibition of RNA synthesis (by actinomycin D) stimulated after addition of prolactin to the medium containing cortisol, also blocks casein synthesis. Hence it was postulated that prolactin acts as an inducer for the mRNA directing casein synthesis (129). RNA synthesis was also measured in isolated mammary cell nuclei incubated *in vitro* under high ionic conditions, which are believed to support RNA polymerase II directed, mRNA synthesis (49), (110). RNA synthesis in isolated nuclei from explants incubated with insulin, cortisol and prolactin was 300% higher than in nuclei isolated from explants incubated with insulin and cortisol. The increase in transcription after addition of prolactin to the medium with insulin and cortisol was also found to correspond with an increase in casein synthesis in the explants incubated under similar condition. Thus, it was postulated, that expression of the casein gene in the mammary cells is regulated by prolactin (129).

While the studies discussed in the preceding paragraphs provided information concerning molecular responses of mammary cells to the hormones, the mechanisms by which prolactin and glucocorticoids regulate synthesis of milk proteins remained obscure. Moreover, results obtained by measuring precursor uptake, sedimentation analysis of the cellular RNA and the influence of inhibitors of macromolecular synthesis failed to establish a specific relationship between the hormone stimulated cellular biosynthesis and production of the milk proteins in the explant. However, results from studies *in vitro* with explants of mammary tissue reiterated the fact that both prolactin and glucocorticoids are involved in the stimulation of RNA and casein synthesis in the mammary cells. At this point it became clear that the elucidation of the mechanisms of the expression of the casein gene requires a direct measure of its hormonal responses.

III. DIRECT MEASURE OF CASEIN mRNA

A. Specific translational activity

Advances of knowledge about eukaryotic mRNAs (19), (83) and of the cellular protein synthesizing apparatus (61), (131) has led to the development of cell-free protein synthesis systems. Soon it became evident that the cell-free protein syntheizing systems derived from homologous or heterologous ribosomes can support faithful translation of eukaryotic mRNAs. Moreover, discovery of the presence of the polyadenylic acid sequence at the 3'-OH end of most eukaryotic mRNAs (83), made it possible to isolate mRNAs from other cellular RNAs by appropriate affinity column chromotography. Furthermore, the polypeptides directed by the mRNAs in the cell-free protein synthesis systems also became analyzable by specific immunoprecipitation. The ascites ribosome cell-free protein synthesizing system originally described by McDowell *et al.* (64) was partially modified in our laboratory (117) by supplementing an Ehrlich's ascites ribosome (S-30) reaction mixture with rabbit reticulocyte initiation factors (0.5 M KCl S-30 wash), and tRNAs to enhance its efficiency for the translation of mouse casein mRNA ($mRNA_{csn}$). Casein among the reaction products was determined by immunoprecipitation with a specific antibody to mouse casein (115). Our demonstration (117) of faithful translation of mouse $mRNA_{csn}$ in the ascites ribosome system, was preceded by a report of the translation of $mRNA_{csn}$ from lactating ewe mammary gland in a reticulocyte lysate system (43). Cell-free translation of $mRNA_{csn}$ from the mammary gland of rabbits and guinea pigs and rats has been accomplished (24), (30), (96).

B. Hormonal regulation of $mRNA_{csn}$ translational activity

Studies in the lactating animal showed (7), (118) that adrenal ablation of the post-partum nursing mouse causes a loss of larger ribosomal aggregates (polysomes) in the mammary cells. The mammary polysomes also fail to support casein synthesis in an *in vitro* protein synthesis system. Injections of cortisol to the animals after adrenalectomy can prevent these adverse effects of adrenal ablation. Thus it became evident that an enriched glucocorticoid environment is required to sustain the mammary cell polysomes, active in $mRNA_{csn}$ activity. These findings are consistent with our earlier observation that loss of casein synthesis, caused by adrenalectomy is accompanied by a loss of rough endoplasmic reticulum (RER) within the mammary cell of lactating mice (8). These observations may thus prompt one to interpret that the role of glucocorticoids in the regulation of casein gene expression is at the cytoplasmic (translational) level of control. Studies in our laboratory have also revealed that in lactating mammary glands of the mouse 6-10 ribosomal aggregates are most active in casein mRNA activity (Lin, F. K. and Banerjee, M. R., unpublished). Thus, it is conceivable that a reduction of cellular concentration of the $mRNA_{csn}$ after adrenal ablation may also cause failure of the ribosomes to constitute larger polysomes active in casein synthesis. Accordingly, influence of the glucocorticoid on cellular $mRNA_{csn}$ activity in the phenol-chloroform extracted RNA (118) was tested by translation in the ascites ribosome cell-free protein synthesis system.

Direct assay of $mRNA_{csn}$ activity determined by specific immunoprecipitation showed that adrenal ablation of the nursing mothers causes a 90% reduction of $mRNA_{csn}$ activity and that cortisol treatment starting immediately after adrenal ablation can prevent this loss. Thus, cell-free translation of the mRNA in the heterologous ribosome protein synthesis system revealed that influence of the glucocorticoid on ribosomal aggregates active in casein synthesis may be a reflection of corticosteroid modulation of cellular accumulation of the $mRNA_{csn}$ itself. This then raises the question whether glucocorticoid action is mediated at the transcriptional level of control. Our earlier studies have further shown that intensity of suckling can also significantly influence $mRNA_{csn}$ activity in the gland (118). Since suckling is known to stimulate synthesis and release of prolactin (71), action of the glucocorticoid in non-hypophysectomized nursing mothers is likely to reflect a synergistic action of the exogenous steroid and the endogenous prolactin.

Although the cell-free translational assays in heterologous ribosome systems provide the information concerning hormonal modulation of the $mRNA_{csn}$ activity, molecular hybridization analysis using a sensitive complementary DNA probe to purified $mRNA_{csn}$ should permit a more precise quantitative assessment. Accordingly a complementary DNA to purified 15S $mRNA_{csn}$ ($cDNA_{csn}$) was synthesized.

IV. PURIFICATION OF CASEIN mRNA AND SYNTHESIS OF COMPLEMENTARY DNA

A detailed account of the purification of the mRNA for mouse casein has been given in earlier reports (9), (42). Briefly, total RNA from lactating mammary glands was extracted by the phenol-chloroform method (79), (118). The RNA solution was then subjected to repeated oligo(dT) cellulose affinity column chromatography (3). Poly(A) RNA obtained by this chromatographic procedure was then sedimented in a 10-30% linear sucrose gradient by centrifugation for 16 hr at 130,000 xg. At each step of fractionation total and casein mRNA activity was assessed by cell-free translation in a wheat germ ribosome assay system (92) optimized for $mRNA_{csn}$ translation (9), (42). Total mRNA activity was measured in trichloroacetic acid precipitable reaction products and casein mRNA activity was determined by specific immunoprecipitation with the antibody to mouse casein. Purification of the $mRNA_{csn}$ was evident from its increase in specific activity at each step of fractionation and RNA sedimenting in the 15S region of the gradient contained 94% casein mRNA activity. The purified 15S casein mRNA after electrophoresis in agarose urea gel resolved as a doublet (42).

^{3}H-DNA complementary to purified 15S $mRNA_{csn}$ was synthesized according to standard procedures, using avian myeloblastosis virus RNA-dependent DNA polymerase (9), (42). After the usual purification by G-50 column chromatography and alkaline hydrolysis of the residual RNA most of the ^{3}H-cDNA sedimented around the 1000-1200 nucleotide region in an alkaline sucrose gradient. The 15S casein mRNA is estimated to have a complexity of 4.0 to 4.5 x 10^{5} and this is expected to correspond to about 1300 nucleotides. Thus the cDNA synthesized represents essentially a complete copy of the 15S casein mRNA. The cDNA hybridized to the 15S $mRNA_{csn}$ 114 fold faster than the total RNA from lactating mammary gland and the hybridization reached 90% completion with a single transition (Fig. 1). Mouse liver RNA failed to hybridize to the cDNA even at $R_{o}t$ values greater than 1000 mol.sec.liter^{-1}. The cDNA to 15S casein mRNA ($cDNA_{csn}$) has been used as a molecular hybridization probe for monitoring the $mRNA_{csn}$ sequences in mammary cell RNA.

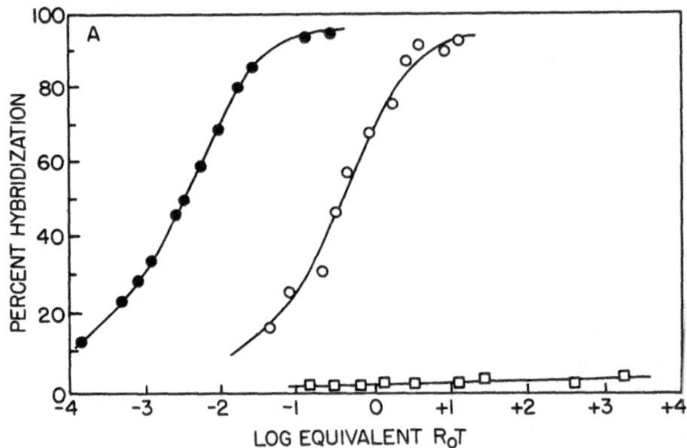

Fig. 1 RNA excess hybridization of the $cDNA_{csn}$ probe. Test RNAs were hybridized to ^{3}H-$cDNA_{csn}$ (500 cpm per reaction) probe at 68°C for varying time periods. After digestion with S1 nuclease (Miles) at 1000 units per ml for 2 hr at 37°C in 0.1 M sodium acetate, pH 4.5/0.2 M NaCl/1.2 mM $ZnCl_2$, cDNA-RNA hybrids were precipitated with trichloroacetic acid on Millipore filters and assayed in a Beckman LS-350 liquid scintillation counter. The 100% hybridization values were determined for each time point and the S1 nuclease resistant background was subtracted from each value. Products of *in vitro* assays were pooled for each determination. $cDNA_{csn}$ hybridized to its own template (●), to total mammary RNA (O), and to total liver RNA of lactating mice (□). From Ganguly *et al.* (42).

V. QUANTITATIVE MEASUREMENT OF CASEIN GENE EXPRESSION BY THE $cDNA_{csn}$

A. Adrenal glucocorticoid influence on casein mRNA accumulation in mammary gland *in vivo*

Molecular hybridization assays of the $cDNA_{csn}$ to mammary gland RNA done in RNA excess conditions failed to show (Fig. 2) a detectable level of $mRNA_{csn}$ in the mammary glands of young virgin mice. In pregnant animals $mRNA_{csn}$ constitutes .09% of total mammary gland RNA and as expected the highest concentration of $mRNA_{csn}$ is present in the lactating mammary gland.

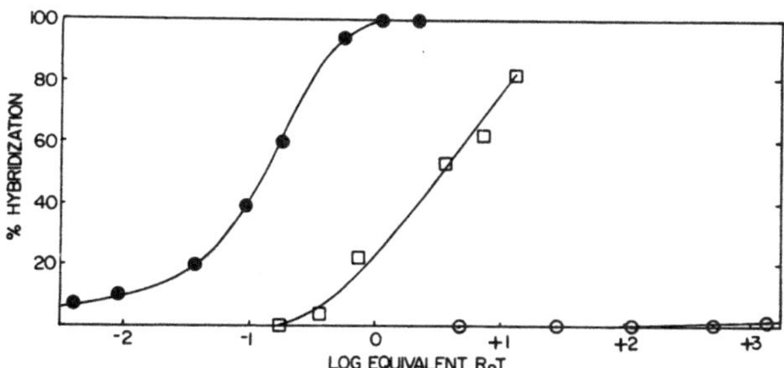

Fig. 2 Casein mRNA levels in mammary glands of BALB/c mice. Total RNA from virgin (O——O), pregnant (▣——▣) and lactating (●——●) mammary glands was hybridized to ^3H-$cDNA_{csn}$ under conditions of RNA excess.

TABLE 1. Influence of Hydrocortisone on Accumulation of the $mRNA_{csn}$ Sequences in Post-Partum Mammary Gland

Animals	% $mRNA_{csn}$	fold increase over 5 day adrenalectomized
10 day lactating	1.56	-
5 days after adrenalectomy	0.25	-
hrs after hydrocortisone injection		
1	0.25	-
3	0.25	-
6	0.74	3.0
12	1.10	4.4
24	0.50	2.0

For each determination, mammary glands from 4-6 animals were pooled, total RNA was extracted and $mRNA_{csn}$ sequences were measured by RNA excess $cDNA_{csn}$ hybridization. (from ref. 42)

Adrenalectomy of the lactating mouse caused a marked reduction of $mRNA_{csn}$ in the total mammary RNA, and this loss is substantially replenished after injections of cortisol starting 5 days after adrenalectomy. Table 1 shows that a single injection of cortisol given 5 days after adrenalectomy, stimulates a 4.4 fold increase of $mRNA_{csn}$ accumulation in the gland of post-partum mice at 12 hr (42). Thus, the quantitative measure of the modulatory influence of glucocorticoids on $mRNA_{csn}$ concentration in the gland corroborates with similar observations obtained by earlier translational assays (118). This then further confirms that the glucocorticoid plays a significant role in regulating cellular accumulation of $mRNA_{csn}$ in murine mammary gland.

B. Measurement of specific casein mRNA transcription

Accumulation of translatable mature messenger RNA in the cellular cytoplasm is believed to require complex post-transcriptional modifications of the primary transcripts (19), (26), (58), (71), (83). Moreover, removal of the intron sequences form the precursor mRNA in the nucleus has been suggested to be a limiting step for maturation of mRNA and its transfer to the cytoplasm (46), (54). It is also becoming apparent that in most eukaryotic cells the initial mRNA transcripts include sequences of both exon-intron segments of the DNA template. Production of the mature $mRNA_{csn}$ thus should require complex processing. Thus a hormonal modulation of post-transcriptional processing (viz., splicing) of the $mRNA_{csn}$ precursor, may also influence cellular concentration of mature $mRNA_{csn}$. The glucocorticoids may regulate cellular accumulation of mature $mRNA_{csn}$ by influencing post-transcriptional processing of the mRNA. On the other hand, a possible regulatory influence of the adrenal steroid hormone at the transcriptional level of control of the casein gene has also been reported (88), although the mechanisms are as yet unclear.

In order to assess the latter possibility, an *in vitro* RNA synthesis system was developed from isolated nuclei of mammary cells (40). At high ionic conditions RNA synthesis in the nuclei *in vitro* remains linear upto 180 min. About 80% of the transcriptional activity is sensitive to α-amanitin, indicating a RNA polymerase II directed DNA dependent RNA synthesis (49). Moreover, portions of the RNA synthesized in the isolated nuclei is polyadenylated *in vitro* and the transcripts include 15S RNA.

To detect the $mRNA_{csn}$ synthesized in isolated nuclei by RNA excess hybridization to the $cDNA_{csn}$, it is necessary to isolate the *in vitro* transcribed RNA from the endogenous nuclear casein mRNA molecules. RNA containing mercurated nucleotides (HgRNA) are known to bind to sulfhydryl agarose or cellulose columns and the HgRNA can be eluted by a mercaptan (40). In several studies of specific gene transcription in isolated nuclei or chromatin, RNA was synthesized *in vitro* in presence of a mercurated nucleotide in the reaction mixture (25), (75), (77), (78), (106). The mercurated RNA synthesized *in vitro*, was separated from the vast excess of endogenous RNAs by SH-agarose or SH-sepharose chromatography. Gene transcription was then measured by hybridization of the HgRNA to specific cDNA probes and the results of these studies have been discussed (22).

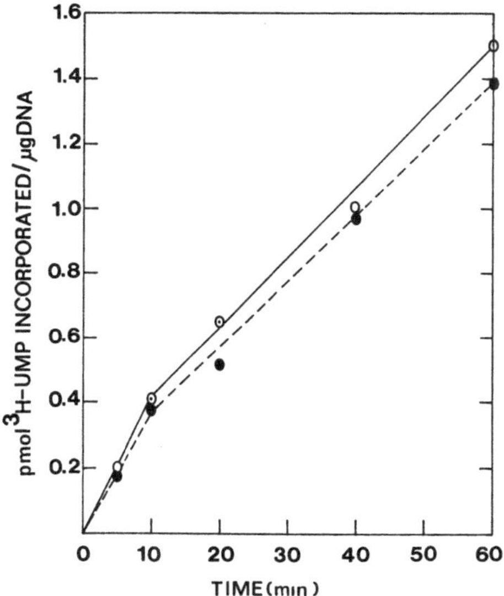

Fig. 3 Kinetics of RNA synthesis in isolated nuclei from mammary cells in presence of unmodified or HgCTP. Nuclei were transcribed for 60 mins in presence of ^{3}H-UTP and in the presence of unmodified CTP (O——O) or HgCTP (●——●). Aliquots were removed for counting at various time points. (from ref. 40)

TABLE 2. RNA Synthesis in Isolated Mammary Cell Nuclei Under Various Assay Conditions in Presence of Hg-CTP

assay conditions[a]	activity[b]	% inhibition
complete	0.31	-
omit HgCTP	0.03	90
+ 10 µg actinomycin D	0.02	94
+ 10 µg α-amanitin	0.10	68

[a] RNA was transcribed for 40 min at 25°C in presence of 20 µg DNA. After the incubation the reaction product was extracted as described by Ganguly *et al.* (40) and radioactivity was determined in toluene-triton X-100 cocktail.

[b] pmol ^{3}H-UMP incorporation/µg DNA. (from ref. 40)

Figure 3 shows that isolated nuclei from mammary cells of lactating glands are capable of synthesizing RNA with equal efficiency in presence of HgCTP or nonmercurated CTP. Synthesis of the HgRNA also remains sensitive to actinomycin D (94%) and α-amanitin (68%), indicating a predominantly DNA-dependent, RNA polymerase II directed HgRNA synthesis *in vitro* (table 2). When the HgRNA synthesized *in vitro* in presence of a high specific activity ^{3}H-labeled nucleotide is passed through SH-agarose column, 70% of the labeled RNA binds to the column and a substantial portion of the bound RNA eluted from the column sediments approximately at 15S region under denaturing conditions in a formamide-sucrose gradient (Fig. 4). In contrast when the mercurated ribonucleotide is omitted from the reaction mixture, 100% of the radioactivity associated with newly synthesized RNA, elutes in the unbound fraction of the SH-agarose column.

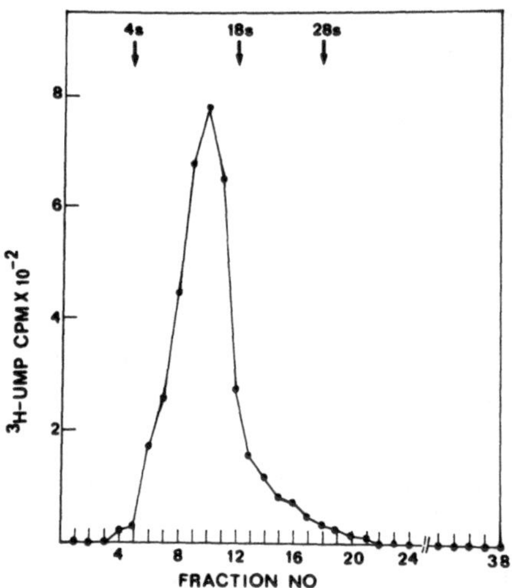

Fig. 4 Formamide-sucrose density gradient sedimentation analysis of the HgRNA synthesized in the isolated nuclei of lactating mammary cells. (from ref. 40)

C. Measurement of casein gene transcription

HgRNA transcripts synthesized in nuclei isolated from lactating mouse mammary gland, were purified from endogenous nuclear RNA by SH-agarose chromatography as described above. HgRNA transcripts were then hybridized to the $cDNA_{csn}$. The HgRNA synthesized in the isolated nuclei from lactating mammary gland hybridized to the $cDNA_{csn}$ at a relatively low $R_{o}t$ value, whereas HgRNA synthesized by liver nuclei under similar *in vitro* conditions failed to hybridize to the $cDNA_{csn}$ probe (Fig. 5). This demonstrates that mammary cell specific casein gene transcription can be measured in HgRNA synthesized in isolated nuclei (42). Quantitative estimates based on the $R_ot_{1/2}$ values showed that 0.09% of HgRNA were $mRNA_{csn}$ specific and estimated levels of $mRNA_{csn}$ in total nuclear RNA of lactating cells was 0.07% (42). The possibility of any endogenous $mRNA_{csn}$ nonspecifically binding to the column and eluting in the bound fraction was further assessed in the following control experiment. Isolated nuclei from lactating mammary cells were incubated in the transcription assay mixture without any ribonucleotides for the usual time period. RNA isolated from the nuclei was then fractionated by SH-agarose chromatography. The "mock" RNA eluting in the bound fraction was incubated with $cDNA_{csn}$ in an hybridization assay condition identical to those used for HgRNA. No significant hybridization was observed (Fig. 5), indicating that the endogenous nonmercurated $mRNA_{csn}$ sequences do not bind to the column nonspecifically and contaminate the HgRNA by eluting in the bound fraction. It was also observed that addition of α-amanitin to the HgRNA synthesizing reaction mixture causes a 85% reduction in hybridizable $mRNA_{csn}$ sequences in the SH-agarose bound fraction (42). This again shows that the hybridizable $mRNA_{csn}$ sequences in the HgRNA are products of *in vitro* DNA dependent RNA polymerase II directed RNA synthesis.

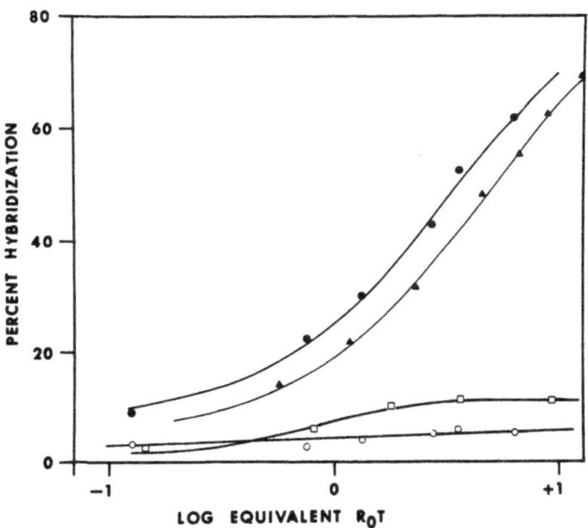

Fig. 5 Hybridization of ^3H-$cDNA_{csn}$ to nuclear RNAs. Hybridization to HgRNA synthesized in isolated lactating mammary cell nuclei (●——●); to HgRNA transcribed in isolated liver cell nuclei of lactating mice (□——□); to total nuclear RNA from lactating mammary cells *in vivo* (▲——▲); and control assay to check for nonspecific binding of non-HgRNA to the SH-agarose column (O——O). (for details see ref. 42)

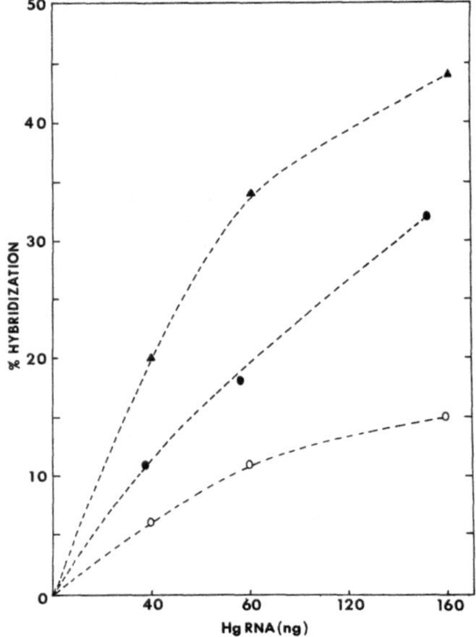

Fig. 6 Effect of adrenalectomy and cortisol treatment on $mRNA_{csn}$ transcription *in vitro*. Hybridization of ^{3}H-$cDNA_{csn}$ to RNA from: 10 day unoperated lactating mice (▲), 5 days after adrenalectomy (O), 5 days after adrenalectomy and 6 hr after single injection of hydrocortisone (●). (from ref. 42)

VI. HORMONAL MODULATION OF CASEIN GENE TRANSCRIPTION

The availability of the hybridizable HgRNA synthesized in the isolated nuclei made it feasible to test the possible influence of the lactogenic hormones on casein gene transcription (42). In one set of these studies lactating mice were adrenalectomized and 5 days later the animals were given a single injection of cortisol. Nuclei isolated from the mammary gland were allowed to synthesize HgRNA *in vitro* as described in the preceding sections. The HgRNA synthesized *in vitro* was then isolated by SH-agarose chromatography. Hybridization of the $cDNA_{csn}$ probe to the purified HgRNA showed that adrenalectomy causes a 75% reduction in $mRNA_{csn}$ sequences in the transcripts as compared to the nuclear transcripts of unoperated control animals (Fig. 6). Six hours after the single injection of cortisol, the $mRNA_{csn}$ sequences in the transcripts increased 2 fold over the nuclei of adrenalectomized mice. These results thus demonstrate that glucocorticoids exert a regulatory influence on the transcription of the casein gene. Hence, influence of the glucocorticoid on increased cellular accumulation of $mRNA_{csn}$ may be mediated through a stimulatory action of the steroid hormone on transcription of the casein gene.

In a second set of studies action of prolactin on transcription of the casein gene was also examined using the specific prolactin inhibitor 2-bormo-α-ergocryptin (CB-154). Serum prolactin levels of the lactating mouse were reduced 80% by injecting the animals with 2-bromo-α-ergocryptin (42). Isolated mammary nuclei from the CB-154 treated and untreated mice were allowed to synthesize HgRNA. After SH-agarose chromatography the purified HgRNA was hybridized to the $cDNA_{csn}$ probe. The CB-154 treatment failed to show a significant alteration of $mRNA_{csn}$ transcription, even though the serum prolactin level in the CB-154 treated mice was reduced 80% (table 3). These results, however, do not permit the conclusion that prolactin exerts little influence on casein gene transcription *in vivo*, because the residual 20% prolactin in CB-154 treated animals may be sufficient to support casein gene transcription in the presence of endogenous glucocorticoids. Circulating levels of prolactin in nursing animals is known to be much higher than what is needed to induce lactogenesis (126), (127). Studies in our laboratory have also shown that intensity of suckling, a stimulus known to stimulate pituitary prolactin synthesis and release (71), also stimulates $mRNA_{csn}$ accumulation in the mammary gland (118).

TABLE 3. Effect of CB-154 Treatment on Serum Prolactin and $mRNA_{csn}$ Level in 10-Day Lactating Mice

animals	serum prolactin ng/ml	% $mRNA_{csn}$
10-day lactating	583.5 ± 81.7	1.56
10-day lactating + CB-154	108.0 ± 23.0	1.16

Total mammary RNA from 4-6 animals in each group was extracted by phenol-chloroform (79) and the level of $mRNA_{csn}$ was assessed by RNA excess-$cDNA_{csn}$ hybridization as described in table 1. Sera from three animals in each determination were assayed by duplicate radioimmunoassay. (from ref. 42)

Therefore, it is likely that responses of the mammary cells to exogenous cortisol treatment is synergistic with endogenous prolactin. The endogenous endocrine environment in the animal is further complicated by the fact that suckling may also stimulate pituitary ACTH release, which in turn elivates serum glucocorticoid levels. Increased glucocorticoid then may also reduce prolactin levels in the animal (127). Thus, the systemic complexities of the endocrine system make it virtually impossible to obtain a reliable assessment of the mechanisms of action of the steroid and the polypeptide hormones regulating a mammary cell specific gene expression

VII. CASEIN GENE EXPRESSION IN MAMMARY TISSUE *IN VITRO*

A. Organ culture of pieces of mammary tissue from pregnant animals

The difficulty of the *in vivo* system was appreciated by earlier investigators studying the complex multihormonal regulation of mammary gland physiology. Accordingly a culture model derived from pieces of mammary tissue from pregnant mice or rats was developed (34), (91). Pieces of mammary tissue from pregnant mice were found to respond to the lactogenic action of cortisol and prolactin eliciting the milk proteins, casein and α-lactalbumin (121), (123), (129) during 48 to 72 hr incubation. This short-term organ culture model derived from pieces of mammary tissue from pregnant animals has been used to study expression of the casein gene (45), (63). Recently, however, important shortcomings associated with the studies using explants of pregnant mammary tissue have been discussed (9), (123). Mammary glands of pregnant mice and rats contain substantial amounts of casein and its mRNA (96), (115). The active state of the casein gene thus restricts reliable assessment of its hormone responses in explants of pregnancy mammary tissue in short-term cultures. To circumvent this experimental limitation the explants are initially incubated for 48 hr in a prolactin-free medium containing insulin and cortisol and this reduces the endogenous $mRNA_{csn}$ to a near basal level (45), (63). Subsequently, the effect of prolactin on casein mRNA accumulation is measured after 24 hr and 48 hr exposure in a cortisol-free medium. The preincubation of the explant with cortisol introduces the second drawback to this culture model. Pregnancy mammary cells rich in glucocorticoid rcceptor (103), (133) are already exposed to the increased level of circulating glucocorticoid (38), (126) in the pregnant animal. Moreover, the mammary explants can take up glucocorticoid and retain the steroid hormone for several days (17), (109) after the hormone has been removed from the medium. Thus, responses of the explants to hormone(s) added to the medium during the second stage of incubation is likely to reflect an influence of the residual glucocorticoid in the explant.

B. The whole mammary organ in culture

From the preceding discussion it is clear that a more reliable *in vitro* model is needed for the elucidation of the mechanisms of multiple hormone regulation of expression of the casein gene. Studies in our laboratory have shown that a whole mammary organ obtained from an immature female mouse can sequentially mimic the stages of mammogenesis, lactogenesis and alveolar regression in a chemically defined medium, containing an appropriately controlled hormone environment (7), (134).

Since the initial report by Ichinose and Nandi (47) the unique culture model of the whole mammary organ has been extensively described (13), (60), (104), (134). Briefly, as a prerequisite of the culture procedure (47), (104),

3-4 week old BALB/c female mice (used in our studies) are primed by daily injections of a mixture of estradiol-17β and progesterone for 9 days. The whole second thoracic mammary gland from these animals is excised on a dacron raft under sterile conditions. The gland resting on the raft is then transferred into a plastic petri dish containing Waymouth's synthetic medium, supplemented with appropriate combinations of hormones. The glands are then incubated at 37°C in an atmosphere of 95% oxygen and 5% carbon dioxide in a humidified chamber (89). As illustrated in figure 7, incubation of the gland first in a mammogenic hormone containing medium induces full lobuloalveolar morphogenesis within 5-6 days. The parenchyma containing the secretory structures during subsequent culture in medium containing insulin, prolactin and cortisol elicits abundant milk-like secretory material, including casein (115). Later cultivation in a prolactin-free regression medium causes the alveolar structures to undergo complete regression leaving only the ductal parenchyma. The combinations of polypeptide and steroid hormones needed to obtain alveolar mammogenesis, lactogenesis and alveolar regression *in vitro* have been described in detail (7), (13).

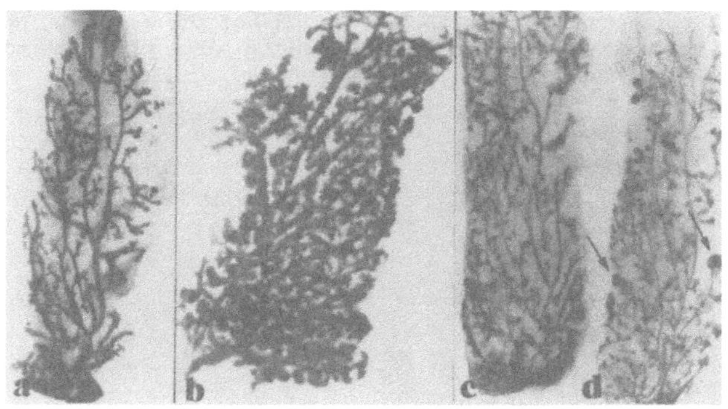

Fig. 7 The mammary gland at different stages of development in culture of the whole organ. a. The ductal gland at 0 time of culture, b. The lobuloalveolar gland after 5 days of culture with the mammogenic hormones, c. The glands after alveolar regression in a prolactin defficient medium containing insulin and aldosterone, d. A regressed gland showing nodule-like alveolar lesions after treatment with 7,12-dimethylbenz[a]anthracene. (for details see ref. 13 and 60)

VIII. CASEIN GENE EXPRESSION IN A TWO-STEP CULTURE MODEL OF THE WHOLE MAMMARY ORGAN

A. Measured by translational assay

For measurement of casein gene expression the whole mammary gland organ culture was modified to a sequential two-step model (115). In step I the immature parenchyma develops pregnancy-like, lobuloalveolar structures after 6 days incubation in a corticosteroid-free medium containing insulin, prolactin, growth hormone, estrogen and progesterone. During step II the lobuloalveolar glands are incubated in a medium containing the lactogenic hormone mixture, insulin, prolactin and cortisol. Histolobically (Fig. 8), no secretory material is detectable in the lobuloalveolar glands after 6 days of incubation in the corticosteroid-free, step I mammogenic medium (Fig. 8a). In step II, abundant milk-like material is present (Fig. 8b) in the alveolar lumen after 6 days of incubation (with insulin, prolactin and cortisol). Thus, the two-step mammogenesis-lactogenesis culture model segregates the developmental stages of lobuloalveolar morphogenesis of the gland into the two distinct non-overlapping compartments. Absence of cortisol in the medium seems to accomplish this separation. In the animal, however, mammogenesis overlaps with lactogenesis during the latter half of the gestation period and this also corresponds with the increase in the serum glucocorticoid level of the animal (126), (127).

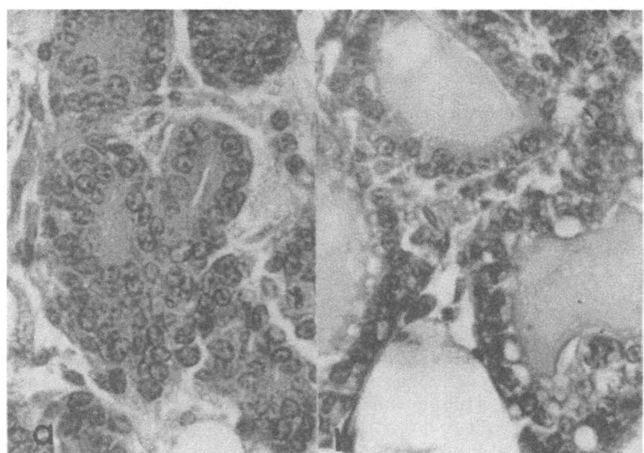

Fig. 8 Histology of the mammary gland after organ culture. a. Six days in the step I medium with insulin, prolactin, growth hormone, estradiol-17β and progesterone. b. After additional 6 days in the step II medium with insulin, prolactin and cortisol. X 400 (for details see ref. 116)

The two-step culture model of the whole mammary organ thus presents suitable conditions for the following studies on the prolactin and cortisol action in stimulating the onset of expression of the casein gene. The glands were incubated in step I culture with insulin, prolactin, growth hormone, estrogen and progesterone for 6 days. The lobuloalveolar glands obtained after step I culture, were then incubated with insulin, prolactin and cortisol for a further 6 days in step II culture. RNA extracted from these glands was then analyzed in the ascites cell-free translational system (117). Results showed virtually no $mRNA_{csn}$ activity in the RNA of glands after step I culture, even though the glands contained the lobuloalveolar secretory units. RNA from the glands after 6 days of step II culture with insulin, prolactin and cortisol showed abundant immunologically determined $mRNA_{csn}$ activity (Fig. 9). Consistent with the results of the translational assays, radioimmunoassay of tissue extracts with antibody to mouse casein also failed to show any measurable casein in the gland after step I culture, whereas abundant casein was present in the gland at the end of step II culture (116).

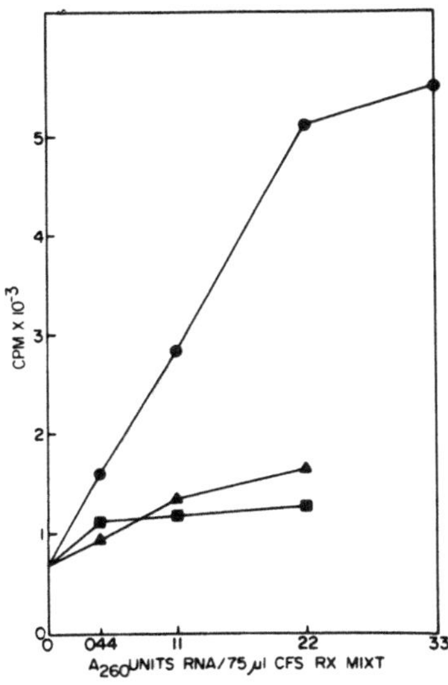

Fig. 9 Determination of casein mRNA activity in total RNA of mammary glands by translation in a cell-free system. After 12 days of priming with estrogen and progesterone (■). After six days in step I medium with insulin, prolactin, growth hormone and estradiol-17β (▲). After six days in the step II medium with insulin, prolactin and cortisol (●). (for details see ref. 116)

B. Measured by molecular hybridization with $cDNA_{csn}$ probe

The cell-free translation assays described above showed that prolactin in the corticosteroid-free mammogenic medium fails to stimulate expression of the casein gene in the whole mammary organ *in vitro*, but prolactin in combination with insulin and cortisol stimulates appearance of $mRNA_{csn}$ activity. These results obtained by the translation assays, however,

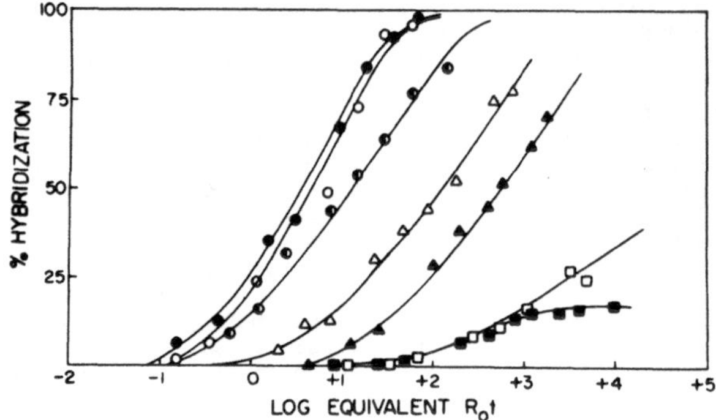

Fig. 10 Hybridization of $cDNA_{csn}$ to total RNA from glands at different stages of organ culture. RNA from glands of nonprimed virgin mice (■), RNA from glands of primed mice (□), RNA from glands after 6 days of culture in step I mammogenic medium (▲), RNA from glands after 1 day (Δ), 3 day (◐), 6 day (O) and 9 day (●) in step II culture medium with insulin, prolactin and cortisol. (for details see ref. 69)

fail to provide an accurate quantitative measure of this stimulatory action. Therefore, in the next set of studies (69) the more sensitive molecular hybridization assays were done using the $cDNA_{csn}$ probe. Figure 10 shows that the $cDNA_{csn}$ fails to detect a measurable level of $mRNA_{csn}$ in RNA from mammary glands of the estrogen-progesterone primed animals. RNA from the lobuloalveolar glands obtained after 6 days of incubation in the step I corticosteroid-free mammogenic medium, hybridized to the $cDNA_{csn}$ to above the 50% level but at relatively high R_ot values. The concentration of $mRNA_{csn}$ sequences in total RNA of these glands was only 0.0067% (table 4). Quantitative estimates of the $mRNA_{csn}$ sequences in these glands further revealed a concentration of only 147 molecules of $mRNA_{csn}$ per epithelial cell. This low level of $mRNA_{csn}$ remains virtually unaltered after subsequent 3 days of incubation in prolactin or ovarian steroid deficient step I medium (9), (69). Thus, 147 molecules/cell appears to represent a basal level of $mRNA_{csn}$ concentration in the lobuloalveolar glands in the corticosteroid-free mammogenic medium, and this level of the mRNA is not influenced by the absence of prolactin or the ovarian steroids in the medium. The basal level of 147 molecules of $mRNA_{csn}$/cell in the lobuloalveolar mammary gland in the present culture model is similar to a basal level of 40 and 500 molecules of ovalbumin and conalbumin mRNAs per tubular gland epithelial cell of chick-oviduct (66). The maintenance of basal level of $mRNA_{csn}$ in the lobuloalveolar mammary gland in the corticosteroid-free medium, however, is in contrast with the presence of a relatively high concentration (0.09%) of $mRNA_{csn}$ in the lobuloalveolar glands of mid-pregnant animals. In this context it is relevant to note that the accumulation of $mRNA_{csn}$ corresponds to a

TABLE 4. Number of Casein mRNA Molecules per Cell at Different Stages of Morphogenesis and Differentiation of the Mammary Gland in Culture

culture medium	$R_0t_{1/2}$	% casein mRNA	no. of casein mRNA molecules per cell	fold increase in molecules per cell over IPrlEPGH[a]
6 day IPrlEPGH	524.8	0.00067	147	-
6 day IPrlEPGH + 1 day IPrlF	104.7	0.0033	1,366	9.3
6 day IPrlEPGH + 3 day IPrlF	12.0	0.029	4,826	32.8
6 day IPrlEPGH + 6 day IPrlF	5.1	0.068	23.699	161.2
6 day IPrlEPGH + 9 day IPrlF	3.9	0.09	37,524	255.2

[a] Abbreviations for hormones are as in Fig. 12. (from ref. 69)

rise in the level of circulating glucocorticoids and prolactin during the latter part of pregnancy. The accumulation of $mRNA_{csn}$ sequences in the gland is associated with the presence of a high level of casein. Our studies have also shown that when the mammogenic hormone mixture is supplemented with aldosterone, a mineralocorticoid having some glucocorticoid activity, the gland *in vitro* elicits both $mRNA_{csn}$ and casein (13, 115). Thus, glucocorticoid deficiency of the step I mammogenic medium appears to prevent $mRNA_{csn}$ accumulation in the gland and the presence of prolactin in the medium is not sufficient to stimulate expression of the casein gene.

During step II culture, the lobuloalveolar gland shows a 9 fold-increase of $mRNA_{csn}$ over basal levels within 24 hr in medium with prolactin, cortisol and insulin (table 4). The marked stimulatory action as early as 24 hr also indicates that the antagonistic action of residual progesterone (carried over from step I medium), if any, is of a nonsignificant level. Progesterone has been reported to be antagonistic to lactogenesis and $mRNA_{csn}$ accumulation in the gland *in vivo* (2), (94). During 9 days of incubation of the glands in step II medium containing prolactin and cortisol, accumulation of $mRNA_{csn}$ progressively rises from 0.00067% to 0.09%, of the total RNA of the gland (table 4). The cellular concentration of $mRNA_{csn}$ during the same period rises from 147 molecules to 37,524 molecules per cell, a 255-fold increase (Fig. 11). Since the number of epithelial cells during the same incubation period remains essentially unaltered (Fig. 11), it is conceivable that the enormous increase in the cellular accumulation of $mRNA_{csn}$ from a basal level is the result of *de novo* transcription of the casein gene in the gland. Cortisol in the medium with prolactin thus appears to bring about the onset of mammary

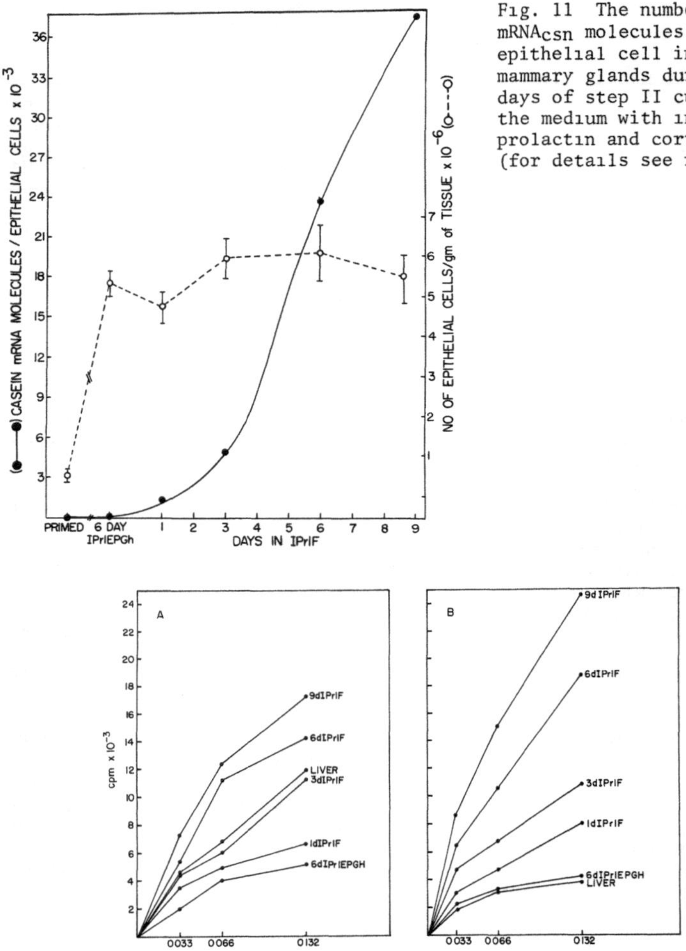

Fig. 11 The number of $mRNA_{csn}$ molecules per epithelial cell in the mammary glands during 0-9 days of step II culture in the medium with insulin, prolactin and cortisol. (for details see ref. 69)

Fig. 12 Total and casein mRNA activity in the glands during the two-step culture. mRNA activity was measured by cell-free translation of total RNA in a wheat germ ribosome system as described (42). a. Acid insoluble reaction product. b. Immunoprecipitable reaction product. I, insulin; Prl, prolactin; GH, growth hormone; E, estradiol-17β; P, progesterone; F, cortisol.

cell specific transcription of the genes for the major milk proteins. Figure 12 shows that specific translational activity of $mRNA_{csn}$ also rises progressively during the same culture period, as assessed in the wheat germ ribosome cell-free protein synthesis system. Thus, it is reasonable to conclude that in the murine mammary gland the requirement of adrenal glucocorticoids is obligatory for the induction of the casein gene in the presence of prolactin. The evidence presented in section IV has shown that within 12 hr after a single injection, hydrocortisone can stimulate a 4-fold replenishment of the loss of $mRNA_{csn}$ in the mammary gland caused by adrenalectomy. This increased accumulation of the $mRNA_{csn}$ is concomitant with glucocorticoid stimulation of specific transcription of the "casein gene".

IX. SIMULTANEOUS OCCURRENCE OF MORPHOGENESIS AND CASEIN GENE EXPRESSION

Results described in section VIII have clearly shown that the lobulo-alveolar mammary gland is capable of accumulating abundant $mRNA_{csn}$ only when exposed to the step II lactogenic medium containing insulin, prolactin and cortisol. However, under physiological conditions lobuloalveolar morphogenesis of the mammary gland in pregnant rats and mice is accompanied by accumulation of $mRNA_{csn}$, indicating that expression of the casein gene ensues prior to parturition (94), (96). Thus, alveolar morphogenesis and functional differentiation of the mammary gland *in vivo* can occur simultaneously, although the maximal production of casein and its mRNA is evident in the gland in post-partum animals.

To assess whether similar simultaneous occurrence of morphogenesis and functional differentiation can be mimicked in the whole mammary organ in culture, the hormone mixture in the medium during these studies was modified to provide a lactogenic hormone environment comparable to that in the pregnant animal (39). Estrogen-progesterone primed mammary glands were incubated in a medium containing insulin, aldosterone, cortisol and growth hormone. In this medium the immature ductal glands develop pregnancy-like lobuloalveolar structures during 6 days of incubation. As the glands progress through morphogenesis *in vitro*, $mRNA_{csn}$ sequences measured (by the $cDNA_{csn}$ probe) in total RNA from these glands appear at an increasing level during the 6 days in culture (Fig. 13a). Moreover, the number of $mRNA_{csn}$ molecules per cell increases 17-fold, whereas the rise in cell number during the same period is only 2-fold (Fig. 13b) indicating a net increase in $mRNA_{csn}$ levels in the glands. Omission of aldosterone from the medium does not alter $mRNA_{csn}$ levels in the gland, showing that the hormone combination of insulin, cortisol and growth hormone is sufficient to maintain the simultaneous occurrence of morphogenesis and functional differentiation of the gland *in vitro* (table 5). Presence of aldosterone in the medium favors increased lobuloalveolar development in the gland (60).

Growth hormone is believed to be nonlactogenic (127). Thus, the accumulation of $mRNA_{csn}$ in the mammary gland in medium with growth hormone and the adrenal steroids may tempt one to interpret that the adrenal steroids in the presence of insulin are stimulatory to casein gene expression. However, the preparation of NIH bovine growth hormone used in these

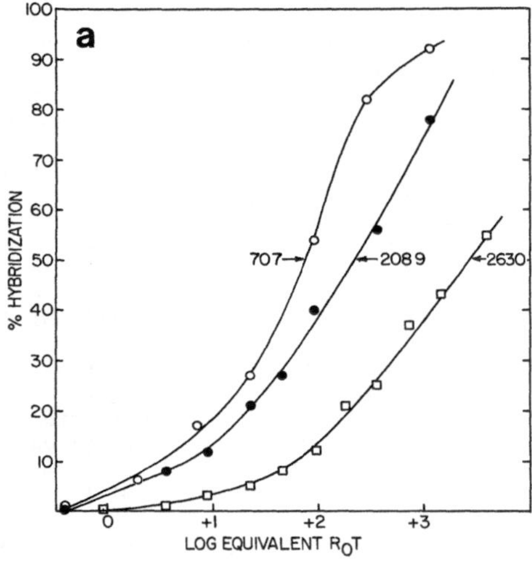

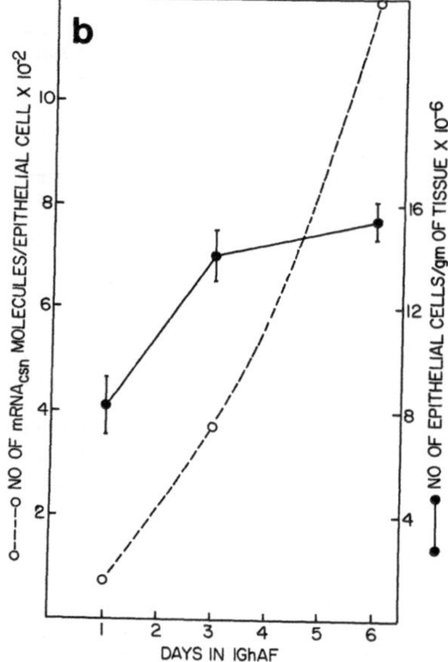

Fig. 13 Casein mRNA accumulation in the glands during 6 days of culture in medium with insulin, prolactin, aldosterone and cortisol. a. Concentration of casein RNA in total RNA of the gland after one day (□——□), 3 days (●——●) and 6 days (O——O) of culture as measured by hybridization to the ^{3}H-cDNA$_{csn}$ probe. b. Molecules of mRNA$_{csn}$ per epithelial cell. (for details see ref. 39)

TABLE 5. $mRNA_{csn}$ Level in the Glands Incubated in Different Hormonal Combinations *In Vitro*

culture condition[a]	$R_ot_{1/2}$[b]	% $mRNA_{csn}$
6 day IGHAF	70.7 ± 3.0[c]	0.005 ± 0.0002[c]
6 day IAF + 80 ng/ml Prl	39.8 ± 2.0	0.0083 ± 0.0004
6 day IGHF	15.9 ± 2.0	0.021 ± 0.003

[a] I, insulin; GH, growth hormone; A, aldosterone; F, cortisol; Prl, prolactin

[b] $R_ot_{1/2}$ of purified $mRNA_{csn}$ = 0.0033 $mol.s.L^{-1}$

[c] mean ± range of duplicate determination (from ref. 39)

experiments contained 1.6% contaminating prolactin and that amounts to 80 ng of prolactin per 5 μg of growth hormone used in the medium. Radioimmunoassay with antibody to bovine prolactin (kindly done by Dr. H. Allen Tucker, Michigan State University, East Lansing) also showed a similar level of contaminating prolactin in the NIH growth hormone preparation. Thus, the expression of the casein gene during morphogenesis in the presence of NIH growth hormone could be due to a synergistic action between the adrenal steroids and the contaminating prolactin present in the growth hormone preparation. To test this possibility the glands were incubated for 6 days in medium containing insulin, aldosterone, cortisol and 80 ng prolactin (39) and a similar level of $mRNA_{csn}$ accumulation was observed in these glands (table 5). Thus, it is probable that expression of the casein gene observed in the glands during alveolar morphogenesis in medium containing NIH growth hormone is due to a synergistic action of the contaminating prolactin and the adrenal steroids. Nonetheless, the results described in this section demonstrate that the simultaneous occurrence of alveolar morphogenesis and casein gene expression as known to occur during pregnancy, can be mimicked in the gland *in vitro*. Again the presence of the glucocorticoid with prolactin appears to be crucial in evoking this response.

X. GLUCOCORTICOID IS OBLIGATORY TO CASEIN GENE EXPRESSION

As indicated in section VII the short-term organ culture model, derived from pieces of mammary tissue from pregnant rats has been utilized to measure hormonal regulation of casein gene expression (45), (63) by a specific $cDNA_{csn}$ probe (to 15S rat casein mRNA). The explants in these studies were routinely preincubated for 48 hr with insulin and hydrocortisone to deplete the high level of $mRNA_{csn}$ in the pregnancy mammary tissue (see section VII). Subsequently 48 hr incubation of the explants in a glucocorticoid-free medium with insulin and prolactin stimulated a pronounced increase of $mRNA_{csn}$ accumulation in the explants, although maximal accumulation required the presence of hydrocortisone in medium in addition to insulin and prolactin. Thus the observations are that (a) 48 hr preincubation with hydrocortisone in a prolactin-free medium causes a reduction of $mRNA_{csn}$ in the explants to a near basal level and (b) subsequent 48 hr incubation with prolactin in medium containing no hydrocortisone stimulates a dramatic rise of the $mRNA_{csn}$. Hence, it has been concluded that prolactin is the hormone required for the induction of the casein gene, and that the presence of hydrocortisone is not necessary for this stimulatory action of the polypeptide hormone.

In the follow-up study (45) the actions of prolactin and hydrocortisone on transcription of the casein gene in explants from rat mammary tissue during pregnancy, was also analyzed in similar short-term organ cultures. Transcription was monitored by the specific cDNA cellulose chromatography procedure (59), (130). Quantitative measurements were obtained by hybridization of ^{3}H-uridine pulse labeled (30 min) RNA to the sepcific casein cDNA-cellulose column. In these experiments pieces of mammary tissue obtained from pregnant rats were preincubated for 48 hr with insulin and hydrocortisone to deplete the endogenous $mRNA_{csn}$ level in the explant. Subsequently, 24 hr incubation in medium with insulin and prolactin was found to stimulate a 4-fold increase of casein gene transcription in the explants. In order to assess whether hydrocortisone may influence the stimulatory action of prolactin, explants were incubated in medium containing the following different combinations of the hormones: (a) insulin alone, (b) insulin and prolactin, (c) insulin and hydrocortisone and (d) insulin, prolactin and hydrocortisone. The results showed that insulin alone is nonstimulatory, and the concentration (0.33%) of $mRNA_{csn}$ transcripts in medium with insulin and prolactin remains essentially similar in the glands regardless of the presence or absence of hydrocortisone in the medium. Thus, the conclusions were made that prolactin induces casein gene transcription, and hydrocortisone does not influence this action of the polypeptide hormone. A 3-fold stimulation of transcription in the presence of insulin and hydrocortisone, over insulin alone was explained as due to a better maintenance of the explants in the presence of the glucocorticoid. Measurement of the turnover of the pulse labeled RNA under a similar experimental protocol, showed that the half-life of $mRNA_{csn}$ in the explants is 5 hr in insulin-hydrocortisone medium and 92 hr in medium with insulin and prolactin. Thus it has been concluded that in addition to its action at the level of transcription, prolactin also regulates degradation of $mRNA_{csn}$ in the explants and that this action of the pituitary hormone presumably favors its increased cellular accumulation.

The conclusions based on the studies described above appear to have overlooked the following limitations of the organ culture model used. Mammary tissue of pregnant rats and mice are rich in glucocorticoid receptor (103), (133). The tissue is exposed to the elevated levels of circulating glucocorticoids in the pregnant animal (127). Mammary glands also have the ability to pick up and retain steroid hormones, including glucocorticoids. Therefore, the explants of pregnancy mammary tissue preincubated in insulin-hydrocortisone medium for 48 hr is likely to retain a substantial amount of residual hydrocortisone. Consequently, the stimulation of the expression (transcription and accumulation of

$mRNA_{csn}$) of the casein gene measured after only 24 hr and 48 hr incubation in medium with insulin and prolactin is likely to reflect a combined effect of prolactin and residual glucocorticoid, rather than the action of the peptide hormone alone. A recent study using a similar experimental protocol has indicated that explants from pregnant rats after 48 hr preincubation with insulin and cortisol can retain the residual steroid hormone for up to 4 days (17). Synthesis of casein (measured by ^{32}P-orthophosphate uptake into Ca^{++} rennin precipitate) in the explants during subsequent incubation with insulin and prolactin has been shown to be influenced by the residual glucocorticoid retained in the explants. Since ^{32}P-orthophosphate uptake into Ca^{++} rennin precipitate was used as a measure of casein synthesis, the significance of these findings has been considered difficult to assess (93). Nevertheless, the preliminary report by Bollander and Topper (17) does point to an important shortcoming of the culture model which requires preincubation of the pregnancy mammary tissue with hydrocortisone to deplete the high level of endogenous $mRNA_{csn}$.

It has been described in section VIII that the whole mammary organ in the two-step culture model can develop pregnancy-like lobuloalveolar structures in corticosteroid-free step I culture medium. Therefore, no residual glucocorticoid is expected to be present when the lobuloalveolar glands are transferred to the step II lactogenic culture medium. Moreover, presence of only a basal level of $mRNA_{csn}$ in the lobuloalveolar gland at the end of step I culture, also eliminates the preincubation step with insulin and cortisol needed with explant cultures of pregnancy tissue to deplete the endogenous $mRNA_{csn}$. Thus, the two-step culture model of the whole mammary organ provides the conditions suitable for the assessment of the role of prolactin and cortisol on the expression of the casein gene under an appropriately controlled *in vitro* hormone environment. Accordingly the following studies were done (42).

As usual the immature whole mammary glands obtained from estrogen-progesterone primed young virgin mice (BALB/c) were incubated, initially for 6 days in step I mammogenic medium containing insulin, prolactin, estradiol, progesterone and growth hormone. The lobuloalveolar glands obtained after step I culture in the corticosteroid-free medium, contains only a basal level of $mRNA_{csn}$ as measured by the $cDNA_{csn}$ probe (69). When these lobuloalveolar glands were transferred to step II medium containing insulin and prolactin or insulin and cortisol, no increase in $mRNA_{csn}$ over basal levels was observed. However, the glands remained competent to respond to the full lactogenic hormone mixture because subsequent 3 day incubation in the presence of insulin, cortisol and prolactin stimulated a significant increase in the level of $mRNA_{csn}$ in the same glands (table 6). This shows that neither prolactin nor cortisol alone can induce expression of the casein gene even though functionally responsive structures are present in the gland.

Table 7 shows that when incubation of the lobuloalveolar glands for 3 days with insulin and prolactin was followed by a further 3 days in medium with insulin and cortisol, $mRNA_{csn}$ levels in the glands also remained at a similar basal level (table 6). On the other hand, when

TABLE 6. Level of $mRNA_{csn}$ in the Lobuloalveolar Glands Incubated with Different Hormonal Combinations

culture condition[a]	$R_ot_{1/2}$[b]	% $mRNA_{csn}$
6 day IPrlEPGH	417	0.0009
3 day IF	832	0.0005
3 day IF → 3 day IPrlF	5.02	0.076
3 day IPrl	N.M.[c]	N.M.
3 day IPrl → 3 day IPrlF	10	0.038

[a] I, insulin (5 μg/ml); Prl, prolactin (5 μg/ml); E, estradiol-17β (0.001 μg/ml); P, progesterone (1 μg/ml); GH, growth hormone (5 μg/ml); F, cortisol (5 μg/ml). Bovine growth hormone was a gift from the National Pituitary Agency of the National Institute of Arthritis, Metabolism and Digestive Diseases. All the glands were incubated for first six days in IPrlEPGH medium. The concentration of each hormone used during subsequent incubation was the same as described above.

[b] $R_ot_{1/2}$ of purified $mRNA_{csn}$ is 0.0038 $mol.s.L^{-1}$.

[c] not measurable (from ref. 41)

TABLE 7. Effect of Preincubation of the Lobuloalveolar Galnds with Cortisol or Prolactin on the Accumulation of $mRNA_{csn}$ Sequences After Subsequent Incubation in Prolactin or Cortisol Containing Medium

culture condition[a]	$R_ot_{1/2}$[b]	% $mRNA_{csn}$
3 day IPrl	N.M.[c]	N.M.
3 day IPrl → 3 day IF	316.0	0.0012
3 day IF	832.0	0.0005
3 day IF → 3 day IPrl	23.4	0.016

[a] All the glands were first incubated for 6 days in the mammogenic medium for lobuloalveolar development. Subsequently these glands were incubated with different hormone combinations as indicated. The concentration of each hormone was the same as described in table 6.

[b] $R_ot_{1/2}$ of pure $mRNA_{csn}$ is 0.0038 $mol.s.L^{-1}$.

[c] not measurable

incubation of the lobuloalveolar glands in step II culture with insulin and cortisol was followed by incubation with insulin and prolactin, a 18-fold increase in $mRNA_{csn}$ levels was observed (table 6). This increase cannot be attributed to a stimulatory action of prolactin alone, because the glands fail to accumulate $mRNA_{csn}$ above basal levels when incubated in a step II medium containing insulin and prolactin (table 6). Therefore, one may ask whether the stimulatory action of the polypeptide hormone is synergistic with residual cortisol retained in the lobulo-alveolar gland during prior 3 day incubation with the steroid hormone.

The hypothesis was tested (41) using an experimental protocol similar to that used for the short-term culture of explants of mammary tissue from pregnant rats (38, 45, 63). At the end of the 6 day step I culture of the whole mammary gland, the pregnancy-like lobuloalveolar glands were incubated for 48 hr in medium with insulin and cortisol. One batch of the glands during this culture period were incubated in the presence of ^{3}H-cortisol during the last 24 hr. The glands were then transferred to a medium with insulin and prolactin. The glands exposed to ^{3}H-cortisol were collected at different times and the level of residual cortisol in the gland during incubation with insulin and prolactin was measured. The glands cultured with unlabeled cortisol were used for assessment of $mRNA_{csn}$ levels. Measurement of ^{3}H-cortisol radioactivity showed that a measurable level of the steroid hormone is retained in the lobuloalveolar gland in the medium containing insulin and prolactin, although the rate of depletion of the residual cortisol was somewhat rapid (Fig. 14). The concentration of $mRNA_{csn}$ in the glands in parallel cultures increased from 0.006% to 0.016% during the initial 2 days in the insulin-prolactin medium. Corresponding to the loss of residual cortisol, $mRNA_{csn}$ concentrantion in the glands also declined during the 6 day culture period. However, when the glucocorticoid was added to the medium with insulin and prolactin, $mRNA_{csn}$ levels showed a dramatic 25-fold increase after a 3 day incubation.

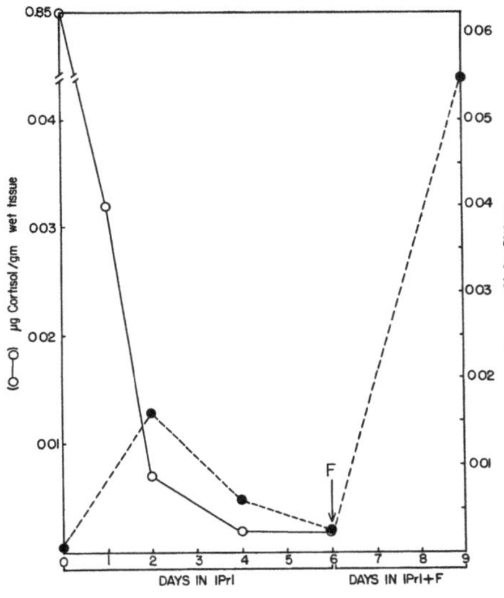

Fig. 14 Relationship between residual cortisol retained and the $mRNA_{csn}$ accumulation in the glands. (for details see ref. 41)

The preceding observations obtained under a controlled hormonal environment thus clearly demonstrate that: (a) neither prolactin nor glucocorticoid alone is sufficient to initiate expression of the casein gene in murine mammary gland, (b) mammary glands take up and retain cortisol for a prolonged period of time, (c) the residual cortisol can influence $mRNA_{csn}$ accumulation in medium with prolactin alone, and (d) the glucocorticoid in the presence of prolactin is essential for induction of casein gene expression in murine mammary gland. The results also reiterate the point that preincubation of the explants with cortisol introduces the artifact of residual steroid hormone action during subsequent incubation.

XI. NEGATIVE INFLUENCE OF PROGESTERONE ON CASEIN GENE EXPRESSION

The ovarian hormone, progesterone, is also known to be involved in the regulation of functional differentiation of mammary cells (127). Unlike the positive action of adrenal steroids, the ovarian steroid hormone is antagonistic to lactogenesis and casein production in the mammary gland (2). Recent reports have indicated that the antagonistic action of progesterone may be mediated by a negative influence on the action of prolactin (93). However, the fact that the ability of the mammary gland to produce casein-like protein in ovariectomized pregnant rats is blocked when the animals are also adrenalectomized (126), (127), suggesting that progesterone may interfere with the lactogenic action of adrenal glucocorticoids. In pregnant animals serum progesterone levels remain reasonably high through most of the gestation period (127). The circulating levels of the adrenal steroid(s) also rise progressively with the advance of pregnancy (127). Thus, it is conceivable that the maintenance of a restricted level of lactogenic activity, including expression of the casein gene, in the prepartum mammary gland may reflect a negative interaction of progesterone with adrenal glucocorticoids. This possibility appears likely since progesterone competes for the cytoplasmic glucocorticoid receptor in the mammary cells (103). This possible mode of action for progesterone inhibition of $mRNA_{csn}$ accumulation, was assessed in the two-step culture model of the whole mammary organ of the mouse.

The second thoracic mammary gland of estrogen-progesterone primed virgin BALB/c mice were initially incubated for 6 days in the step I mammogenic medium to obtain the usual lobuloalveolar structures as described in section VIII. The lobuloalveolar glands were then incubated in the step II culture for another 3 or 6 days in the same mammogenic hormone mixture containing cortisol, with or without progesterone. RNA isolated from these glands was assessed for the level of $mRNA_{csn}$ by the $cDNA_{csn}$ probe. Figure 15 shows that when cortisol is present in the mammogenic medium without progesterone, the $mRNA_{csn}$ increases as a function of time and its level remains essentially similar in medium with 1 µg or 5 µg/ml of cortisol. In contrast, when cortisol is added to the complete mammogenic medium (i.e. mammogenic medium containing progesterone) the concentration of $mRNA_{csn}$ is significantly lower. This suggests that while cortisol is capable of supporting casein gene expression in the mammogenic

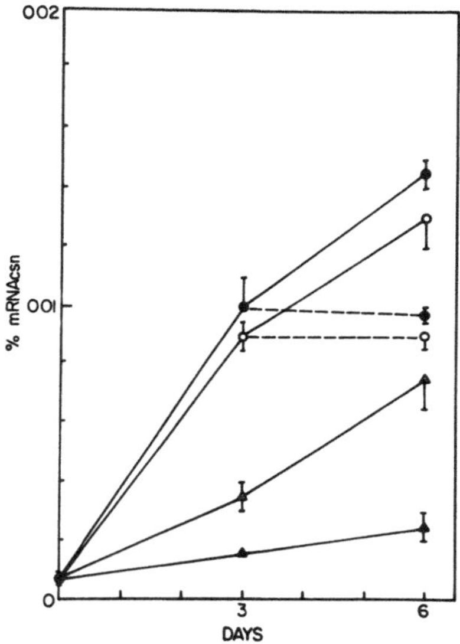

Fig. 15 Casein mRNA levels in the glands incubated in culture medium with insulin, prolactin, growth hormone, cortisol, estrogen and with or without progesterone. The glands were initially cultured in the cortico-steroid-free step I mammogenic medium (insulin, prolactin, growth hormone, estrogen and progesterone) for 6 days to obtain the lobuloalveolar structures. The concentration of $mRNA_{csn}$ in the glands was measured by the cDNAcsn probe. Broken lines show the $mRNA_{csn}$ level after addition of progesterone in the medium. (●) 1 µg/ml cortisol, (O) 5 µg/ml cortisol of medium, (▲) 1 µg cortisol + 1 µg progesterone, (Δ) 5 µg cortisol + 1 µg progesterone per ml of medium.

medium, the presence of progesterone can restrict the stimulatory action of the glucocorticoid.

Figure 15 also shows that the continuous rise in the level of $mRNA_{csn}$ as a function of the incubation time in progesterone-free, cortisol containing medium, can be interrupted by addition of progesterone. The level of $mRNA_{csn}$ in the glands increases approximately 45% between the 3rd and the 6th day of culture in progesterone-free, mammogenic medium containing cortisol. This increase of $mRNA_{csn}$, however, is blocked when progesterone is added to the medium on the 3rd day during a total of 6 days of incubation, indicating a progesterone mediated reduction in $mRNA_{csn}$ accumulation in the lobuloalveolar glands. However, the ovarian steroid fails to reduce the $mRNA_{csn}$ level in the gland to a basal

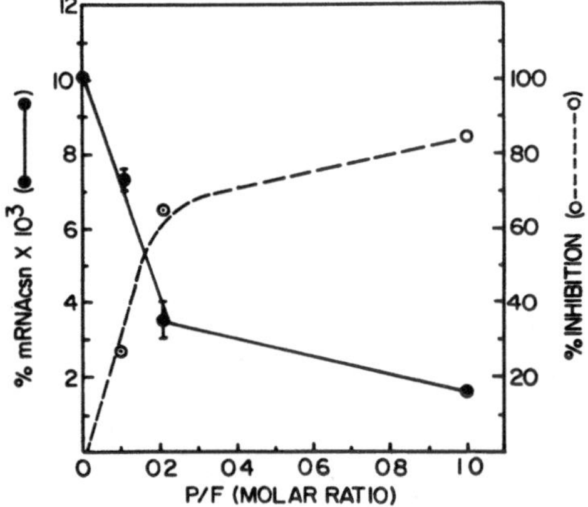

Fig. 16 Relationship between molar ratio of progesterone to cortisol in the medium and $mRNA_{csn}$ accumulation in the gland. The glands were initially incubated in the standard step I mammogenic medium for lobulo-alveolar development and then for additional 3 days in the mammogenic medium with different concentrations of progesterone and cortisol. In the absence of progesterone (P/F = 0), the concentration of cortisol in the medium was 3 μM. $mRNA_{csn}$ sequences were measured by the $cDNA_{csn}$ probe.

condition and this may be due to the continued stimulatory action of cortisol in the medium. This possibility can be tested by measuring the rates of transcription and turnover of the $mRNA_{csn}$ in presence or absence of progesterone. Figure 16 shows that the mammary gland cultured in medium with 3 μM cortisol and no progesterone elicits 0.01% $mRNA_{csn}$ after 3 days of incubation. However, $mRNA_{csn}$ levels in the glands progressively decrease as the P/F ratio is increased in the medium. At equimolar concentration (P/F = 1) the level of inhibition reaches 85%. These results clearly show that the extent of the antagonistic effect of progesterone is limited by the concentration of glucocorticoid present in the medium. Thus, it appears that the inhibitory action of progesterone on expression of the casein gene is due to a negative interaction of the ovarian steroid with the stimulatory function of glucocorticoid. The earlier interpretation (114) that the antagonistic action of progesterone on casein gene expression is due to an inhibitory action of the ovarian steroid on prolactin function appears to have been influenced by the conclusion (85) that prolactin is the hormone required for the regulation of the casein gene. However, studies using the two-step culture model of the whole mammary gland have demonstrated that both prolactin and glucocorticoid are required (41) and neither prolactin nor cortisol alone can induce expression of the casein gene. Addition of an excess

(5 μg/ml) amount of cortisol in the prolactin containing medium stimulates $mRNA_{csn}$ accumulation in the gland in the presence of progesterone. This strongly suggests that the negative action of progesterone is directed towards the stimulatory action of the glucocorticoid. The mechanism of this negative interaction may be related to the competitive affinity of the ovarian and adrenal steroid hormones for the same cytoplasmic receptor protein in the mammary cells.

Future studies on the consequence of the progesterone-glucocorticoid receptor interaction, on the nuclear translocation of the glucocorticoid receptor complex, and the transcriptional response of the casein gene should provide further insight into the molecular mechanisms of the progesterone mediated, negative regulation of the casein gene and mammary cell differentiation.

XII CLONING OF $cDNA_{csn}$

It is clear from the preceding discussions in this chapter that both cortisol and prolactin are required for casein gene expression. However, the molecular hybridization assays using the $cDNA_{csn}$ probe in most of the studies measured only the accumulation of $mRNA_{csn}$ in the gland. Therefore, the possibility remains open that the steroid or the polypeptide hormone alone may act at the transcriptional level of control of the casein gene, the glucocorticoid and/or prolactin may then influence post-transcriptional processing and cytoplasmic stabilization of the $mRNA_{csn}$ allowing its cellular accumulation. Accordingly, extensive measurement of the transcriptional response of the casein gene in the presence of different hormone combinations will need to be done in furture studies. Highly sensitive and reliable assay systems will be required for these studies. While the HgRNA synthesis system in isolated nuclei (9), (42) or hybridization of pulse labeled RNA by specific casein cDNA cellulose chromatography (45) may allow measurement of casein gene transcription, a number of technical complexities associated with these procedures (22) limit their use to an appreciable extent.

Reliable measurement of specific transcription of the casein gene, however, is feasible in hybridization assays using radioactive RNAs (transcripts) and unlabeled excess cDNA probe (32), (67), (125). These experiments require the availability of abundant amounts of $cDNA_{csn}$. Recent advances in plasmid recombinant DNA technology has made it possible to obtain amplification of the cDNAs by bacterial cloning (100). Accordingly bacterial cloning of $cDNA_{csn}$ was undertaken.

The cloning of the $cDNA_{csn}$ and the subsequent screening of the bacterial clones were carried out in collaboration with Drs. Robert B. Helling and Raafat El-Gewely at the Department of Biological Sciences, University of Michigan, Ann Arbor. The cloning experiments were done under P_2 containment conditions as required by NIH guidelines for recombinant DNA research.

The starting material for the cloning experiments was purified 15S casein mRNA (9), (42), which was used as a template for synthesis of the single stranded complemetnary $cDNA_{csn}$ using AMV reverse transcriptase. The reaction mixture generally employed contained 50 mM Tris-HCl, pH 8.3; 10 mM dTT, 6 mM $MgCl_2$, 5 μg/ml oligo$(dT)_{12-18}$, 40 μg/ml actinomycin D, 1% ethanol, 100 μM each of dATP, dCTP and dGTP, 200 μM dTTP, 5 μM [5-^{3}H]dCTP (15-30 Ci/mmol), 50 μg/ml template RNA (purified 15S casein mRNA) and 150 units/ml of AMV reverse transcriptase. The reaction mixture was incubated at 46°C for 15 mins. The RNA remaining in the RNA-cDNA hybrid was hydrolyzed by incubation of the mixture in 0.1 N NaOH at 66°C for 2 hrs. The $cDNA_{csn}$ molecules larger than 800 N were collected by sedimentation on an 8-18% alkaline sucrose gradient. Starting with 25-30 μg of purified 15S casein mRNA the reaction yielded 2 μg of single stranded $cDNA_{csn}$ ($sscDNA_{csn}$).

The bacterial (*E. coli*) DNA polymerase I was used for synthesis of the second DNA strand (32). The reaction mixture for the preparation of double stranded $cDNA_{csn}$ ($dscDNA_{csn}$) was essentially similar to that used for synthesis of the first strand, except that the Mg^{++} concentration was reduced to 4.5 mM, actinomycin D was omitted from the reaction mixture

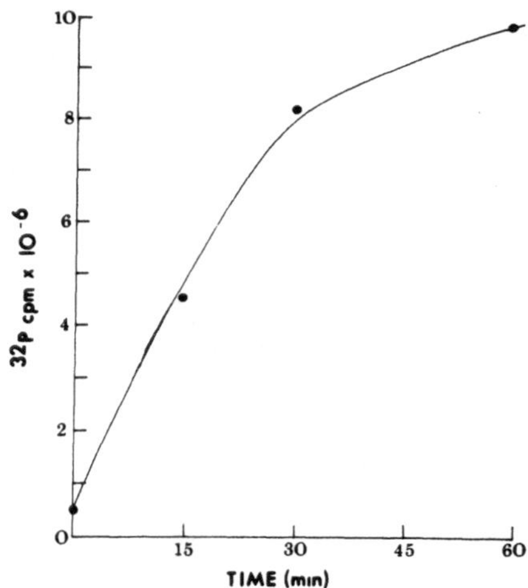

Fig. 17 Kinetics of $dscDNA_{csn}$ synthesis. Single stranded $cDNA_{csn}$ molecules ranging in size form 800-1300 N were converted to the double-stranded form by incubation in 50 mM Tris-HCl pH 8.3, 9 mM $MgCl_2$, 10 mM dTT, 500 μm/ml each of ATP, dCTP, dGTP, TTP, 50 μCi/ml α-^{32}P dATP (380 Ci/mmol, 25 units/ml of *E. coli* DNA polymerase I and 20 μg/ml of single stranded $cDNA_{csn}$. The reaction was done for 60 min at 30°C. 2 μl aliquots were taken at various time points during the incubation and the TCA precipitable radioactivity determined.

mixture and ^{32}P-dATP was used as the labeled isotope. The reaction was carried out for 60 mins at 37°C using 50 units of DNA polymerase I/µg $sscDNA_{csn}$ (Fig. 17). Starting with about 2 µg of $sscDNA_{csn}$ the reaction yielded nearly 0.75 to 1 µg of $dscDNA_{csn}$.

The double stranded DNA was then treated with S_1 nuclease (20,000 units/µg $dscDNA_{csn}$) in order to remove the looped structure at the 5' end of the DNA as well as any single strands remaining after the reaction (105).

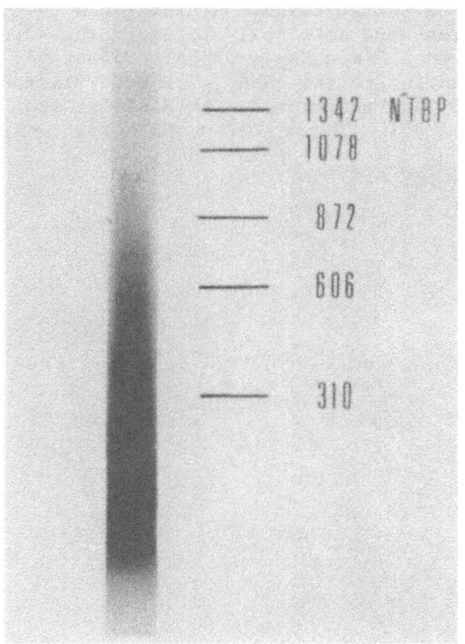

Fig. 18 Size determination of $dscDNA_{csn}$ on agarose gels. The DNA was electrophoresed on 1.5% agarose gels in Peacock's buffer at 175 V for 2 hr. The DNA was visualized by autoradiography for 1 hr using Kodak XR-5 film. The nucleotide base pairs indicated were determined by running Hae III digested ϕX 174 RF DNA on an adjacent lane and staining with 2 µg/ml ethidium bromide.

Electrophoresis of the S_1 nuclease digested $dscDNA_{csn}$ in 1.5% agarose preparative gels (Fig. 18) revealed that the S_1 nuclease resistant $dscDNA_{csn}$ consisted of molecules ranging in size from 1500 to about 100 nucleotide base pairs (NTBP). The portion of the gels containing molecules between 600 to 1500 NTBP were excised, homogenized and DNA was eluted by overnight incubation in 10 mM Tris-HCl (pH 7.6), 0.2 M NaCl, 1 mM EDTA (105). The 600-1500 NTBP long $dscDNA_{csn}$ was then linked to a Hind III restriction endonuclease specific decanucleotide linker molecule [d(C-C-A-A-G-C-T-T-G-G) Collaborative Research] using T_4 DNA ligase, in a buffer containing 50 mM Tris-HCl pH 7.5, 10 mM $MgCl_2$, 10 mM dTT (102). The linkers were then cleaved with Hind III (in a buffer containing 20 mM Tris-HCl, pH 7.5, 7 mM $MgCl_2$, 60 mM dTT) in order to generate the Hind III specific "sticky ends" at either end of the $dscDNA_{csn}$ molecule.

The plasmid pBR322 (18), linearized by digestion with Hind III, was mixed together with the linker-ligated $dscDNA_{csn}$ in the presence of T_4 DNA ligase, under conditions of plasmid excess. The plasmid pBR322 carries the genes for resistance to ampicillin (Ap) and tetracycline (Tc). The restriction endonuclease Hind III cleaves the plasmid pBR322 only at the promoter region for the Tc resistance gene (18). Insertion of the $dscDNA_{csn}$ molecules into the plasmid DNA thus makes the plasmid Ap^+Tc^-. The hybrid plasmids were then used to transform *E. coli* strain K12 RN202 which is Ap^-Tc^- (1). Bacterial cells having picked up hybrid plasmid molecules were then scored by plating first on ampicillin containing plates and then by "replica" plating on tetracycline containing plates. A total of 64 Ap^+Tc^- bacterial colonies were obtained. Tc^- colonies were screened by colony hybridization (44) to a ^{32}P-$cDNA_{csn}$ probe. Colony no. 51 (pCSN-51) showed positive hybridization to the $cDNA_{csn}$ probe. Plasmid DNA from this colony was isolated (33) and restricted with Hind III and then electrophoresed on a 1.5% agarose gel. The migration patterns

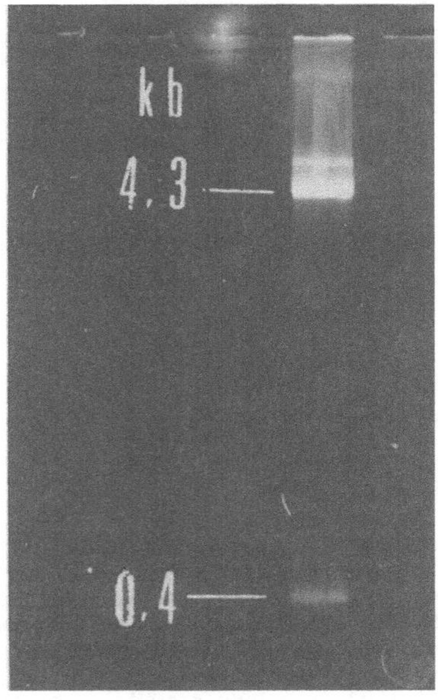

Fig. 19 Hind III restriction of recombinant plasmid pCSN 51 and electrophoresis of the fragments. 10 µg pCSN 51 was digested with 50 units of Hind III in 20 mM Tris-HCl pH 7.5, 7 mM $MgCl_2$, 60 mM NaCl for 2 hrs at 37°C. Electrophoresis was done in 1.5% agarose gels. Hae III digested ϕX 174 RF DNA and Hind III digested phage λ DNA were run on parallel lanes and the sizes indicated were determined from these markers. Staining was with ethidium bromide (2 µg/ml) for 30 mins.

in the gels showed that an inserted DNA fragment of about 400 NTBP was excised from the plasmid DNA by the Hind III treatment (Fig. 19). Southern blotting (107) of the gel bands to nitrocellulose and subsequent hybridization to the ^{32}P-cDNA$_{csn}$ probe further confirmed that the 400 NTBP fragment contained casein DNA sequences (Fig. 20).

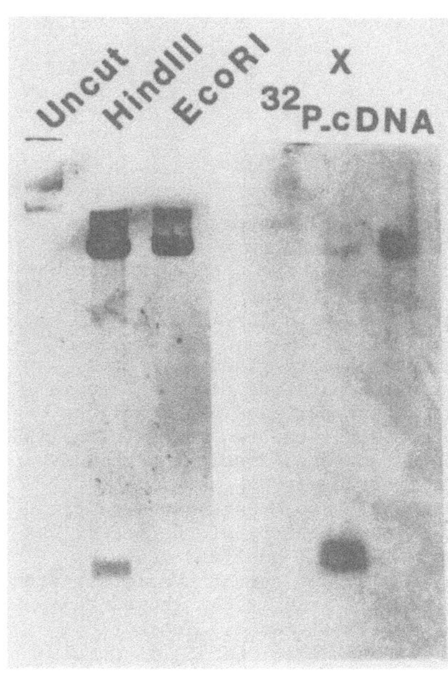

Fig. 20 Southern hybridization of recombinant plasmid pCSN 51. Left Panel: Electrophoresis of pCSN 51 DNA either without digestion or after digestion with Hind III and Eco RI. Staining is with ethidium bromide. Right Panel: Autoradiograph of the gel pattern in the left panel after Southern blotting and hybridization to ^{32}P-cDNA$_{csn}$.

A preliminary attempt to characterize the inserted DNA in pCSN-51 by digestion with various restriction enzymes (viz. EcoRI, Ave I, Pst I, Hind III, Taq I, Bam HI) revealed that only Pst I generates a single cut yielding two 174 and 226 NTBP fragments. Further confirmation that the inserted DNA indeed contains casein sequences was obtained by hybridization of the inserted 400 NTBP DNA to ^{32}P-cDNA$_{csn}$ in solution (table 8). Control assays were done using salmon sperm DNA. The hybridization reactions were carried out in 0.6 M NaCl at 68°C under conditions where the unlabeled DNA was in excess (52). At 6 hours the insert DNA was able to protect 16.3% of the ^{32}P-cDNA$_{csn}$ from S_1 nuclease digestion, whereas only 1.5% of the ^{32}P-cDNA$_{csn}$ was protected by the salmon sperm control DNA. Hybridization for periods longer than 6 hours also showed essentially similar results. The 16.3% hybridization of the ^{32}P-cDNA$_{csn}$ to the insert DNA is somewhat close to the expected results because: (a) the cDNA$_{csn}$ represents a mixture of the sequences for the two 15S casein mRNAs and also some 12S casein mRNA sequences. Therefore, the insert,

TABLE 8. Insert Hybridization to ^{32}P-cDNA$_{csn}$

time	counts hybridized to pCas51	% hybrid	counts hybridized to salmon DNA	% hybrid
0 H	90	3.0	39	1.3
3 H	145	4.8	34	1.1
6 H	487	16.3	43	1.5
6 H control	2,987		2,938	

being a single DNA species, is likely to be complementary to only one of the three mRNAs, unless all three mRNAs have extensive regions of sequence homology. (b) Since the average size of the cDNA$_{csn}$ molecules is 1000 N and the insert DNA only 400 NTBP long, less than half of the ^{32}P-cDNA$_{csn}$ is expected to be in a hybrid form with the insert DNA.

Recently 3 individual casein mRNAs of mouse mammary gland have been isolated and purified in our laboratory by preparative electrophoresis in 1.5% agarose gel. Electrophoresis of these purified RNA fractions on an analytical agarose gel (Fig. 21), showed that the two mRNAs in the 15S fraction (mRNA$_{csn}$ α, mRNA$_{csn}$ β) have been separated from each other as well as from the casein mRNA in the 12S fraction (mRNA$_{csn}$ γ). The additional band in the 12S fraction apparently represents a non-casein RNA. In order to determine the sequence complementary of the insert DNA (obtained from pCSN-51) it was hybridized to the 3 purified mRNA$_{csn}$ fractions, (mRNA$_{csn}$ α, mRNA$_{csn}$ β, mRNA$_{csn}$ γ). Subsequent hybrid arrested translation (81) in a rabbit reticulocyte cell-free system showed that (table 9) the translation of mRNA$_{csn}$ β was almost totally inhibited. Therefore, we conclude that a 400 NTBP insert DNA in pCSN-51 is complementary to mouse mRNA$_{csn}$ β. The pCSN-51 thus provides a specific hybridization probe for measuring the transcriptional response of the gene for mRNA$_{csn}$ β induced by different hormonal stimulation. Meanwhile, studies are underway to isolate bacterial clones carrying DNA sequences complementary to the other 2 casein mRNAs.

XIII. MAMMARY NEOPLASIA AND CASEIN GENE EXPRESSION

Pathogenesis of neoplasia is characterized by the escape from normal regulatory forces on steady-state conditions of cell proliferation, cellular immune responses and expression of differentiation. The diverse nature of these abnormalities is likely to involve alteration of various metabolic processes including cellular gene expression. Accordingly, assessment of tissue-specific gene expression during neoplastic transformation is of interest, particularly with respect to the search for tissue specific markers of transformation. Developmental processes in most endocrine target organs are characterized by hormone-inducible modifications of the cellular mRNA population with resultant production of specialized proteins (111). Therefore, neoplastic transformation in endocrine target organs presents the conditions suitable for monitoring possible alterations in tissue specific gene expression.

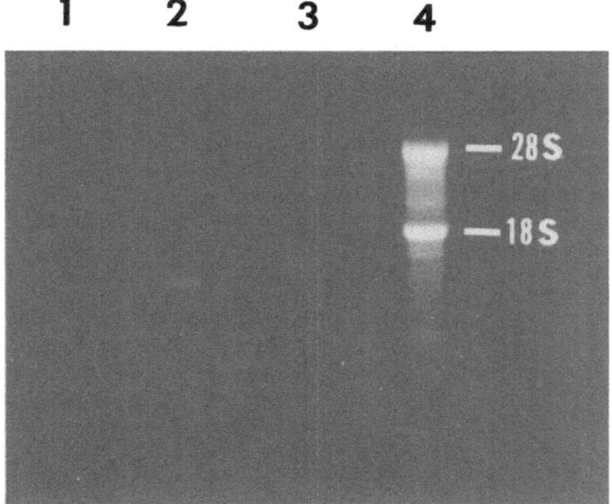

Fig. 21 Electrophoresis of purified casein mRNAs on 1.5% agarose gels. Oligo(dT) bound RNA from 7-12 day lactating mammary gland was first electrophoresed on a preparative agarose gel. 50 µg of RNA was applied to each of twelve lanes after heat denaturation at 70°C for 10 mins. The bands were visualized by staining with ethidium bromide and bands corresponding to the three casein RNAs were excised from the gel and the RNA was eltued.

Aliquots of each purified RNA were then heat denatured a second time and re-electrophoresed on analytical agarose gels. 10 µg of total RNA has been electrophoresed on an adjacent lane (lane 4) to indicate the positions of the 28S and 18S ribosomal RNAs and the relative positions of the casein mRNAs. Lanes 1-3 show the purified mRNA bands of γ, β and α casein, respectively.

TABLE 9. Hybrid-Arrested Translation of Purified Casein Messenger RNAs

samples	counts/min	CPM - background	% inhibition
casein mRNA α	29,610	21,540	6.2
casein mRNA α control	31,030	22,960	
casein mRNA β	9,600	1,530	92.0
casein mRNA β control	27,750	19,680	
casein mRNA γ	40,060	31,990	19.0
casein mRNA γ control	47,850	39,780	
background without added mRNA	8,070		

The multistep neoplastic transformation of murine mammary gland is characterized by preneoplastic precursor lesions generally referred to as hyperplastic alveolar nodules (HAN), with mammary neoplasms appearing more frequently in the outgrowths of HAN tissue (16), (29), (68), (73). Hence HANs inducible in mouse mammary gland by the murine mammary tumor virus, chronic hormone stimulation, and oncogenic chemicals are designated as preneoplastic (68). Similar putative preneoplastic lesions, generally referred to as "carcinoma *in situ*" or "precancerous cystic hyperplasia" are also observed in humans (21), (36), (132). As altered pattern of response of the epithelial cells in HAN tissue to the hormonal regulation of morphogenesis and DNA, RNA (including HnRNA) synthesis is well documented (68), (73). An unregulated expression of differentiation, as evidenced by the unscheduled presence of casein and α-lactalbumin has also been observed in mammary neoplasms in rodents and humans (84), (85). As indicated in the preceding sections of this chapter, it is now clear that expression of the casein gene is dependent upon stimulation by the lactogenic hormones, prolactin and glucocorticoid. The hormone-dependent expression of the gene for these major milk-proteins thus provides a distinct marker to monitor possible alterations of this mammary cell specific expression in preneoplastic and neoplastic mammary cells.

A. In mammary cells transformed *in vivo*

The studies so far reported are rather limited. Specific translational assays or molecular hybridization analysis using the $cDNA_{csn}$ probe have been used to monitor the level of accumulation of the $mRNA_{csn}$ in the transformed tissues. Cell-free translational assays in a wheat germ ribosome system led to the observation that the rat mammary carcinoma line R3230AC is responsive to prolactin treatment and the cells elicit $mRNA_{csn}$, but the level of the mRNA remains limited to only 1% of total mRNA activity (74). In another study (95) $mRNA_{csn}$ accumulation was measured by a $cDNA_{csn}$ probe and it was observed that 22 out of 31 7,12-dimethylbenz[a]anthracene (DMBA)-induced rat mammary tumors, elicit a detectable but insignificant level of $mRNA_{csn}$. The levels of $mRNA_{csn}$ sequences in these tumors were less than 10% of those present in the normal 8 day lactating glands. Hormone treatment with a combination of prolactin and estradiol, was more stimulatory than estradiol alone to casein gene expression in the tumors carried in ovariectomized rats. Failure of estradiol to stimulate $mRNA_{csn}$ accumulation in the tumors is rather curious, as estradiol action is likely to provide increased prolactin stimulation through its well known stimulatory action on pituitary prolactin synthesis and release (127). The same study also analyzed 3 DMBA-induced mammary tumors of BALB/c mice. These tumors generally referred to as hormone-independent, failed to elicit any measurable amount of $mRNA_{csn}$ in host animals treated with a combination of prolactin and estradiol.

Since mammary tumors in mice appear more frequently in HAN tissue, assessment of casein gene expression in this preneoplastic tissue may provide clues concerning evolution of the altered hormone response of the neoplastic tissue. A recent study (82) has examined two groups of HAN tissues. One group referred to as D-series HAN was derived from mammary glands of old BALB/c females chronically hyperstimulated with hormones. The second batch was obtained from mammary glands of BALB/c female mice treated with DMBA (73). The level of $mRNA_{csn}$ in these HAN tissues and in their mammary tumors was measured by titrating the specific $cDNA_{csn}$ (to 15S mouse casein mRNA) with vast excess of test RNA samples. Treatment of the host animals with a combination of 500 µg prolactin and 100 µg dexamethasone stimulated only a modest accumulation of $mRNA_{csn}$ in the HAN tissue, but the mammary tumors in general failed to respond to the lactogenic hormones. The ability of the different HAN tissue to respond to lactogenic hormones by expressing the casein gene (although at a very modest level) failed to show any correlation with the tumorigenicity of the different HANs.

B. In mammary cells transformed *in vitro*

Recently our laboratory has introduced a new *in vitro* carcinogenesis model in organ culture of the whole mammary gland of the female mouse (9), (114). A variety of carcinogenic chemicals including hydrocarbons, amines and amides have been observed to induce transformation of epithelial cells eliciting nodule-like alveolar lesions (see Fig. 7d section VII-B) in the glands *in vitro* (9), (14), (57), (60), (120). The epithelial cells

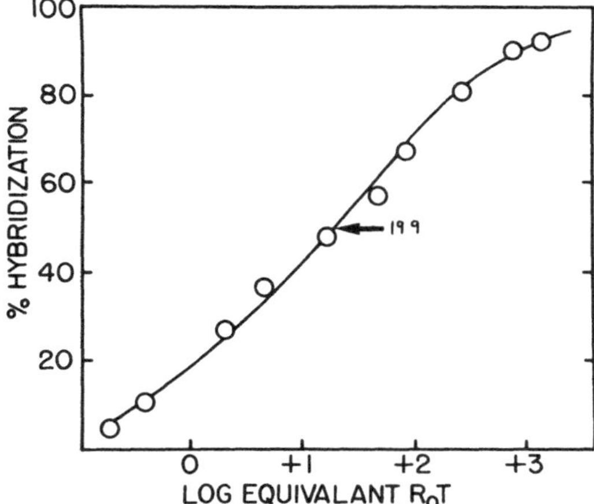

Fig. 22 Hybridization of the $cDNA_{csn}$ probe to the total RNA extracted from the whole mammary gland cultivated *in vitro*. Second thoracic mammary glands of estrogen-progesterone primed immature BALB/c female mice were incubated for six days in a medium containing insulin, prolactin, aldosterone and cortisol. Total RNA extracted from these glands by phenol-chloroform emthod (40), (79) was hybridized to the $cDNA_{csn}$ probe.

transformed *in vitro* by DMBA, after transplantation into gland-free mammary fat pads (inguinal) of syngeneic virgin hosts, produce serially tansplantable lobuloalveolar outgrowths of mammary hyperplasias (MH). Like in the lobuloalveolar outgrowths of HAN tissue, MH tissue also produces mammary carcinomas (48), (114). Thus MH lines derived from mammary epithelial cells transformed *in vitro* are preneoplastic and analogous to the preneoplastic HAN tissue of the mouse mammary gland *in vivo* (48). Three of these DMBA-induced MH lines (MH1, MH5, MH9) and 2 D series HAN lines (HAN-D1 and HAN-D8) and the mammary tumors obtained from these preneoplastic tissues were analyzed for casein gene expression in virgin and lactating hosts. Expression of the casein gene was assessed by measuring cellular accumulation of $mRNA_{csn}$ sequences with the $cDNA_{csn}$ probe (to 15S mouse $mRNA_{csn}$).

Since incubation of the glands in medium containing insulin, prolactin and aldosterone is conducive to the transforming aciton of DMBA (9), (14) the level of expression of the casein gene in the presence of the same mixture of hormones was determined. Figure 22 shows that $mRNA_{csn}$ constitutes 0.19% of the total RNA of the mammary gland after incubation for 6 days in insulin, prolactin, aldosterone and cortisol containing medium. Since virtually no $mRNA_{csn}$ is measurable in the immature mammary gland of virgin mice, the high level of $mRNA_{csn}$ accumulation in this tissue is likely to be due to hormonal induction of the casein gene in the gland *in vivo*. These results also indicate that the mammary epithelial cells were in an active state of casein gene transcription when the glands were exposed to the transforming action of DMBA. Table 10 shows that MH1 and MH5 lines fail to show a measurable level of $mRNA_{csn}$ in virgin hosts. However, when exposed to the hormone environment of the lactating host $mRNA_{csn}$ sequences become measurable in both of these preneoplastic tissues, although concentrations of the $mRNA_{csn}$ in total RNA of MH1 (0.0044%) and MH5 (0.0014%), are variable. This indicates that while the casein gene in both of this transformed tissues are responsive to the host's lactogenic hormone stimulus, the level of this response remains much lower than what is present in the lactating host's own mammary glands (2.5%). MH9 on the other hand showed a relatively high concentration (0.022%) of $mRNA_{csn}$ in virgin hosts and an essentially similar level (0.017%) was also present in the lactating host (table 10). This reveals that the epithelial cells in MH9 are capable of expressing the casein gene, and the relatively high level is not dependent upon the modulatory influence of the host's hormone environment. In contrast the mammary tumors derived from MH9 failed to elicit a detectable expression of the casein gene both in virgin and lactating hosts (table 10). Mammary neoplasms from MH1 and MH5 could not be analyzed because no mammary tumors appeared in these lines at the time of these studies. However, both of these MH lines have subsequently produced mammary tumors (48).

Table 10 shows that among the two hormone-induced HAN lines examined, HAN-D1 failed to show a measurable level of $mRNA_{csn}$ sequences in virgin hosts. In lactating host RNA from the same tissue showed a 35% hybridization to the $cDNA_{csn}$ but only at a very high $R_{o}t$ value. Moreover, the concentration of $mRNA_{csn}$ remained nonsignificant for a quantitative estimate, which requires at least a 50% level of hybridization. Mammary

TABLE 10. Levels of $mRNA_{csn}$ in Different MH, HAN and Mammary Tumors

RNA source	% $mRNA_{csn}$ host mice virgin	pregnant	lactating	*in vitro*
MH1 outgrowth	N.M.[a]	-	0.0044	-
MH5 outgrowth	N.M.	-	0.0014	-
MH9 outgrowth	0.022	-	0.017	-
MH9 tumor	N.M.	-	N.M.	-
HAN-D1 outgrowth	N.M.	-	N.M.	-
HAN-D1 tumor	N.M.	-	-	-
HAN-D8 outgrowth	N.M.	-	0.006	-
HAN-D8 tumor	N.M.	-	-	-
normal mammary gland (lactating)	N.M.	0.09	2.5	-
organ culture[b] mammary gland	-	-	-	0.019

[a] N.M., not measurable

[b] Immature virgin mammary gland was grown to lobuloalveolar structure after incubating for 6 days in medium containing insulin, prolactin, aldosterone and cortisol, as described previously (60).

tumors produced by this HAN tissue failed to elicit any $mRNA_{csn}$. These obsertavions are consistent with earlier reports (14). HAN-D8, however, showed a relatively high level of $mRNA_{csn}$ in lactating hosts, although $mRNA_{csn}$ sequences were nonmeasurable in virgin hosts (table 10). Mammary tumors obtained from HAN-D8 tissue failed to show any $mRNA_{csn}$ regardless of the hormone environment of the host animals.

The results obtained from preneoplastic and neoplastic mammary cells transformed by DMBA *in vitro*, thus seem to exhibit a pattern essentially similar to the HAN tissue induced by the same carcinogenic chemicals or hormones in the mammary gland *in vivo*. However, it is interesting that although the cells in these lesions exhibit an altered expression of the casein gene, the pattern of the alteration is variable among the different preneoplastic tissues. It is also of interest to note that although the transformation was induced by the same agent the pattern of alteration, particularly with respect to hormonal responses, appears to be different. This suggests that the tissues may be composed of different cell types within the individual lines as well as among the different lines of preneoplastic outgrowths irrespective of the etiology. It is also apparent from these limited studies that while expression of the casein gene in preneoplastic and neoplastic mammary tissues presents an altered response to exogenous or endogenous hormones, the patterns of these alterations are variable. Comments with respect to the significance of the alterations need further analysis of the tissues. At this time it is also not clear whether the alterations are at the transcriptional or post-transcriptional level of control. Nonetheless, from the limited data so far available it appears that transformation does cause an alteration of the pattern of the mammary cell specific expression of the casein gene.

XIV. SUMMARY AND COMMENTS

It is evident from studies discussed in this chapter that lactogenesis in the mammary gland is accompanied by increased cellular RNA content, formation of larger ribosomal aggregates (polysomes) and accumulation of casein in the gland. The activation of these macromolecular events is influenced by prolactin and adrenal glucocorticoid(s) indicating that the cellular protein synthesis apparatus becomes responsive to the modulatory actions of the lactogenic hormones. Casein synthesis in mammary explants *in vitro* is also dependent upon increased RNA synthesis stimulated by the lactogenic hormones, suggesting a hormonal induction of the mRNA for the milk-protein. In recent years, application of the knowledge and technology of molecular biology has allowed acomplishment of faithful translation of the casein mRNA in cell-free protein synthesis systems, purification of the mRNA and synthesis of cDNA to casein (15S) mRNA. Utilization of these tools then facilitated a direct measure of hormonal modulation of expression of the casein gene. Results of translational assays revealed that $mRNA_{csn}$ level in the lactating mammary gland is influenced by the adrenal glucocorticoid, as well as by intensity of suckling, a stimulus believed to provide increased prolactin stimulation. Quantitative analysis obtained by molecular hybridization of the cellular RNA to the $cDNA_{csn}$ probe also showed that cortisol exerts a pronounced regulatory influence on $mRNA_{csn}$ accumulation in the lactating gland.

In organ culture studies using pieces of mammary tissue from pregnant rats it was observed that prolactin in presence of insulin stimulates casein gene transcription and $mRNA_{csn}$ accumulation in explants preincubated with insulin and cortisol. Based on these observations it has been concluded that expression of the casein gene is regulated by prolactin, and that the presence of the glucocorticoid is not necessary for the action of the polypeptide hormone, although the adrenal steroid hormone may potentiate the action of prolactin. However, recent reappraisal of these studies strongly indicate that the stimulatory action of prolactin in the explants preexposed to the cortisol reflects a synergistic action of prolactin in the medium and the residual steroid hormone retained in the explant. The failure to consider this important limitation of the experimental protocol thus appears to have led to the erroneous conclusion that prolactin is the hormone regulating casein gene expression in the mammary gland. Corticosterone, in presence of prolactin and insulin also has been found to be an absolute requirement for production of α-lactalbumin in cultures of mammary epithelial cells from pregnant rats (86), (87).

Studies using organ culture of the whole mammary gland have also demonstrated that prolactin in a corticosteroid-free mammogenic medium stimulates pregnancy-like alveolar morphogenesis with no $mRNA_{csn}$ accumulation. Subsequent incubation of the lobuloalveolar glands with prolactin, cortisol and insulin stimulates an enormous accumulation of $mRNA_{csn}$. Using the organ culture model of the whole mammary gland it has been also demonstrated that neither prolactin nor cortisol alone can stimulate casein gene expression in presence of insulin. However, when preincubation of the galnd with cortisol is followed by incubation with prolactin abundant $mRNA_{csn}$ accumulates in the gland in presence of insulin. The accumulation of $mRNA_{csn}$ in the glucocorticoid-free medium with prolactin in presence of insulin has been demonstrated to be the result of the synergistic action of the polypeptide hormone and the residual steroid hormone retained in the tissue. The organ culture model of the whole mammary gland also demonstrated a simultaneous occurrence of lobulo-alveolar morphogenesis and casein gene expression in the medium containing prolactin and the adrenal steroid hormones. Thus it is clear that expression of the casein gene as measured by the accumulation of $mRNA_{csn}$ requires both prolactin and adrenal glucocorticoid(s). However, the studies so far have not ruled out the possibility that prolactin or glucocorticoid alone may initiate transcription of the casein gene, and post-transcriptional processing and cytoplasmic stabilization of the mature $mRNA_{csn}$ may be regulated by the polypeptide and/or the steroid hormones. An understanding of these mechanisms will require measurement of $mRNA_{csn}$ sequences in (a) short-term pulse labeled RNA and/or (b) in labeled RNA synthesized in isolated mammary cell nuclei obtained from glands incubated with appropriate hormone mixture.

The unique culture model of the whole mammary organ should provide reliable conditions for proper hormonal stimulation under controlled conditions. The availability of abundant copies of casein cDNA probe by the recombinant DNA technology should permit the sensitive hybridization analysis under DNA excess conditions. These techniques are likely to provide an improved understanding of the complex mechanisms of the multiple hormonal regulation of the mammary cell specific gene expression. Specific receptors for prolactin and glucocorticoid also may play a regulatory role. In the mammary gland, adrenal glucocorticoid has been reported to exert a significant influence on the level of prolactin receptors (96), (97). Little is known about a correlation between receptor-hormone interaction and specific responses of the mammary cells. Again the whole mammary gland organ culture model should permit such studies under reliable experimental conditions. It is anticipated that the studies during the next few years will provide significant advances to our understanding of the specific role of prolactin and adrenal glucocorticoid in regulation of expression of functional differentiation of the mammary cells.

ACKNOWLEDGMENTS

We thank Dr. Y. N. Sinha, Scripps Clinic and Research Foundation, LaJolla, California for determining the serum prolactin level shown in table 3. We also thank Arvilla Kirchhoff for secretarial assistance and Linda Crump for technical assistance. The work was supported by grants CA11058-12 and CA25304-02 from the National Cancer Institute. We also thank Dr. Michael Antoniou for his careful reading of the manuscript.

REFERENCES

1. Adams J, Kinney T, Thompson S, Rubin L, Helling B. Frequency-dependent selection for plasmid-containing cells of *E. coli*. Genetics 91: 627-637, 1979.

2. Assairi L, Delouis C, Gaye P, Houdebine LM, Olliver-Bousquet M, Denamur R: Inhibition by progesterone of the lactogenic effect of prolactin in the pseudopregnant rabbit. Biochem J 144: 245-252, 1974.

3. Aviv H, Leder P. Purification of biologically active globin messenger RNA by chromatography on oligo thymidylic acid cellulose. Proc Natl Acad Sci USA 69: 1408-1412, 1972.

4. Banerjee DN, Banerjee MR. Rapidly labeled RNA synthesis in pre-lactating and lactating mammary gland. J Endocrinol 56: 145-154, 1973.

5. Banerjee DN, Banerjee MR, Mehta RG. Hormonal regulation of rapidly labeled RNA synthesis in normal mammary gland, preneoplastic mammary nodules and mammary tumors of BALB/c mice with or without MTV. J Natl Cancer Inst 51: 843-849, 1973.

6. Banerjee DN, Banerjee MR, Wagner JE. Regulation of DNA-polymerase activity in mouse mammary gland by ovarian steroids. J Endocrinol 51: 259-264, 1971.

7. Banerjee MR. Responses of mammary cells to hormones. Int Rev Cytol 46: 1-97, 1976.

8. Banerjee MR, Banerjee DN. Hormonal regulation of RNA synthesis and membrane ultra structure in mouse mammary gland. Exp Cell Res 64: 307-316, 1971.

9. Banerjee MR, Ganguly N, Mehta NM, Iyer AP, Ganguly R. Functional differentiation and neoplastic transformation in an isolated whole mammary organ *in vitro*. pp 485-516 in Cell Biology of Breast Cancer, eds C McGrath, M Brennan, M Rich, Academic Press, New York, 1980.

10. Banerjee MR, Rogers FM, Banerjee DN. Hormonal regulation of RNA and protein synthesis in the mouse mammary gland before and during lactation. J Endocrinol 50: 281-291, 1971.

11. Banerjee MR, Terry PM, Sakai S, Lin FK. Regulation of mRNA and specific milk protein in mammary gland. J Toxicol & Environ Health 3: 281-308, 1977.

12. Banerjee MR, Terry PM, Sakai S, Lin FK, Ganguly R. Hormone regulation of casein messenger RNA (mRNA). In Vitro 14: 128-139, 1978.

13. Banerjee MR, Wood BG, Lin FK, Crump LR. Organ culture of the whole mammary gland of the mouse. vol 2 pp 457-462 in Tissue Culture Assoc Manual, Tissue Culture Assoc, Rockville, Maryland, 1976.

14. Banerjee MR, Wood BG, Washburn LL. Chemical carcinogen-induced alveolar nodules in organ culture of mouse mammary gland. J Natl Cancer Inst 53: 1387-1393, 1974.

15. Barnawell EB. A comparative study of the responses of mammary tissues from several mammalian species to hormones *in vitro*. J Exp Zool 160: 189-206, 1965.

16. Bern HA, Nandi S. Recent studies of the hormonal influence in mouse mammary tumorigenesis. Prog Exp Tumor Res 2: 91-145, 1961.

17. Bolander EF Jr, Nicholas KR, Topper YJ. Retention of glucocorticoid by isolated mammary tissue may complicate interpretation of results from *in vitro* experiments. Biochem Biophys Res Commun 91: 245-252, 1979.

18. Bolivar F, Rodriguez RL, Greene PJ, Betlach MC, Heynecker HL, Boyer HW, Crosa JH, Falkow S. Construction and characterization of new cloning vehicles. II. A multipurpose cloning system. Gene 2: 95-113, 1977.

19. Brawerman G. Eukaryotic messenger RNA. Annu Rev Biochem 43: 621-642, 1974.

20. Breathnach R, Mandel JL, Chambon P. Ovalbumin gene is split in chicken DNA. Nature (Lond) 270: 314-319, 1977.

21. Cardiff RD, Wellings SR, Faulkin LJ Jr. Biology of breast preneoplasia. Cancer 39: 2734-2743.

22. Chambon P. The molecular biology of the eukaryotic genome is coming of age. Cold Spring Harbor Symp Quant Biol 42: 1209-1234, 1977.

23. Cowie AT, Tindal JS. in The Physiology of Lactation, Arnold, London, 1971.

24. Craig RK, Brown PA, Harrison OS, MacIlreavy D, Campbell PN. Guinea pig milk protein synthesis. Biochem J 160: 57-74, 1976.

25. Dale RMK, Livingston DC, Ward DC. The synthesis and enzymatic polymerization of nucleotides containing mercury: Potential tools for nucleic acid sequencing and structural analysis. Proc Natl Acad Sci USA 70: 2238-2242, 1973.

26. Darnell JE, Jelinek W, Malloy GR. Biogenesis of mRNA: Genetic regulation in mammalian cells. Science 181: 1215-1221, 1973.

27. Denamur R. Hormonal control of lactogenesis. J Dairy Res 38: 237-264, 1971.

28. Denamur R. Ribonucleic acids and ribonucleoprotein particles of the mammary gland. vol 1 pp 414-465 in Lactation, a Comprehensive Treatise, eds BL Larson, VR Smith, Academic Press, New York, 1974.

29. DeOme KB. The mammary tumor system in mice. A brief review. pp 127-137, ed J Burdette, Univ of Utah Press, Salt Lake City, 1966.

30. Devinoy E, Houdebine LM, Delouis C. Role of prolactin and glucocorticoids in the expression of casein gene in rabbit mammary gland organ culture, quantification of mRNA. Biochim Biophys Acta 517: 360-366, 1978.

31. Edstrom JE, Lambert B. Gene and information diversity in eukaryotes. Prog Biophys Mol Biol 30: 57-82, 1975.

32. Efstratiadis A, Kafatos FC, Maxam AM, Maniatis T. Enzymatic *in vitro* synthesis of globin genes. Cell 7: 279-285, 1976.

33. El-Gewely MR, Helling RB. Preparative separation of DNA-ethidium bromide complexes by zonal density gradient centrifugation. Anal Biochem 102: 423-428, 1980.

34. Elias JJ. Effect of insulin and cortisol on organ cultures of adult mouse mammary gland. Proc Soc Exp Biol Med 101: 500-502, 1959.

35. Elias JJ. The role of prolactin in normal mammary gland growth and function. pp 37-74 in Hormonal Proteins and Peptides, ed Ch Li, Academic Press, New York, 1980.

36. Farber E, Sporn MB. Early lesions and the development of epithelial cancer. Cancer Res 36: 2475-2706.

37. Forsyth IA. Organ culture techniques and the study of hormone effects on the mammary gland. J Dairy Res 38: 419-444, 1971.

38. Gala RR, Westphal U. Corticosteroid binding activity in serum of mouse, rabbit and guinea pig during pregnancy and lactation: Possible involvement in the initiation of lactation. Acta Endocrinol 55: 47-61, 1965.

39. Ganguly, N., Ganguly R, Mehta NM, Crump LR, Banerjee MR. Simultaneous occurrence of pr-gnancy-like lobuloalveolar morphogenesis and casein gene expression in a culture of the whole mammary gland. In Vitro 17. 55-60, 1980.

40. Ganguly R, Banerjee MR. RNA synthesis in isolated nuclei of lactating mammary cells in presence of unmodified and mercury-labeled CTP. Nucleic Acids Res 5: 4463-4477, 1978.

41. Ganguly R, Ganguly N, Mehta NM, Banerjee MR. Absolute requirement of glucocorticoid for expression of the casein gene in presence of prolactin. Proc Natl Acad Sci USA 77: 6003-6006, 1980.

42. Ganguly R, Mehta NM, Ganguly N, Banerjee MR. Glucocorticoid modulation of casein gene transcription in mouse mammary gland. Proc Natl Acad Sci USA 76: 6466-6470, 1979.

43. Gaye P, Houdebine L, Denamur R. Isolation of active messenger RNA for α-s casein from bound polyribosomes of mammary gland. Biochem Biophys Res Commun 51: 637-644, 1973.

44. Grunstein M, Hogness DS. Colony hybridization: A method for the isolation of cloned DNAs that contain a specific gene. Proc Natl Acad Sci USA 72: 3961-3965, 1975.

45. Guyette WA, Matusik RJ, Rosen JM. Prolactin mediated transcriptional and post-transcriptional control of casein gene expression. Cell 17: 1013-1023, 1979.

46. Hammer DH, Leder P. SV40 recombinant carrying a functional RNA splice function and polyadenylation site from chromosomal mouse β^{maj} globin gene. Cell 17: 737-747, 1979.

47. Ichinose RR, Nandi S. Influence of hormones on lobuloalveolar differentiation of mouse mammary gland *in vitro*. J Endocrinol 35: 331-340, 1966.

48. Iyer AP, Banerjee MR. Sequential expression of preneoplastic and neoplastic characteristics of mammary epithelial cell transformed in organ culture. J Natl Cancer Inst (in press), 1981.

49. Jacob ST, Sajdel EM, Macke W, Munro HM. Soluble RNA polymerases in rat liver nuclei: Properties, template specificity and amanitin responses *in vitro* and *in vivo*. Cold Spring Harbor Symp Quant Biol 35: 681-691, 1970.

50. Jeffreys AJ, Flavell RA. The rabbit β-globin gene contains a large insert in the coding sequence. Cell 12: 1097-1108, 1977.

51. Jenness R. The composition of milk. vol 3 pp 3-107 in Lactation, a Comprehensive Treatise, eds BL Larson, VR Smith, Academic Press, New York, 1974.

52. Jenkins JR, Bishop JO, Butterworth PHW. Molecular cloning of three major sequence species from rainbow trout protamine mRNA. Nucleic Acids Res 6: 3805-3820, 1979.

53. Juergens WG, Stockdale FE, Topper YJ, Elias JJ, Hormone dependent differentiation of mammary gland *in vitro*. Proc Natl Acad Sci USA 54: 629-634, 1965.

54. Kantor JA, Turner PH, Nienhuis AW. Beta thalassemia: Mutations which affect processing of the β-globin mRNA precursor. Cell 21: 149-157, 1980.

55. Karlson P. New concepts on the mode of action of hormones. Perspective Biol Med 6: 203-314, 1963.

56. Kraminsky GP, Clarck WC, Estelle R, Gietz D, Sage BA, O'Conner JD, Hodgetts RB. Induction of translatable mRNA for dopa carboxylase in drosophila. An early response to ecdysterone. Proc Natl Acad Sci USA -7: 4175-4179, 1980.

57. Kundu AB, Telang NT, Banerjee MR. The binding of 7,12-dimethylbenz-[a]anthracene to mammary cell DNA in organ culture. J Natl Cancer Inst 61: 465-469, 1978.

58. Leder P, Konkel DA, Nishioka Y, Leder A, Homer DH, Kachler M. The organization and evolution of cloned globin genes. Recent Prog Horm Res 36: 241-260, 1980.

59. Levy S, Aviv H. Quantitation of labeled globin messenger RNA by hybridization with excess complementary DNA covalently bound to cellulose. Biochemistry 15: 1844-1847, 1976.

60. Lin FK, Banerjee MR, Crump LR. Cell cycle-related hormone carcinogen interaction during chemical carcinogen induction of nodule-like mammary lesions in organ culture. Cancer Res 36: 1607-1614, 1976.

61. Lodish HF. Translational control of protein synthesis. Annu Rev Biochemistry 45: 39-72, 1976.

62. Lyons WR, Li CH, Cole RD, Johnson RE. The hormonal control of mammary growth and lactation. Rec Prog Horm Res 14: 219-248, 1958.

63. Matusik RJ, Rosen JM. Prolactin induction of casein mRNA in organ culture. J Biol Chem 253: 2343-2347, 1978.

64. McDowell MJ, Jolik WK, Villakomoroff L, Lodish HF. Translation of reovirus messenger RNAs synthesized *in vitro* into reovirus polypeptides by several mammalian cell-free extracts. Proc Natl Acad Sci USA 69: 2649-2653, 1972.

65. McEnzie HA. Whole casein, isolation, properties and zone electrophoresis. vol 2 pp 87-116 in Milk Protein Chemistry and Molecular Biology, ed HA McEnzie, Academic Press, New York, 1971.

66. McKnight GS. The induction of ovalbumin and conalbumin mRNA by estrogen and progesterone in chick oviduct explant cultures. Cell 14: 403-413, 1978.

67. McKnight GS, Palmiter RD. Transcriptional regulation of the ovalbumin and conalbumin genes by steroid hormones in the chick oviduct. J Biol Chem 254: 9050-9058, 1979.

69. Medina D. Preneoplasia in Breast Cancer. vol 2 pp 47-102, ed WL McGuire, Plenum Publishing, New York, 1978.

69. Mehta NM, Ganguly N, Ganguly R, Banerjee MR. Hormonal modulation of the casein gene expression in a mammogenesis-lactogenesis two-step culture model of whole mammary gland of the mouse. J Biol Chem 255: 4430-4434, 1980.

70. Mehta RG, Banerjee MR. Action of growth promoting hormones on macromolecular biosynthesis during lobuloalveolar development of the entire mammary gland in organ culture. Acta Endocrinol 80: 501-516, 1975.

71. Mena F, Enjalbert L, Carbonell M, Priam M, Kordan C. Effect of suckling on plasma prolactin and hypothalamic monoamine levels in the rat. Endocrinology 99: 445-451, 1976.

72. Nandi S. Hormonal control of mammogenesis and lactogenesis in C3H/HeCrgl mouse. Univ Calif Publ Zoo 65: 1-129, 1959.

73. Nandi S, McGrath CS. Mammary neoplasia in mice. Adv Cancer Res 17: 353-414, 1973.

74. Nardacci NJ, McGuire WL. Casein and α-lactalbumin mRNA in experimental breast cancer. Cancer Res 37: 1186-1190, 1977.

75. Nguyen-Huu MC, Sippel AA, Hynes NE, Groner B, Schutz G. Preferential transcription of the ovalbumin gene in isolated hen oviduct nuclei by RNA polymerase B. Proc Natl Acad Sci USA 75: 686-690, 1978.

76. O'Malley BW, Roop DR, Lai EC, Nordstrom J, Callerall JF, Swaneck DA, Colbert M, Tsai J, Dugaiczyk A, Woo SLC. The ovalbumin gene: Organization structure, transcription and regulation. Rec Prog Hormone Res 35: 1-46, 1979.

77. O'Malley BW, Tsai MJ, Tsai SY, Towele HC. Regulation of gene expression in chick oviduct. Cold Spring Harbor Symp Quant Biol 52: 605-615, 1977.

78. Orkin SH, Swerdlow PS. Globin RNA synthesis *in vitro* by isolated erythroleukemic cell nuclei: Direct evidence for increased transcription during erythroid differentiation. Proc Natl Acad Sci USA 74: 2475-2479, 1977.

79. Palmiter RD. Magnesium precipitation of ribonucleoprotein complexes. Expedient techniques for the isolation of undegraded polysomes and messenger ribonucleic acid. Biochemistry 13: 3606-3615, 1974.

80. Palmiter RD, Moore PB, Mulvihill ER, Emtage S. Significant lag in the induction of ovalbumin messenger RNA by steroid hormones. A receptor translation hypothesis. Cell 8: 557-572, 1976.

81. Paterson BM, Roberts BE, Kuff EL. Structural gene identification and mapping by DNA mRNA hybrid-arrested cell-free translation. Proc Natl Acad Sci USA 74: 4370-4374, 1977.

82. Pauley RJ, Socher SH. Hormonal influences on the expression of casein messenger RNA during mouse mammary tumorigenesis. Cancer Res 40: 362-367, 1980.

83. Perry RP. Processing of RNA. Annu Rev Biochem 45: 605-629, 1976.

84. Pich A, Bussolati G, DiCarlo F. Production of casein and presence of estrogen receptor in human breast cancer. J Natl Cancer Inst 58: 1483-1484, 1977.

85. Qasba PK, Gullino PM. α-lactalbumin content of rat mammary carcinomas and effect of pituitary stimulation. Cancer Res 37: 3792-3795, 1977.

86. Ray DB, Horst IA, Jansen RW, Kowal J. Normal mammary cells in long-term culture: I. Development of hormone dependent functional monolayer cultures and assay of alpha-lactalbumin production. Endocrinology 108: 573-583, 1981.

87. Ray DB, Horst IA, Jansen RW, Mills NC, Kowal J. Normal mammary cells in long-term culture. II. Prolactin, corticosterone, insulin and triodothyronine effects on alpha-lactalbumin production. Endocrinology 108: 584-590, 1981.

88. Ringold GM, Yamamoto KR, Bishop JM, Varmus HE. Glucocorticoid stimulated accumulation of mouse mammary tumor virus RNA: Increased rate of synthesis of viral RNA. Proc Natl Acad Sci USA 74: 2879-2883, 1977.

89. Rivera E. Mammary gland culture. pp 442-471 in Methods in Mammalian Embryology, ed JC Danial, Freeman, San Francisco, 1971.

90. Rivera EM. Hormonal control of cellular events during lactogenesis, some unresolved problems. pp 279-295 in Lactogenic Hormones Fetal Nutrition and Lactation, ed JB Josimovich Jr, Wiley and Sons, New York, 1974.

91. Rivera EM, Bern HA. Infleunce of insulin on maintenance and secretory stimulation of mouse mammary tissue in organ culture. Endocrinology 69: 340-353, 1961.

92. Roberts BE, Paterson BM. Efficient translation of tobacco mosaic virus RNA and rabbit globin as RNA in a cell-free system from commercial wheat germ. Proc Natl Acad Sci USA 70: 2330-2334, 1973.

93. Rosen JM, Matusik R, Richard DA, Gupta P, Rodgers JR. Multihormonal regulation of casein gene expression at the transcriptional and post-transcriptional levels in the mammary glands. Recent Prog Hor Res 36: 157-193, 1980.

94. Rosen JM, O'Neal DL, McHugh JE, Comstock JP. Progesterone mediated inhibition of casein mRNA and polysomal casein synthesis in the rat mammary gland during pregnancy. Biochemistry 17: 290-297, 1978.

95. Rosen JM, Socher SH. Detection of casein messenger RNA in hormone dependent mammary cancer by molecular hybridization. Nature (Lond) 269: 83-86, 1977.

96. Rosen JM, Woo SLC, Comstock JP. Regulation of casein messenger RNA during development of rat mammary gland. Biochemistry 14: 2895-2903, 1975.

97. Sakai S, Banerjee MR. Glucocorticoid modulation of prolactin receptors on mammary cells of lactating mice. Biochim Biophys Acta 582: 79-88, 1979.

98. Sakai S, Enami J, Nandi S, Banerjee MR. Prolactin receptor on dissociated mammary epithelial cells at different stages of development. Mol Cell Endocrinol 12: 285-298, 1978.

99. Schimke RT, McKnight GS, Shapiro DJ, Sullivan D, Palacois R. Hormone regulation of ovalbumin synthesis in chick oviduct. Recent Prog Horm Res 31: 175-211, 1975.

100. Science (issue no. 4286) vol 196, 1977.

101. Shaaya E, Serkeris CE. Ecdysone during insect development. Comp Gen Endocrinol 5: 35-39, 1965.

102. Shine J, Seeburg PH, Martial JA, Baxter JD, Goodman HM. Construction and analysis of recombinant DNA for human chorionic somatomammotropin. Nature (Lond) 270: 494-499, 1977.

103. Shymala G. Specific cytoplasmic glucocorticoid hormone receptors in lactating mammary glands. Biochemistry 12: 3085-3090, 1973.

104. Singh D, Bern HA, DeOme KB. Strain differences in response of the mouse mammary gland to hormones *in vitro*. J Natl Cancer Inst 45: 657-675, 1970.

105. Sippel UE, Land H, Lindenmaier W, Nguyen-Huu MC, Wortz T, Timmis KN, Giesecke K, Schutz G. Cloning of chicken lysozyme structural gene sequences synthesized *in vitro*. Nucleic Acids Res 5: 3275-3294, 1978.

106. Smith MM, Huang RC. Transcription *in vitro* of immunoglobulin kappa light chain genes in isolated mouse myeloma nuclei and chromatin. Proc Natl Acad Sci USA 73: 775-779, 1976.

107. Southern EM. Detection of specific sequences among DNA fragments separated by gel electrophoresis. J Mol Biol 98: 503-517, 1975.

108. Spelsberg TC, Thrall C, Webster G, Pickler G. Isolation and characterization of the nuclear acceptor that binds the progesterone-receptor complex in hen oviduct. pp 309-337 in Hormone Res. eds N Norvell, T Shellenberger, Hemisphere Publishing, Washington, DC, 1977.

109. Strobl J, Lippman M. Prolonged retention of estradiol by human breast cancer cells in tissue culture. Cancer Res 39: 3319-3329, 1979.

110. Tata JR. Hormones and the synthesis and utilization of ribonucleic acid. vol 5 pp 191-250 in Progress in Nucleic Acid Research and Molecular Biology, eds JN Davidson, WE Cohn, Academic Press, New York, 1966.

111. Tata JR. Regulation of protein synthesis by growth and developmental hormones. vol 1 pp 89-133 in Biochemical Actions of Hormones, ed G Litwack, Academic Press, New York, 1970.

112. Tata JR. Expression of the vitellogenin gene. Cell 9: 1-14, 1976.

113. Tata JR, Smith DF. Vitellogenesis: A versatiel model for hormonal regulation of gene expression. Recent Prog Horm Res 35: 47-95, 1979.

114. Telang NT, Banerjee MR, Iyer AP, Kundu AB. Neoplastic transformation of epithelial cells in whole mammary gland *in vitro*. Proc Natl Acad Sci USA 76: 5886-5890, 1979.

115. Terry PM, Ball EM, Ganguly R, Banerjee MR. An indirect radioimmunoassay for mouse casein using ^{125}I-labeled antigen. J Immunol Methods 9: 123-134, 1975.

116. Terry PM, Banerjee MR, Lui RM. Hormone-inducible casein messenger RNA in a serum-free organ culture of whole mammary gland. Proc Natl Acad Sci USA 74: 2441-2445, 1977.

117. Terry PM, Ganguly R, Ball EM, Banerjee MR. Murine mammary gland RNA directed synthesis of casein in a heterologous cell-free protein synthesis system. Cell Differ 4: 113-122, 1975.

118. Terry PM, Lin FK, Banerjee MR. Responses of mouse mammary gland casein mRNA to corticosteroid action and suckling. Mol Cell Endocrinol 9: 169-182, 1977.

119. Tilghman SM, Tiemeier DC, Seidman JG, Peterkin BM, Sullivan M, Meizel GV, Leder P. Intervening sequence of DNA identified in the structural portion of mouse β-globin gene. Proc Natl Acad Sci USA 75: 725-729, 1978.

120. Tonelli QJ, Custer RP, Sorof S. Transformation of cultured mouse mammary glands by aromatic amines and amides and their derivatives. Cancer Res 39: 1784-1792, 1979.

121. Topper YJ. Multiple hormone interaction related to growth and differentiation of mammary gland *in vitro*. Trans NY Acad Sci 30: 869-874, 1968.

122. Topper YJ. Multiple hormone interaction in development of mammary gland *in vitro*. Recent Prog Horm Res 26: 287-308, 1970.

123. Topper YJ, Freeman CS. Multiple hormone interactions in the developmental biology of the mammary gland. Physiol Rev 60: 1049-1106, 1980.

124. Topper YJ, Oka T. Some aspects of mammary gland development in the mature mouse. vol 1 pp 327-348 in Lactation, a Comprehensive Treatise, eds GL Larson, VR Smith, Academic Press, New York, 1974.

125. Tsai MJ, Tsai SY, Chang CW, O'Malley BW. Effect of estrogen on gene expression in the chick oviduct: *In vitro* transcription of the ovalbumin gene. Biochim Biophys Acta 521: 689-707, 1978.

126. Tucker HA, Endocrinology of lactation. vol 3 pp 199-223 in Seminars in Perinatology, eds TK Oliver, TH Kirschbaum, Grune and Stratton, New York, 1979.

127. Tucker HA. General endocrinological control of lactation. vol 1 pp 277-326 in Lactation, a Comprehensive Treatise, eds BL Larson, VR Smith, Academic Press, New York, 1974.

128. Turkington RW. Multiple hormonal interaction. vol 2 pp 55-80 in Biochemical Actions of Hormones, ed G Litwack, Academic Press, New York, 1972.

129. Turkington RW, Mazumdar GC, Kadohama N, MacIndoe JH, Frantz WL. Hormonal regulation of gene expression in mammary cells. Recent Prog Horm Res 29: 417-455, 1973.

130. Venetianer P, Leder P. Enzymatic synthesis of solid phase bound DNA sequences corresponding to specific mammalian genes. Proc Natl Acad Sci USA 71: 3892-3895, 1974.

131. Weissbach H, Ochoa S. Soluble factors required for eukaryotic protein synthesis. Annu Rev Biochem 45: 191-216, 1976.

132. Willis RA. in Pathology of Tumors, Butterworth, London, 1967.

133. Wittliff JL. Steroid binding proteins in normal and neoplastic mammary cells. Methods Cancer Res 11: 293-354, 1975.

134. Wood BG, Washburn LL, Mukherjee AS, Banerjee MR. Hormonal regulation of lobuloalveolar growth, functional differentiation and regression of whole mammary gland in organ culture. J Endocrinol 65: 1-6, 1975.

135. Yamamoto R, Albert B. Steroid receptors: Elements for modulation of eukaryotic transcription. Annu Rev Biochem 38: 722-746, 1976.